NEUROECONOMICS

ADVANCES IN HEALTH ECONOMICS AND HEALTH SERVICES RESEARCH

Series Editors: Michael Grossman & Björn Lindgren

ADVANCES IN HEALTH ECONOMICS AND HEALTH SERVICES RESEARCH VOLUME 20

NEUROECONOMICS

EDITED BY

DANIEL HOUSER
Department of Economics and Interdisciplinary Center for Economic Science, George Mason University, USA

KEVIN McCABE
Department of Economics and Center for the Study of Neuroeconomics, George Mason University, USA

Emerald
JAI

United Kingdom – North America – Japan
India – Malaysia – China

JAI Press is an imprint of Emerald Group Publishing Limited
Howard House, Wagon Lane, Bingley BD16 1WA, UK

First edition 2008

Reprints and permission service
Contact: booksandseries@emeraldinsight.com

British Library Cataloguing in Publication Data
A catalogue record for this book is available from the British Library

ISBN: 978-1-84855-304-0
ISSN: 0731-2199 (Series)

CONTENTS

LIST OF CONTRIBUTORS

Gregory S. Berns	Department of Psychiatry & Behavioral Sciences, Emory University School of Medicine, Atlanta, GA, USA
Warren K. Bickel	Center for Addiction Research, Fred & Louis Dierks Research Laboratories, Psychiatric Research Institute, University of Arkansas for Medical Sciences, Little Rock, AR, USA
Sarah F. Brosnan	Departments of Psychology & Neuroscience, and Language Research Center, Georgia State University, Atlanta, GA, USA
C. Monica Capra	Department of Economics, Emory University, Atlanta, GA, USA
Luke J. Chang	Department of Psychology, University of Arizona, Tucson, AZ, USA
Robin Chark	Department of Marketing, Hong Kong University of Science and Technology, Hong Kong
Soo Hong Chew	Department of Economics, Hong Kong University of Science and Technology, Hong Kong; Department of Economics and Department of Business Policy, National University of Singapore, Singapore
Giorgio Coricelli	Institut des Sciences Cognitives, Centre de Neurosciences Cognitives, Bron, France

Daniel Houser	Department of Economics and Interdisciplinary Center for Economic Science, Fairfax, VA, USA
Ming Hsu	Beckman Institute of Advanced Science and Technology, University of Illinois at Urbana-Champaign, Urbana, IL, USA
King King Li	Department of Economics, Hong Kong University of Science and Technology, Hong Kong
Hung-Tai Lin	Department of Agricultural and Consumer Economics, University of Illinois at Urbana-Champaign, Urbana, IL, USA
Anup Malani	University of Chicago Law School, Chicago, IL, USA
Paul E. McNamara	Department of Agricultural and Consumer Economics, University of Illinois at Urbana-Champaign, Urbana, IL, USA
Mircea Miclea	Department of Psychology, Babeş-Bolyai University, Cluj-Napoca, CJ, Romania
Andrei C. Miu	Department of Psychology, Babeş-Bolyai University, Cluj-Napoca, CJ, Romania
Sara Moore	Department of Psychiatry & Behavioral Sciences, Emory University School of Medicine, Atlanta, GA, USA
Lisbeth Nielsen	Division of Behavioral and Social Research, National Institute on Aging, Bethesda, MD, USA
Charles Noussair	Department of Economics, Emory University, Atlanta, GA, USA and Department of Psychiatry & Behavioral Sciences, Emory University School of Medicine, Atlanta, GA, USA

John W. R. Phillips	Division of Behavioral and Social Research, National Institute on Aging, Bethesda, MD, USA
K. Richard Ridderinkhof	Department of Psychology, Amsterdam Center for the Study of Adaptive Control in Brain and Behavior (Acacia), University of Amsterdam, Amsterdam, The Netherlands
Martin Salm	Department of Econometrics and Operations Research, Tilburg University, The Netherlands
Alan G. Sanfey	Department of Psychology, University of Arizona, Tucson, AZ, USA
Daniel Schunk	Institute for Empirical Research in Economics, University of Zurich, Switzerland
Mirre Stallen	Erasmus Research Institute of Management (Erim), Erasmus University, Rotterdam, The Netherlands and Radboud University, Nijmegen, The Netherlands
Frans van Winden	CREED, Department of Economics, University of Amsterdam, Amsterdam, The Netherlands and Tinbergen Institute, Amsterdam, The Netherlands
Erte Xiao	Department of Social and Decision Sciences, Carnegie Mellon University, Pittsburg, PA, USA
Richard Yi	Center for Addiction Research, Fred & Louis Dierks Research Laboratories, Psychiatric Research Institute, University of Arkansas for Medical Sciences, Little Rock, AR, USA
Songfa Zhong	Department of Economics, Hong Kong University of Science and Technology, Hong Kong

ACKNOWLEDGMENTS

Daniel Houser, senior editor for this volume, thanks the participants of the 2008 Arne Ryde symposium on Neuroeconomics at which chapters included herein were discussed. He is grateful to this series' general editors Björn Lindgren (organizer of the Arne Ryde symposium) and Michael Grossman for the opportunity. Tyler Cowen and Vernon Smith provided valuable input at this project's early stages. Li Hao provided outstanding editorial assistance, and Alana Mistretta demonstrated excellence in proof-reading. The International Foundation for Research in Experimental Economics provided financial support. His wife and son, Patty Houser and Daniel J. Houser, provided support in ways of even greater importance.

Kevin McCabe would like to acknowledge the early financial support of the National Science Foundation and the International Foundation for Research in Experimental Economics which made his research in Neuroeconomics possible. He would also like to acknowledge the academic support by his many colleagues who helped make his research interesting. Finally, he would also like to acknowledge the personal support of his wife, Kathy McCabe, and his sons Brian McCabe and Tim McCabe, who gave his research meaning.

INTRODUCTION TO NEUROECONOMICS

INTRODUCTION

Neuroeconomics is the study of how the brain makes economic decisions. By its nature neuroeconomics studies the mechanisms of decision-making, assumed to be computational, in order to better understand the strategies people use and the choices that people make. The focus of this book is how neuroeconomics connects to health economics in a way that improves our understanding of health care and treatment decisions. This is natural for several reasons. First, the brain and the body are intimately connected to each other and the health of one depends on the other. Second, the health system is inherently about decisions. Decisions to stay healthy, decisions to diagnose illness, decisions to treat, decisions to invest in new treatments, decisions to insure, and decisions to pay. Finally, these decisions can be difficult, as the media's consistent attention to this area attests. In light of this, for this volume we chose to include chapters that review basic research on emotion or social preference that have direct relevance to decisions in health economics. We have also included chapters that refer more specifically to some aspect of people's health care or treatment decisions. In the following we indicate the chapters within each topic area. Although many chapters could arguably fit in multiple categories, we have listed each chapter only once and without particular order.

EMOTION AND DECISION

Emotion is an important component of health care decisions, at least in part because decisions regarding health care often involve pain management. The contribution by Gregory S. Berns, C. Monica Capra, Sara Moore, and Charles Noussair discusses the authors' recent neuroeconomics research that connects emotion and decisions involving pain. They discuss the neural foundations of "dread," an emotion experienced when subjects anticipate future pain. The authors point out that "dread" results in people preferring to experience pain sooner rather than later. At the same time, the authors identify neural systems connected to rejoice in avoiding pain, as well as the regret associated with making a decision that leads to pain. Their discussion highlights the importance of studying behavior when pain is chronic, and is an important first step in understanding how anticipation of acute pain affects decisions.

Anticipation also plays a prominent role in the chapter by Luke J. Chang and Alan G. Sanfey, which examines the role of the emotions in supporting a dual-system interpretation of decision-making in the human brain. They observe that emotions can be either expected or immediate. Expected emotions, including regret, arise in the future as a consequence of our decisions. On the other hand, one experiences immediate emotions, such as fear and disgust, at the time of decision. The authors examine the neural correlates of expected and immediate emotions in various individual choice, game theoretic, and moral decision experiments. The findings of this chapter challenge scholars to provide specific computational neuroeconomics models of emotions, and further to demonstrate the role these computations play in the formation and execution of individuals' decision strategies.

In their contribution, Andrei C. Miu, Mircea Miclea, and Daniel Houser draw attention to the importance of individual differences, particularly trait anxiety, in affecting individual decision strategies. Trait anxiety is at the frontier of the psychobiology of personality. Its importance enhanced because it is significantly genetic in nature and also seems tightly connected to risks for negative health outcomes (such as anxiety and affective disorders.) The Miu et al. chapter provides a comprehensive review of the neurobiology and cognitive effects of trait anxiety within a neuroeconomics perspective. Their survey makes a compelling case that taking the step from emotional states to individual differences in emotion allows one both to extend emotion's neurobiological foundations as well as strengthen its clinical relevance.

OTHER-REGARDING PREFERENCES: ORIGINS, NEUROECONOMIC MODELING, AND IMPLICATIONS

The health of one person can affect the health of a nearby other, meaning that other-regarding preferences necessarily play a central role in health care policy and treatment choices. Fundamental questions remain, however, regarding the origin, modeling, and implications of such preferences. In her contribution to this volume, Sarah F. Brosnan reviews the steps she has taken with various colleagues towards addressing these fundamental issues. She chooses to focus on inequity responses by capuchin monkeys and chimpanzees. One reason to use this unique subject pool is that the experimenter has precise knowledge about the monkey's social interaction outside of the experiment. Another reason is the absence of cultural artifacts that can at times complicate inferences from human experiments. These twin advantages, among others, have allowed Brosnan and her colleagues to explore systematically the effect of key social differences (including gender, dominance, and length of social interaction) on inequity responses. Interesting findings emerging from this agenda are that these monkeys share with humans an ability to recognize, react to, and potentially rectify inequity. Future research might profitably exploit the available detailed data on social interaction to develop formal models to shed light on the emergence of social ties.

A comprehensive discussion of one promising model of social ties appears in the contribution by Frans van Winden, Mirre Stallen, and K. Richard Ridderinkhof. The importance of social ties to health outcomes is clear, as it has long been recognized that people without social attachments are more prone to depression and anxiety, and are less likely to report being happy. Moreover, social attachment seems to promote other-regarding preferences which have impact in a wide variety of domains. In light of its evident importance, it is surprising that very little is understood about the process by which social attachment emerges. Van Winden et al., discuss recent efforts in modeling the emergence of social ties, with particular emphasis on the dual-system model of Van Dijk and Van Winden (1997). Moreover, they use the model as a foundation for speculation on the neural foundations of attachment. Their research represents a useful first step towards developing frameworks that draw neuroeconomic connections among social ties, addiction, and norm-obedient behaviors. Future research in this area might profitably focus on age-related changes in social attachment and the corresponding effects on health and economic well-being.

The chapters by Van Winden et al. and Brosnan provide evidence that social ties are inherently connected to emotional responses. In her contribution, Erte Xiao focuses on the human desire to express aroused emotions. The desire for emotion expression is connected to health outcomes, and Xiao has discovered that opportunities to express emotions can promote fair and efficient economic exchange. One reason these findings are important is that, unlike difficult-to-control emotional experiences, people have greater ability to control the way they express emotion. Moreover, institutions can be designed either to limit or encourage various forms of emotion expression. Finding the right balance in this regard is an important task for future institution design research, particularly in that cycles of excessively negative emotional expressions could lead to downward spirals in cooperation, reduce economic efficiency, and have detrimental effects on a variety of health-related outcomes.

HEALTH CARE DECISIONS: AGE AND RISK

How people make decisions regarding health care, and how age and attitudes towards risk affects those decisions, are key questions addressed by the chapters in this section. Soo Hong Chew, King King Li, Robin Chark, and Songfa Zhong discuss the "source-preference" model of risk and ambiguity. This model captures situations where identically distributed risks arising from different sources of uncertainty can lead to distinct preferences among decision makers. Moreover, they design an imaging experiment to test the source-preference model, and provide new evidence that the risk-ambiguity distinction can be assumed by a source-preference model. The source-preference model of decisions under uncertainty may contribute to our understanding of health care choices in general, and might be especially powerful to the extent that one discovers systematic changes in source-preference over the life cycle.

Ming Hsu, Hung-Tai Lin, and Paul E. McNamara focus on puzzling data indicating low rates of purchases of long-term care (LTC) insurance. Such insurance provides services that assist people with limitations they might have in their ability to perform activities of daily living as a result of chronic illness or disability. They point to several reasons for under-purchase behavior, including risk seeking over losses, ambiguity preferring over losses, or hyperbolic discounting. The aging process, however, receives special attention by the authors, as they note that age is associated with changes in both brain tissue as well as cognitive abilities. Understanding the effects of aging on LTC decisions is important for practical purposes, and can also shed light on general decision-making deficits that may emerge during the aging process. Such research takes on special importance in light of the ongoing changes in the population age distribution towards older ages.

The contribution by Lisbeth Nielsen and John W.R. Phillips also considers health care decisions in aging populations. The authors note that older adults face many complex problems directly affecting their health and well-being, including LTC insurance, prescription drug plans, and end of life care. These decisions are complicated by the fact that older adults face well-known age-related declines in cognition (see also Hsu et al.), and also develop distinct affect-processing profiles. Nielsen and Phillips review what is known about psychological differences between younger and older adults that might impact economic behavior, and also survey what is known about the neurobiological correlates of these differences. In light of the health challenges facing the elderly, this chapter offers a timely neuroeconomic perspective on determinants of health-economic behaviors and decisions over the life cycle.

While the first two chapters in this section discuss how age-related decline in cognition can affect health decisions, in their contribution Martin Salm and Daniel Schunk ask rather how decline in health during one's youth might affect one's ability to develop cognitive skill. In particular, using data from German elementary school entrance examinations, their analysis sheds light on the role of child health for the intergenerational transmission of human capital. They find that children in poor health (say because they are obese or have severe respiratory problems) are also substantially less ready for schooling than their more healthy peers. This can be important because key determinants of a brain's architecture that persist into adulthood develop during childhood. A possibility suggested by this research is that by enriching existing knowledge of the neural basis of economic behavior of adults with models of brain development during youth we might be better able to understand, model and positively influence the process of human capital formation.

HEALTH TREATMENT DECISIONS

In their chapter, Warren K. Bickel and Richard Yi propose a new conceptual model of addiction involving the dopamine reward system as well as the areas of prefrontal cortex involved in executive functions (which refers to those functions that produce self-directed behavior intending to change the self's future behavior in order to attain more preferred outcomes). The model stipulates that addiction is a result of an overactive stimulus-impulse system combined with an underactive executive system.

Such a system would explain the effectiveness of behavioral therapeutic efforts that combine contingency management (to reinforce abstinence) with cognitive-based therapy (to improve executive control) and could also explain why such therapies sometimes fail. A valuable next step, and one that would seem especially useful to health care professionals, would be to formalize the Bickel and Yi model so that it could be used to predict the likelihood of addiction as well as the effectiveness of various treatment options.

Decision-making by health care professionals is considered by Giorgio Coricelli. In particular, his contribution explores how models of regret processing in the human brain can lead to a better understanding of physician decisions. Coricelli argues that physicians tend to overprescribe standard treatments in order to avoid regret associated with not having done enough to promote a patient's good health. At the same time, physicians tend to underprescribe novel treatments, perhaps because of a perception of a heightened risk that the patient might be harmed. Coricelli hypothesizes that a physician's brain processes regret in the same way as the patient who might experience the consequences. This study furthers our understanding of such empathetic processes, an area where little is currently known. For the study of health care, knowing more about how delegated parties make decisions for others (the so-called "principal agent problem") is critical to understanding the relationship between patients, caregivers, and the resulting decisions.

Placebo effects are at the nexus of economics and health research and have especially important implications for treatment decisions. A placebo effect is a change in health outcome due to a change in beliefs about the value of a treatment. They are important to economics because they are believed to be connected to expectations, so understanding the source of placebo effects can usefully inform the modeling of expectations and their effects on decisions. In turn, placebo effects are clearly important to the field of medicine and health policy. For example, it has been argued that it might be more cost-effective for the healthcare system to encourage physicians to induce positive expectations about an inexpensive inert substance rather than to prescribe the more expensive active medication. With their contribution to this volume, Anup Malani and Daniel Houser argue that expectations play an important role in placebo effects beyond their role in affecting decisions. In particular, their evidence suggests that expectations may mediate non-behavioral, brain-modulated neural mechanisms that underlie changes in health outcomes.

SUMMARY

Neuroeconomics has quickly attracted the attention of economists, psychologists, and neuroscientists. These scholars have joined to combine experimental methods and mathematical models from which novel results on brain and behavior have emerged. In this book the authors, who represent the cutting edge of this new discipline, draw connections between research in neuroeconomics and health economics. Moreover, they direct interested readers to a goldmine of additional references. Much of the research discussed here offers more questions than answers, and many of the answers are tentative first steps at a new understanding. It is precisely this that fuels our excitement about neuroeconomics.

Daniel Houser
Kevin McCabe
Editors

THREE STUDIES ON THE NEUROECONOMICS OF DECISION-MAKING WHEN PAYOFFS ARE REAL AND NEGATIVE

Gregory S. Berns, C. Monica Capra, Sara Moore and Charles Noussair

ABSTRACT

Purpose – *We summarize three previous neuroeconomic studies with two features that distinguish them from most others in experimental economics: (1) the use of physical pain to induce incentives and (2) acquisition of data on brain activation levels. By correlating behavior when payoffs are painful with brain activation, we are able to test for the neurobiological relevance of important phenomena previously observed in experimental studies that are at odds with classical economic theories of decision-making. These specific phenomena are (a) negative discounting of future payoffs; (b) nonlinear probability weighting; (c) the experience of regret and rejoice when making a decision under risk.*

Methodology/approach – *The expectation of pain is created through the use of mild electric shocks to the top of the foot. Pain confers disutility, so decisions are made in the domain of losses relative to the status quo.*

Neuroeconomics
Advances in Health Economics and Health Services Research, Volume 20, 1–29

ISSN: 0731-2199/doi:10.1016/S0731-2199(08)20001-4

Simultaneous with these decisions, brain activation data is acquired through functional magnetic resonance imaging (fMRI).

Findings – *We find evidence for negative time discounting of electric shocks. Participants who exhibited the most extreme forms of this discounting were distinguished by early and robust activation of a subset of the cortical pain matrix. We also find evidence for probability weighting in the domain of electric shocks, which is manifest at the neural level. We find evidence both behaviorally and neurally for regret and rejoice functions for painful outcomes.*

Originality/value of chapter – *Previous experimental economic studies in the domain of losses have typically used monetary rewards. Here, we report behavioral effects and neural correlates using pain.*

1. INTRODUCTION

In this chapter, we summarize three neuroeconomic studies previously reported in (Berns et al., 2006; Berns, Capra, Moore, & Noussair, 2007; Berns, Capra, Chappelow, Moore, & Noussair, 2008) and Chandrasekhar, Capra, Moore, Noussair, and Berns (2008). There are two features that distinguish these three studies from most others in the experimental economic literature. The first feature is that in these studies we use physical pain to induce incentives. Pain is created by applying mildly painful electric shocks to participants. In contrast, almost all other experimental economic studies use monetary incentives, either real or hypothetical. The second feature is that in addition to recording decisions, we acquire data on brain activation levels. By correlating behavior when payoffs are painful and real with brain activation, we are able to test for the neurobiological relevance of important phenomena previously observed in experimental studies that are at odds with classical economic theories of decision-making. These specific phenomena are (a) negative discounting of future payoffs; (b) nonlinear probability weighting; and (c) the experience of regret and rejoice when making a decision under risk.

In the research described here, participants made decisions in the domain of losses relative to the status quo. This is a feature of many situations of interest in economics, but it is difficult to study in control environments. Consider, for example, a patient who is diagnosed with a serious health problem and must decide between alternative risky treatments. The best possible outcome under any treatment is the restoration of a status quo level of health. All other outcomes involve unfavorable results, such as failure of the treatment, emergence of uncomfortable side effects, or protracted morbidity. Another example is a defendant in a criminal court case faced with the choice of accepting a plea bargain or going to trial. The plea bargain offers a fixed jail sentence, whereas the trial is a lottery in which the best possible outcome is avoidance of prison. Note that in these two examples, the decisions are made over non-monetary variables, health level, and prison time. In contrast, previous experimental economic studies of decisions in the domain of losses have typically used monetary reward media. In the research that we report here, all outcomes are also in terms of a non-monetary medium, electric shock voltage.

It is reasonable to argue that using electric shocks to induce incentives results in decisions that are exclusively in the domain of losses, since the only possible outcomes are the receipt of a shock or the avoidance of a shock. The reason is that unless special experimental procedures are employed to habituate participants to receiving electric shocks, the status quo can be assumed to be the absence of a shock. In addition to providing a means of inducing non-monetary incentives, the use of electric shocks allows us to mitigate a methodological problem that arises in the study of decisions in the domain of losses. Because of the difficulty of inducing voluntary participation in studies where individuals can lose money, monetary losses have been studied with two techniques intended to circumvent the problem. The first technique is to have individuals make hypothetical decisions. The drawback of this technique is that it may fail to induce incentives to make decisions in accordance with one's true preferences, since there are no direct payoff consequences that result from the decisions. The second technique is to give individuals an initial endowment of cash at the beginning of or before the experimental session, from which losses incurred over the course of a session are subtracted. This second procedure, while creating incentives to make meaningful decisions, also has a drawback. Using this procedure, it is unclear whether decisions can be truly considered as taking place in the domain of losses relative to the status quo. While observed decisions under such a protocol do differ from those obtained when individuals are accumulating positive earnings over the course of an experimental session, it is unknown whether they reflect the same principles of decision-making as are present outside the laboratory when decisions involve losses relative to the status quo.

Physical pain satisfies non-satiation and dominance, the two precepts proposed by Smith (1982) concerning the appropriateness of the medium whereby incentives are induced in an experiment. Non-satiation is the property that the utility of a participant is monotonic in the level of the medium received. This allows an experimental researcher to have confidence that individuals are optimizing the value of the intended objective function by maximizing or minimizing the amount of the reward medium they receive. Non-satiation is satisfied in the studies described here since higher voltage or longer shocks yield more disutility than lower voltage and shorter shocks (indeed, the results of participant self reports confirm this). Dominance means that the difference in the quantity of the incentive medium received between alternative decisions outweighs the decision cost associated with trying to achieve higher or lower levels of the medium. For the studies described in this chapter, dominance is satisfied if the electric shocks are administered in large enough voltage gradations that the incentive to minimize the voltage received exceeds the cost of the decisions required. As will be seen in the three studies, it can be comfortably assumed that dominance is satisfied.

Physical pain also has several other properties that confer advantages over the use of cash payments for certain types of experiments. One feature is that pain is consumed immediately. This is typically not the case with money, since money may only be spent (i.e., translated into consumption) after the experimental session is over. When control over the timing of consumption is important, cash payments may not be appropriate. For example, it is not clear to us how the negative discounting experiment described in section two could be performed with monetary incentives. Another advantage of pain is that, unlike money, it is not transferable to other individuals, and thus must be consumed by the participant in the experiment himself. Finally, pain is of independent interest due to the fact that it is a consideration in many actual decisions that individuals face, such as the health levels and jail times examples explained earlier.

The first study focuses on the nature of negative time discounting. Negative discounting (see Lowenstein, 1987, or Caplin & Leahy, 2001) is a formulation of the intuition that an individual at times may wish to bring forward an adverse experience to "get it over with," or to postpone a favorable experience as if they wish to "savor" it. The study described in Section 2, also reported in Berns et al. (2006), considers the motivation behind the negative discounting of losses, with a focus on the existence and the nature of *dread*, a disutility associated with the anticipation of a future negative event. Traditional experimental economic methods, which record decisions, can accumulate evidence consistent with the existence of dread by showing that individuals try to avoid it. However, there are alternative explanations for decision patterns, which are consistent with negative discounting but exclude dread. One of these alternative explanations is that the disutility of the outcome itself increases with the length of time an individual waited for it (Ji, Kohno, Moore, & Woolf, 2003), and an individual seeks to bring the aversive outcome forward in time to lower the disutility when it is realized. That is, rather than focusing on the anticipation of the outcome, it focuses on the outcome itself.

Because fMRI technology provides information about process, it allows researchers to establish whether there is really an aversive experience associated with dread. In addition, it is possible to study the time profile of the aversive experience as the unpleasant outcome approaches. Characterization of the time profile would permit the researcher to distinguish between the two explanations of negative discounting described earlier. The use of painful shocks is particularly well suited to studying the existence of dread. Indeed, dread is defined only over outcomes that yield negative payoffs relative to the status quo, and so negative payoffs must be induced. In addition, the fact that in this particular experiment the researcher must exercise precise control over the timing of consumption of the incentive medium means that monetary payments cannot be used, but electric shocks can be an effective reward medium.

The second study, presented in Section 3 and also reported in Berns et al., (2007, 2008), concerns probability weighting. This is the notion that individuals make decisions as if they transform probabilities by a function $\pi(p)$, where p is the probability of an event. Probability weighting is a well-documented empirical phenomenon (see Starmer, 2000, for a survey) and is one of the core assumptions of prospect theory (Kahneman & Tversky, 1979). This contrasts with expected utility theory, which assumes that individuals choose between lotteries over uncertain outcomes using the objective probabilities of each outcome as the weight they place on each potential outcome. Prospect theory assumes that decisions are consistent with maximization of the average utility of outcomes, but with a transformation of the probabilities of each outcome used to calculate the average. Most of the empirical evidence suggests that $\pi(p)$ has an inverted S form, involving the overweighting of moderately small probabilities and the underweighting of relatively large ones. In the domain of losses, this pattern of inverted S-shaped probability weighting has only been established in experimental studies with hypothetical monetary lotteries, and with real losses that are subtracted from a fixed endowment of money. The use of electric shocks as a stimulus permits the realization of outcomes that are clearly inferior to the status quo. The use of neuroeconomic methods allows one to consider whether probability weighting originates at the stage of decision-making or whether it occurs in the absence of choice. This is because fMRI technology registers the response to the display of the lottery, in the absence of any decision.

The third experiment that we review concerns the nature of regret and rejoice (or rejoicing), and will be referred to as the "regret experiment" to facilitate exposition. Regret occurs when a choice an individual makes yields a payoff that is lower than an alternative choice would have yielded. Rejoicing occurs when an outcome of an individual's decision yields a higher payoff than would have resulted from an alternative decision. Regret and rejoice are ex-post phenomena experienced after a decision is made. This means that in decision-making experiments, their existence is inferred indirectly. While regret can be created in the domain of positive payoffs with the inducement of opportunity costs of foregone rewards, it is of special interest to study regret in the domain of negative payoffs. One reason for this is that making a decision that results in an outcome worse than the status quo typically results in real costs rather than opportunity costs. Thus, there may be more scope for regret – or for rejoicing at avoiding an adverse outcome – to exert a powerful effect when the decision is taken in the domain of losses. The use of neuroeconomic methods allows us, at least in principle, to identify whether the experience of an outcome is different when there is reason to believe that regret and rejoicing are occurring, and whether what is experienced in a situation where regret (rejoicing) is present is unpleasant (pleasant).

2. WHY DO PEOPLE WANT TO GET AN ADVERSE EXPERIENCE OVER WITH AS SOON AS POSSIBLE?

The experiment described in this section (see Berns et al., 2006 for more detail) was designed to distinguish between two potential explanations for why observed decisions might be consistent with negative discounting. One possibility is that, in addition to the utility of the outcome, the anticipation of the outcome may yield utility in itself. For impending negative outcomes, this means that an experience would be felt of "dread," a disutility incurred while waiting for the outcome. This disutility can be reduced if the time of the outcome is brought forward. In this account, waiting for an adverse experience is unpleasant for an individual, so it is optimal to get the experience behind him. A second possibility is that waiting for the outcome increases the disutility of the outcome itself. A bad outcome "hurts" more when it arrives because one waited longer for it. This would also account for a willingness to bring adverse outcomes forward in time, if possible. In the experiment described here, these two explanations imply a different time course of activation in the pain matrix, a network of brain regions associated with unpleasant or noxious stimuli (Ploghaus et al., 1999; Koyama, McHaffie, Laurienti, & Coghill, 2005; Raij, Numminen, Narvanen, Hiltunen, & Hari, 2005; Tracey, 2005; Craig, 2003; Peyron et al., 2000). Measuring the time profile of activation allows us to distinguish between the two explanations.

The pain matrix includes the following regions: the primary somatosensory cortex (SI), the secondary somatosensory cortex (SII), and the posterior insula, all of which are associated with the somatosensory experience of pain. Activity in the anterior insula, the rostral ACC, and the amygdale, has been linked to the visceral and emotions aspects of pain. Preparation for a withdrawal response has been linked to activity in mid-ACC and supplementary motor area (SMA). We take measures of activation of these regions as a measure of disutility, in an analogous manner to authors who have interpreted activation of other regions as a measure of positive utility (Camerer et al., 2005; Glimcher, 2002; Hsu, Bhatt, Adolphs, Tranel, & Camerer, 2005; Huettel, Stowe, Gordon, Warner, & Platt, 2006; Knutson, Taylor, Kaufman, Peterson, & Glover, 2005; Preuschoff, Bossaerts, & Quartz, 2006).

The experiment consisted of two phases, and each phase was divided into a sequence of trials. In each trial, cutaneous electrical shocks were delivered using a Grass SD-9 stimulator (West Warwick, RI) through shielded, gold electrodes placed 2–4 cm apart on the dorsum of the left foot. Each shock was a monophasic pulse of 10–20 ms duration. The Grass stimulator was modified by attaching a servo-controlled motor to the voltage potentiometer. The motor allowed for computer control of the voltage level without compromising the safety of the electrical isolation in the stimulator. The motor was controlled by a laptop through a serial interface. During the experiment, individuals were lying down in an fMRI scanner, and their skin conductance was registered. Scanning was conducted with a Siemens 3T Trio wholebody scanner. After acquisition of a high-resolution T1-weighted scan, fMRI of the BOLD response was performed (TR = 2350 ms, TE = 30 ms, 64 × 64 matrix, 35 axial slices, 3 mm cubic voxels). To prevent electrical artifacts in the fMRI signal due to shock deliveries, the latter occurred during a 50 ms pause after each volume, yielding an effective TR = 2,400 ms.

Prior to scanning, the voltage range was titrated for each participant. The detection threshold was determined by delivering pulses starting at zero volts and increasing the voltage until the individual indicated that he could feel them. This minimum perception threshold is denoted here as V_{min}. The voltage was increased further, while each participant was instructed, "When you feel that you absolutely cannot bear any stronger shock, let us know – this will be şet as your maximum; we will not use this value for the experiment, but rather to establish a scale. You will never receive a shock of maximum value." This maximum is denoted as V_{max}. The purpose of this procedure was to control for the heterogeneity of the skin resistance among subjects and to administer potentially painful stimuli in an ethical manner. Admittedly, this is an imperfect procedure in that some participants may not have indicated their maximum value, introducing another source of heterogeneity between subjects (willingness to reveal their maximum). We index the strength of the shock administered to an individual by s, where the associated voltage for an individual is $V_s = s * V_{max} + (1\ s) * V_{min}$. For the experiment, s took on values of 10%, 30%, 60%, and 90%. The stimuli in the experiment were of the form (s_t, d_t) where s_t is the shock strength at time t, and d_t is the delay between when the stimulus is shown and when the shock occurs.

In the first phase of the experiment each of 32 individuals participated in the 96 trials that constituted the Passive Phase of the experiment. Each trial began with the presentation of a cue that indicated both the voltage level and the amount of time one would have to wait for the outcome. The displays and timing are illustrated in Fig. 1. Shocks were delivered to the dorsum of the left foot on a 100% reinforcement schedule. After this was completed, the Active Phase of the experiment took place. The neural activation patterns were registered as the voltage delay combinations were displayed, and as individuals waited for the shock. After the realization of the outcome, the subject was required to rate the experience of the trial, in a range between "very unpleasant" and "very pleasant." To indicate his rating, he marked a location on a visual analog scale (Noussair, Robin, & Ruffieux, 2004) using a cursor operated with his hand control.

After the Passive Phase ended, the Active Phase took place. In this phase, participants were presented in a series of trials with pairs of voltage and delay: for example, a 90% voltage shock in 3 sec and a 60 percnt shock in 27 sec. Individuals were required to choose which of the two options they would prefer to receive. The shock was then administered in accordance with the choice of the participant. Choosing the shorter delay could not speed up the experiment, as each trial lasted the length of the longer of the two choices (when the shorter duration was chosen, the extra time was added to the interval between the shock and the next trial).

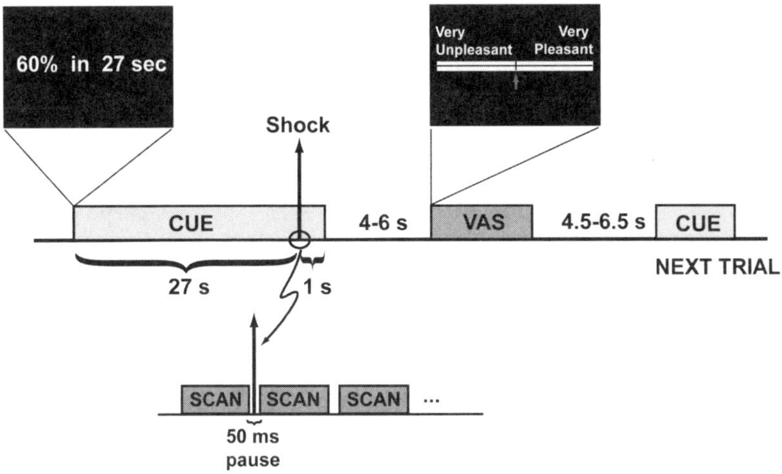

Fig. 1. Timing and Displays of a Trial, Dread Experiment.

In the Active Phase, in trials when the voltages were identical and the delays differed, 78.9% of the choices were in favor of the shorter delay, which is consistent with negative discounting. 27 of the 32 individuals chose the shorter delay in a majority of trials. Some individuals were even willing to accept a larger shock if it were administered sooner. The participants were classified into 23 mild and nine extreme dreaders. The extreme dreaders were those individuals who preferred more voltage sooner to less voltage later, and the mild dreaders were those who dreaded only to the extent of shortening the delay at a given voltage but were not willing to take more voltage just to get the shock over with. These classifications were consistent with individuals' self reports. Extreme dreaders reported a worse experience when they had to wait longer for the shock.

We examined the fMRI response to the shock itself and identified brain regions sensitive to shock amplitude by a linearly increasing contrast across voltage levels. We then selected 12 subregions of this map that intersected the pain matrix. A voltage-weighted contrast on the instantaneous response to the shock revealed a map consistent with previous reports of the pain matrix. Although a significant effect of the length of delay was observed in the right SII, the predominant pattern in the pain matrix was that waiting did not change the response to the shock itself; also, there was not a differential voltage sensitivity between mild and extreme dreaders. Therefore, whatever differentiated the two groups must have occurred during the waiting period, and it does not appear that the preference for expediting negative outcomes results from any impact of waiting on the utility of the outcome itself. Fig. 2 illustrates the activation as a function of voltage and delay for several regions for the mild and extreme dreaders separately.

To study differences between mild and extreme dreaders during the waiting period, we performed a time-series analysis on the regions of interest (ROIs). We used Loewenstein's (1987) model for the utility of anticipation to test the hypothesis that the distinguishing characteristic between mild and extreme dreaders lies in the prospective response to future outcomes. In this model, the present value of a delayed act of consumption is divided into two components: (a) the utility from consumption and (b) the utility from anticipation (dread). Assuming instantaneous consumption at the time (T) of shock delivery, the present value at time (t) of a future act of consumption is the utility of consumption U discounted by an exponential function with

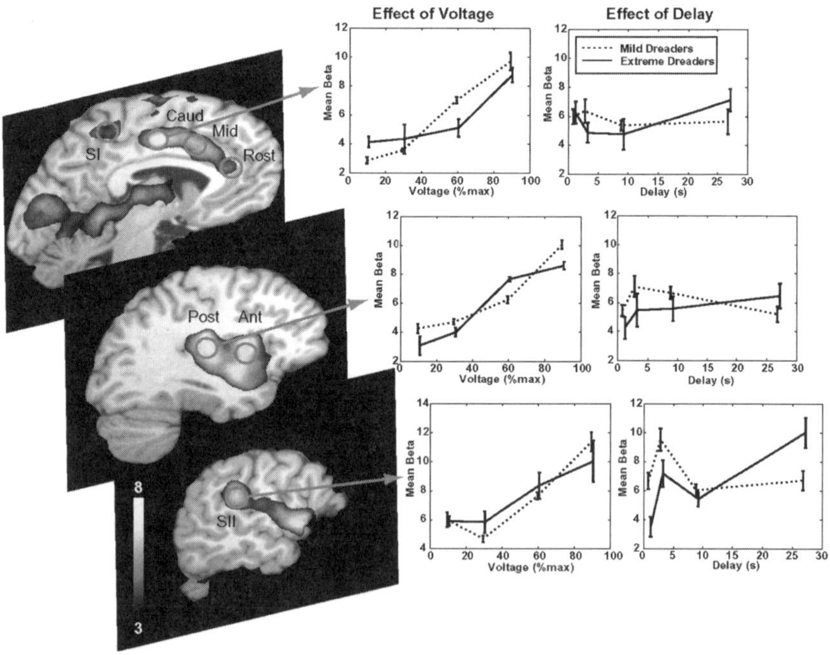

Fig. 2. Activation of Selected Brain Regions as a Function of Voltage and Delay, Dread Experiment.

rate $r = Ue^{-r(T-t)}$. In addition to the discounted consumption utility, anticipation (dread) also yields utility. For simplicity, we assumed that the instantaneous intensity of dread was constant and that the present value was this constant, a, multiplied by the time remaining until the shock. The constant a is referred to as the dread factor. Thus, combining the terms for dread and discounted consumption, the present value of future utility at time t, $U(V,t) = U(V) * [a(T-t) + e^{-r(T-t)}]$, where $U(V)$ is the utility of the shock with voltage V occurring at time T, a is the dread factor, and r is the discount rate. Differences in the utility of dread are reflected as differences in the dread factor a.

We observed that all of the contralateral (right hemisphere) regions of interest and the caudal ACC displayed time courses with dread factors significantly different from zero, but this was an effect observed primarily in the extreme dreaders and not the mild dreaders. Both SI and SII showed marked elevations in activity after the presentation of the cue – an elevation which continued to increase in advance of the shock. But the initial elevation in SI, SII, and right posterior insula, which was measured by the dread factor, was significantly greater in the extreme dreaders. The time course in the caudal ACC displayed a significant dread factor for only the extreme dreaders. The right amygdala had a significant dread factor for both groups, but was not significantly different between mild and extreme dreaders. From the time course of the response in these regions, coupled with its predominance in individuals who showed the most extreme behavioral evidence of not wanting to wait, we conclude that the component of anticipation that can be specifically attributed to dread appears in the posterior elements of the cortical pain matrix (SI, SII, the posterior insula, and the caudal ACC) and not the anterior ones (the anterior insula and the rostral ACC).

Both SI and SII have generally been associated with the physical intensity of noxious stimulation (Tracy, 1999; Craig, 2003; Petrovic, Petersson, Hansson, & Ingvar, 2002; Bentley et al., 2004), whereas the caudal ACC has been associated with the attentive component of pain (Vogt, 2005; Bentley, Derbyshire, Youell, & Jones, 2003). The localization of dread to the posterior elements of the matrix suggests that dread has a substantial attentive component. Both the mild and extreme dreaders displayed time courses of activity in SI, SII, the caudal ACC, and the posterior insula that were consistent with the utility-based theory of dread. The more anterior, emotional components of the pain matrix (e.g., the anterior insula, the rostral ACC, and the amygdala) did not have such time courses, indicating that dread is not primarily fear of the outcome. Moreover, it was the significantly different dread factor in the posterior divisions that most clearly distinguished mild from extreme dreading behavior when individuals subsequently had to make decisions regarding wait times. With regard to nociceptive inputs, both SI and SII receive afferent signals from the posterior portion of the ventromedial nucleus of the thalamus, whereas the ACC receives input from the mediodorsal nucleus (Craig, 2003). As the terminal fields from the spinothalamic system, these regions naturally show activations that track stimulation voltage. The amygdala, whose role in aversive conditioning is well known (Phelps, 2006), displayed a significant dread response on the right side, but this was not significantly different between the mild and extreme dreaders.

3. PROBABILITY WEIGHTING

A similar methodology to the one described earlier was used to consider the issue of probability weighting. In this second study, a total of 37 (20 female, 17 male) people were scanned using fMRI (28 were used for the analysis due to signal artifacts for nine subjects). The general framework and voltage setting procedure were similar to the experiment described in Section 2, except that the shocks were delivered probabilistically and all shocks occurred with the same delay. The study is reported in more detail in Berns et al. (2007) and in Berns et al. (2008).

After the voltage titration, the experiment began, and was divided into two phases. The first phase of the experiment, again called the Passive Phase, consisted of 120 trials. At the beginning of each trial, each participant was presented with a pie chart that conveyed both the voltage of the impending shock and the probability with which it would be received. The display thus defined a lottery consisting of a shock with voltage level, s, and a probability, p, in trial t, (s^t, p^t). The size of the pie chart indicated the strength of the shock that might be applied in the current trial, with the area of the pie chart equaling s times the area of the outer reference circle (denoting $V_{\max}$). The percentage of the inner circle that was filled in red indicated the probability with which the shock was to be administered. The possible probabilities were 1/6, 1/3, 2/3, 5/6, and 1. With the four voltage levels, this yielded 20 voltage-probability combinations, each of which was presented six times during the 120 trials that made up the passive phase of a session.

In the second phase, the Active Phase, each individual faced a sequence of 60-pairwise choices from the set of probability/shock combinations presented in the passive phase. In each round, two lotteries appeared side by side, and subjects were required to choose one of them, using the keypad provided to them. The experimenter chose the pairs so that in every trial one alternative always specified both a higher voltage shock as well as lower probability than the other alternative. In other words, if s^t_A and s^t_B are the strengths of the shocks that may be applied under choices A and B respectively in trial t, it was always the case that $s^t_A > s^t_B \leftrightarrow p^t_A < p^t_B$, where p^t_A is the probability that a shock is applied under choice A in trial t. Subjects received a shock with the voltage specified by their choice and with the indicated probability.

In the passive phase, a well-defined network of brain regions was active in response to the cue, and the pattern of activation could be largely dissociated into magnitude-sensitive and probability-sensitive regions. The probability-sensitive regions are given in Table 1. Some of these regions were clearly related to the low-level processing of visual stimuli (e.g., visual cortex). Other regions, however, encoded aspects of the anticipated voltage and/or probability. The probability of receiving a shock was most significantly correlated with activity in the bilateral inferior parietal cortex, near the temporal–parietal–occipital junction, whereas the magnitude of the impending shock was correlated with bilateral activity in the insula/superior

Table 1. Probability Sensitive Regions, Probability Weighting Experiment.

Region	MNI Coordinates	*T*-Statistic	NPRR(1/6) > 1/6?
Probability sensitive regions (Positive correlation)			
R Cingulate Gyrus (BA 24)	9, −18, 39	5.88	N
L Inferior Parietal Gyrus (BA 40)	−57, −57, 42	4.98	N
R Superior Temporal Gyrus (BA 22)	63, −48, 12	4.97	Y
R Superior Frontal Gyrus (BA 6)	9, 3, 63	4.92	Y
R Inferior Parietal Gyrus (BA 40)	66, −36, 30	4.91	N
L Cingulate Gyrus (BA 24)	−6, 0, 45	4.89	N
L Postcentral Gyrus (BA 7)	−9, −57, 69	4.64	Y
Probability sensitive regions (Negative correlation)			
L Visual Cortex (BA 18)	−30, −96, 6	5.58	N
L Posterior Cingulate (BA 29)	−12, −51, 6	4.66	Y
R Lingual Gyrus (BA 19)	18, −57, −3	4.30	N
L Anterior Cingulate (BA 24)	−6, 21, −3	4.05	Y
R Thalamus	21, −30, −3	4.03	Y
L Middle Temporal Gyrus (BA 37)	−48, −60, −3	4.00	Y

temporal cortex, precuneus, cerebellum, and a region of the precentral gyrus associated with the foot. Many other regions, including the caudate/subgenual ACC, displayed negative correlations with the impending magnitude of the outcome or the probability of receiving a shock. There was very little anatomical overlap between the magnitude and probability maps, with the exception of the ACC and supplementary motor area dorsal to it, in which interaction of the two dimensions was observed.

The ACC has been previously implicated in modulating decision weights for risky financial decisions (Paulus & Frank, 2006; Knutson et al., 2005). However, unlike Paulus and Frank, we found no significant correlation between individuals' levels of ACC activation and the curvature of their probability weighting implied by their lottery choice decisions. One possible reason is that the activation we measured represented a passive response in the absence of a decision. The ACC is a prime candidate for the integration of magnitude and probability information – even in the absence of a required response, because of its role in integrating the affective system and the motor response system (Botvinick, Braver, Barch, Cohen, & Carter, 2001; Critchley, Mathias, & Dolan, 2001; Miller & Cohen, 2001). Although prospect theory assumes functional separability of probability and utility functions, the multiplication of these two dimensions must occur somewhere. The ACC is an integral component of the cortical pain matrix, and current evidence suggests that the ACC integrates several dimensions of the subjective pain experience, including emotional and attentional components (Craig, 2003; Ploghaus et al., 1999; Vogt, 2005).

In order to determine a probability weighting function with fMRI measurements, we define a neurobiological probability response ratio (NPRR). This is the ratio of (i) the activation level associated with a lottery with two possible outcomes, a non-null outcome denoted by x, and a null outcome, and (ii) the non-null outcome with certainty. The activation associated with the null outcome, the non-null outcome, and the lottery are denoted by y_0, $y(x,1)$, and $y(x,p)$ respectively. The NPRR is given by:

$$\mathrm{NPRR}(x,p) = \frac{[y(x,p) - y_0]}{[y(x,1) - y_0]}$$

We choose y_0 as the activation associated with $p = 1/3$ for our study in light of an extensive behavioral literature on probability weighting in the financial domain suggesting that the probability weighting function crosses the diagonal in the vicinity of $p = 0.4$ (Abdellaoui, 2000; Kahneman & Tversky, 1979; Tversky & Kahneman, 1992; Wu & Gonzalez, 1996). In our experiment, the probability prospect that came closest to meeting these requirements was $p = 1/3$. Thus, for purposes of our analysis we employ:

$$\text{NPRR}(x, p) = \frac{2}{3}\frac{[y(x, p) - y(x, 1/3)]}{[y(x, 1) - y(x, 1/3)]} + \frac{1}{3}$$

Although this formula can be applied to all probabilities in the interval [0,1], its validity for probabilities less than 1/6 was untested in this experiment. We note, for example, that $p = 0$ may be a case that is treated categorically different by the brain. Because of deviations from normality in the distributions of NPRR, we used the median of the means of the three highest voltages value at each probability to estimate the central tendency. 95% confidence intervals of the median were computed according to this formula: $[(N+1)/2] \pm 1.96 * (\sqrt{N})/2$, which corresponded to subjects 9 and 20 in an ordered listing of the 28 participants. To test the null hypothesis of linear probability weighting, and thus the expected utility hypothesis, we used the 95% confidence intervals at $p = 1/6$, 2/3, and 5/6. Because previous behavioral evidence suggests non-linear probability weighting has an inverted S-shaped functional form, overweighting low-probability and underweighting high-probability events, we were particularly interested in whether NPRR(1/6) > 1/6, NPRR(2/3) < 2/3, and NPRR(5/6) < 5/6.

Our fMRI data, however, are consistent with a biological bias toward non-linear weighting of probabilities. Fig. 3 illustrates the activation of several of the regions of interest as a function of probability. In most cases, including in all of the regions shown in the figure, the NPRR displayed an inverted-S shape, which is characteristic of the behavioral probability weighting function hypothesized in prospect theory. As shown in the last column of Table 1, the majority of regions have the property that NPRR(1/6) is significantly different from (greater than) 1/6. The majority of regions also have the properties that NPRR(2/3) < 2/3, and NPRR(5/6) > 5/6 (results are available from the authors). Although we did not find significant departures from linearity for each probability value for each brain region, most regions displayed a significant departure from linearity for one of the probabilities. Importantly, when such a departure from linearity was observed, it was always in the direction predicted by prospect theory.

Regions that have been previously associated with probabilistic decision-making, notably in the parietal cortex (Huettel et al., 2006; Platt & Glimcher, 1999; Shadlen & Newsome, 2001; Glimcher, Dorris, & Bayer, 2005), showed significant forms of nonlinearity. We found maps for both probability and magnitude adjacent to each other near the temporo-parietal

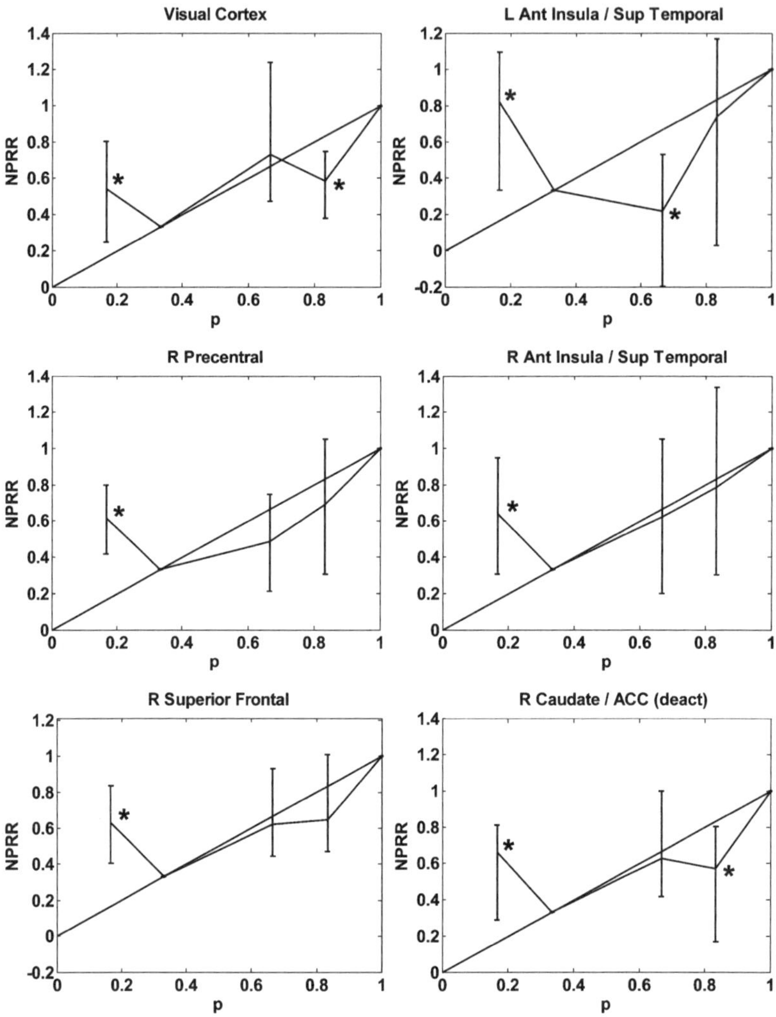

Fig. 3. Activation of Selected Brain Regions as a Function of Probability, Probability Weighting Experiment.

junction. The temporo-parietal junction, including both the inferior parietal lobule and superior temporal gyrus, has been implicated in at least one previous study of risky financial decision-making (Paulus & Frank, 2006). This region has also been conjectured to play a critical role in the judgment of true and false beliefs originating from other people (Grezes, Frith, & Passingham, 2004; Saxe & Kanwisher, 2003; Sommer et al., 2007) as well as attention shifting (Shulman, Astafiev, McAvoy, d'Avossa, & Corbetta, 2007). Its role in our experiment may operate similarly, if more generally outside the specific circumstance of decision-making: judging the likelihood of receiving and avoiding an aversive outcome (Mitchell, 2007).

Another region that showed non-linear weighting of probabilities was a large bilateral cluster encompassing the anterior insula and the superior temporal gyrus. The anterior insula, in particular, has been previously associated with anticipatory responses to painful stimuli (Craig, 2003; Koyama et al., 2005; Ploghaus et al., 1999; Tracey, 2005). Although this region was identified by its monotonically increasing response to expected magnitude, it also showed a significantly non-linear NPRR, suggesting that the distortion of probabilities becomes intertwined with representations of the likelihood of subjective states. Notably, we did not find significant activations of the amygdala, which has previously been associated with learning associations between cues and shocks. However, this could be due to the extended nature of the cues we used, or to the tendency of the amygdala to be activated transiently during cue acquisition (LaBar, Gatenby, Gore, LeDoux, & Phelps, 1998).

To test whether participants' decisions are consistent with non-linear probability weighting (see Berns et al., 2007, for more detail), we estimated values for γ in a standard specification for non-linear weighting (Tversky & Kahneman, 1992):

$$V(L) = \sum_i -\lambda \frac{p_i^\gamma}{(\sum_i p_i^\gamma)^{1/\gamma}} |x_i|^\alpha$$

Across all 37 subjects, the estimated median value was 0.685 for γ and was thus consistent with an inverted S-shaped probability weighting function, and with previous studies. We also considered the incidence of common-ratio-violations. In our experiment, common-ratio-violations were observed when the lottery (V_h, $p_l = 1/6$) was chosen over (V_l, $p_h = 2/6$), but (V_l, $p_h = 4/6$) was chosen over (V_h, $p_l = 2/6$), or vice versa. Out of six possible instances in which each individual could commit a common-ratio-violation, the average number of violations was 1.95, which was significantly different from zero. In general, the directions of the violations were consistent with fanning out of indifference curves.

The main conclusion of the experiment is the existence of a consistent form of non-linearity observed in neurobiological probability response ratios that parallels the type of nonlinearity observed behaviorally. When observing choice behavior alone, the source of this nonlinearity is unknowable. Individuals, for example, might distort probabilities only when they make a decision. Our data, however, suggests that these distortions occur even in the absence of choice and thus are a property of a more fundamental process of how the brain transforms representations of probabilities into biological responses.

4. REGRET AND REJOICING

In regret theory, regret and rejoicing affect the value of a lottery (Bell, 1982, 1983; Gilovich, Medvec, & Kahneman, 1998; Loomes & Sugden, 1987), and influence decisions between risky lotteries. A number of experimental studies have found that regret does influence decision-making (Cooke, Meyvis, & Schwartz, 2001; Janis & Mann, 1977; Sorum et al., 2004; Wolfson & Briggs, 2002; Zeelenberg, 1999; Zeelenberg, Beattie, van der Pligt, & de Vries, 1996) and can explain various economic phenomena (Smith, 1996; Tsiros & Mittal, 2000; Braun & Muermann, 2004; Dodonova & Khoroshilov, 2005; Muermann, Mitchell, & Volkman, 2006; Cooke et al., 2001).

A few neuroeconomic studies have investigated the neural correlates of regret when payoffs are monetary (Coricelli et al., 2005; Lohrenz, McCabe, Camerer, & Montague, 2007). These studies find that activity in the medial orbitofrontal cortex (OFC), anterior cingulate cortex (ACC), and right hippocampus is positively correlated with the magnitude of financial regret. Patients with damage to the OFC neither reported regret nor anticipated negative consequences associated with their actions (Camille et al., 2004). How this activation affects decision-making remains unknown, but one possibility is through the propagation of fictive error signals in the ventral striatum (Lohrenz et al., 2007) when the outcome is better than anticipated, or activation in the orbitofrontal cortex when the outcome is worse that expected (Liu et al., 2007).

Thirty-six right-handed volunteers (21 females and 15 males; 18–38 years of age with a mean of 21.64 years) participated in the study. Due to scanner gradient malfunctions, the data from six subjects were only partially acquired, leaving 30 subjects (17 females and 13 males; 18–38 years of age with a mean of 21.3 years) for the data analysis. Each participant was paid USD 40 for her participation. The experiment consisted of 100 trials. At the beginning of each trial, subjects were shown a display containing three doors on a screen located inside the scanner. In each trial, the subject's task was to select one of the doors, which would then be opened. Responses were registered with a fiber optic button-box, placed in the subject's right hand. At the beginning of each trial, the number of doors that contained shocks was indicated at the top of the display. The number ranged from zero to three. The conditions with zero or three shocks served as control conditions with no uncertainty, and we denote these as the no-rejoice and the no-regret conditions respectively. The other two conditions, with shocks behind one or two of the doors, allowed for regret and rejoice to be experienced. After a delay of 6.2–9.8 sec after the decision was made, all of the doors were opened. At the same time that the doors were opened, and depending upon whether a shock was associated with the door selected, the subject was either shocked once or not shocked. After the doors were opened, subjects were required to rate their experience on a horizontal visual analog scale (VAS), as in the experiments described in Sections 2 and 3. The study is described in more detail in Chandresakhar et al. (2008).

We assumed that in trials where the subjects received a shock, they would experience more regret when the probability of the shock was 1/3, followed by 2/3, and by 1 (i.e., monotonic). Similarly, in trials where subjects avoided a shock, they would experience rejoicing. The rejoicing would be strongest when the prior probability of a shock was 2/3, followed by 1/3, and then by 0. We measured fMRI BOLD responses to categorize the regions involved in the experience of regret, of rejoice, and of both experiences. Indeed, the results of the self-reports indicated that participants experienced different levels of regret, as well as different levels of rejoice, in a pattern consistent with our assumptions. Shocks were rated as more unpleasant the less likely they were to be received, and avoidance of a shock was rated more favorably the more likely the shock had been.

Analysis of the fMRI data indicated that individuals experienced a different pattern of brain responses associated with regret and rejoice, and these responses correlated with the degree of the two experiences. A within-subjects ANOVA of the fMRI activation revealed that several regions activated with an intensity modulated by the level of regret (obtained from the interaction term where receiving a shock interacted with the ex-ante probability of it being received). A region was classified as related to regret if it exhibited a pattern of decreasing activity from higher regret to higher rejoice conditions. The set of regret-related brain regions included the left thalamus, left middle occipital cortex, left inferior temporal cortex, right angular gyrus, left precuneus, left superior frontal cortex, and medial orbitofrontal cortex. Activation in the medial orbitofrontal cortex, the left thalamus, the left superior frontal cortex, and the right angular gyrus was greater in high regret than in no regret, as well as greater in no rejoice than in high rejoice. These areas are illustrated in Fig. 4.

A different network of brain regions was modulated by the level of rejoice. This network consisted of the bilateral ventral striatum, right caudate, left hippocampus, mid-brain/brain-stem, right supramarginal gyrus, right lingual gyrus, left calcarine, bilateral anterior insula, rostral anterior cingulate cortex, and the superior medial frontal cortex. These rejoice-related brain regions showed decreasing activity from higher rejoice to higher regret conditions. A subset of these regions also displayed greater activation with the highest level of rejoice than under no rejoice, as well as greater activation under no regret than the high regret. The subset consisted of the left hippocampus, left ventral striatum, rostral anterior cingulate, and mid-brain. The activation patterns in these regions are displayed in Fig. 5.

Other brain regions exhibited activation levels that increased with both the levels of regret and rejoice. This pattern of activation can be thought of as related to "surprise." As can be seen in Fig. 6, the right inferior orbitofrontal cortex, pre-supplementary motor area, dorsal anterior cingulate, and the posterior cingulate all displayed this type of pattern. They activated more strongly the lower the prior likelihood of the outcome that was eventually realized, whether the outcome was a shock or no shock. The right amygdala (identified from the main effect of levels) displayed a pattern of activity that did not fit into any of the above classifications. It had greater activation when the possibility of a shock existed. That is, it activated identically under every condition except for the one in which there was zero probability of a shock, in which it exhibited a lower level of activation.

Areas showing the strongest relationship included visual processing regions (middle occipital cortex and precuneus), which most likely reflected a shift in visual attention that scaled with the number of alternative outcomes. The thalamus, also associated with visual attention (Kastner & Pinsk, 2004), showed a similar increase in both higher regret and higher rejoice conditions. The other areas associated with regret but not with rejoice included the right angular gyrus, left superior frontal cortex, and the medial orbitofrontal cortex. In a previous study of regret using monetary outcomes, the medial orbitofrontal cortex was implicated in the experience of regret (Coricelli et al., 2005). This study also found that the presence of regret activated the inferior parietal lobule, a region that partially overlapped the area of regret-related activity we observed in the angular gyrus. Liu et al. (2007) found a similar pattern of activation in the

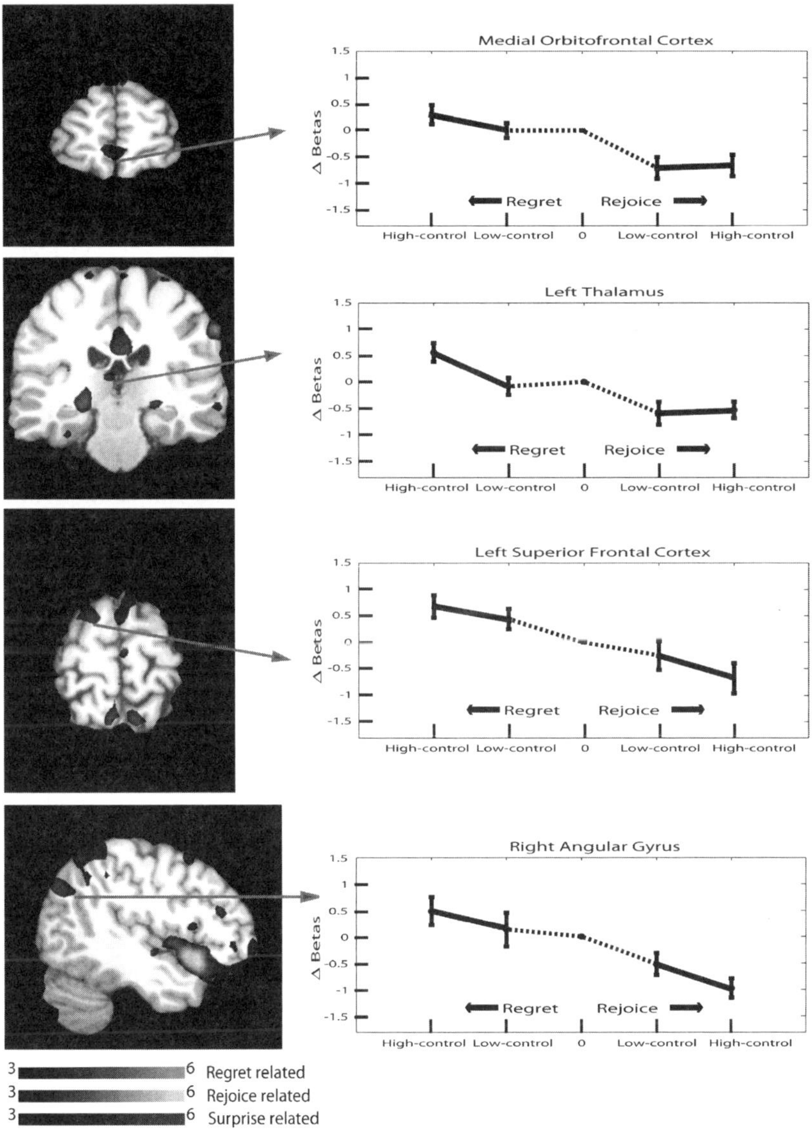

Fig. 4. Activation of Regret-Related Regions, Regret Experiment.

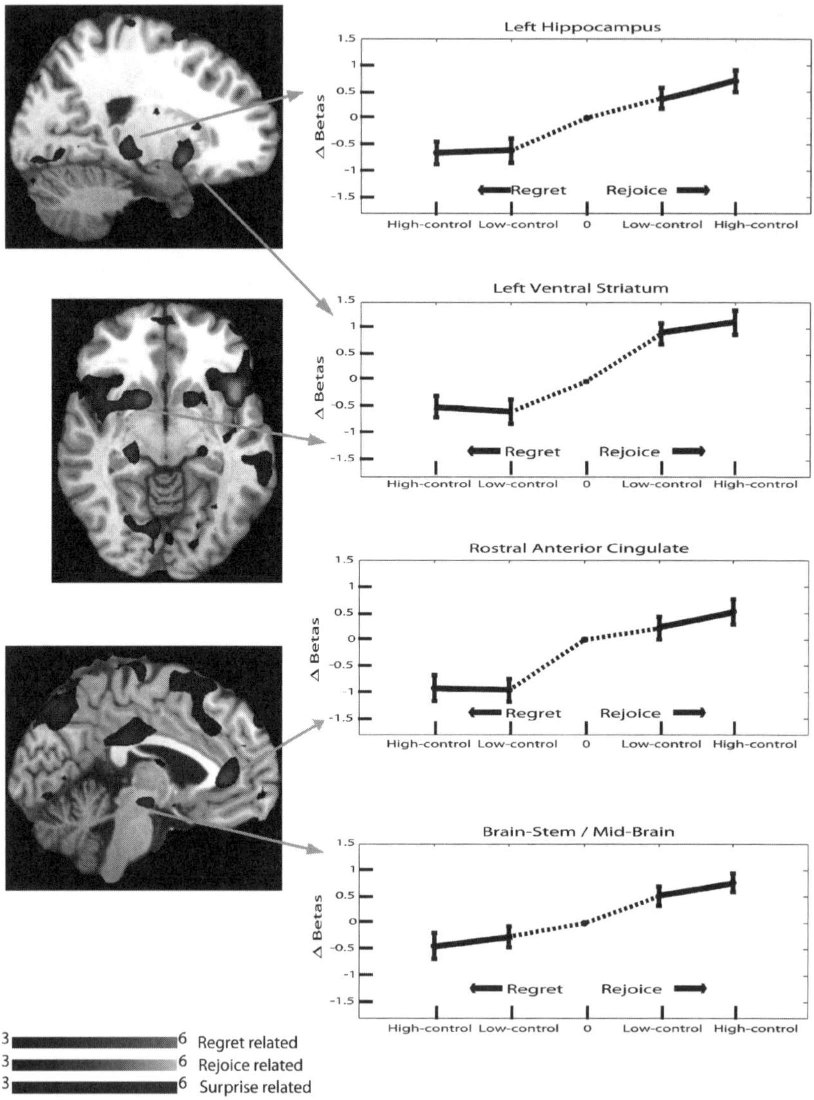

Fig. 5. Activation of Rejoice-Related Regions, Regret Experiment.

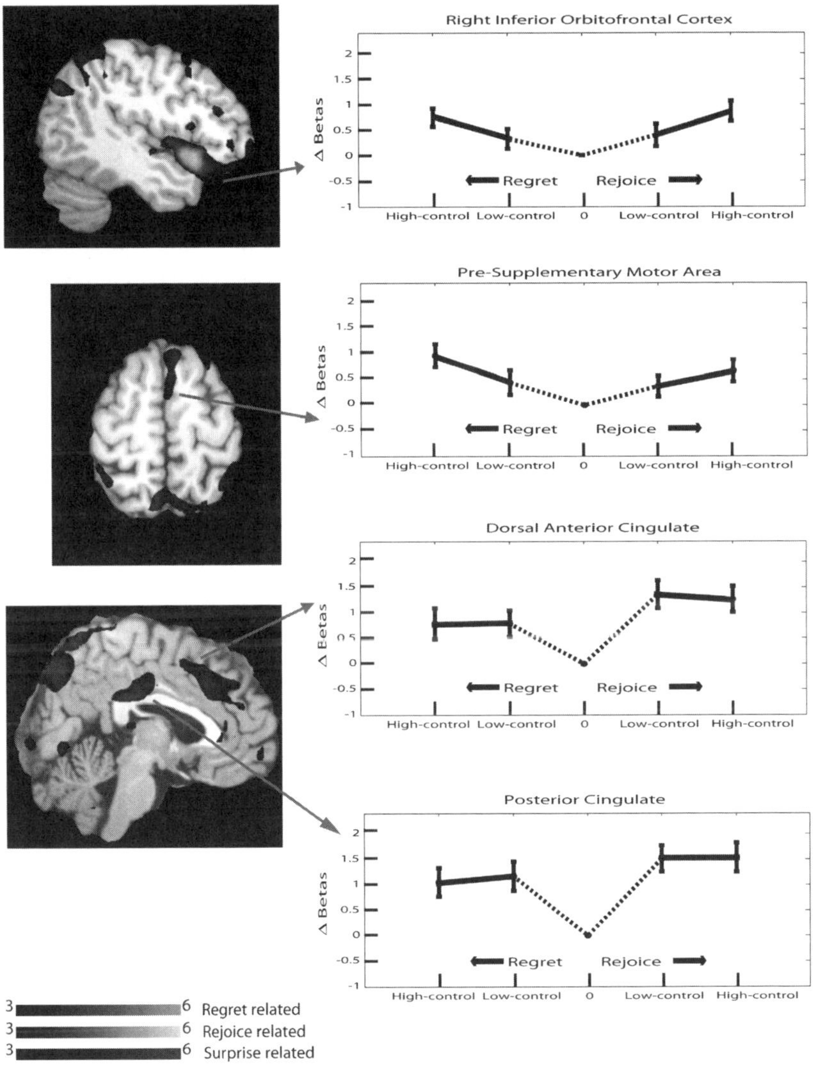

Fig. 6. Activation of Surprise-Related Regions, Regret Experiment.

orbitofrontal cortex when the outcome was worse than anticipated and striatum when better than anticipated. Thus, it indicates that the activation of some of the regret-related regions, notably the OFC, are robust with respect to a completely different incentive medium – electrical shocks.

Moreover, the creation of regret can also occur through variation in ex-ante probability in addition to the variation in magnitude of alternative outcomes.

Avoidance of a shock, leading to the experience of a degree of rejoice, was associated with a distinct network from regret. Surprisingly, the bilateral anterior insula showed the strongest relationship to the degree of rejoice. Although the insula has been linked with painful outcomes (Berns et al., 2006; Brooks & Tracey, 2005; Koyama et al., 2005; Peyron et al., 2000; Ploghaus et al., 1999), its anterior extensions have been characterized as relating to the anticipated emotional state of something potentially painful (Craig, 2003). Its role in rejoice here may reflect the tracking of the ex-ante probability of receiving a shock. More specific to the positive valence of avoiding a shock was the increasing rejoice-related activity of the left hippocampus and bilateral ventral striatum. The striatum, in particular, is generally accepted as playing a key role in reward-prediction errors (Berns, McClure, Pagnoni, & Montague, 2001; McClure, Berns, & Montague, 2003; Montague, King-Casas, & Cohen, 2006; O'Doherty, Dayan, Friston, Critchley, & Dolan, 2003; O'Doherty et al., 2004; Pagnoni, Zink, Montague, & Berns, 2002; Schultz, Dayan, & Montague, 1997; Yacubian et al., 2006). Since we manipulated regret/rejoice through probability, the more likely the anticipated shock, the greater the reward-prediction error when it was avoided. The fact that we observed increasing striatal activity with rejoice only, and not decreasing activity with regret, suggests that the ventral striatum may be involved in only one side of the regret/rejoice continuum. This finding is consistent with a recent study using financial markets which found that this same region computed only positive "fictive error" and not negative ones (Lohrenz et al., 2007). Thus, our finding can be viewed as an extension of this result to non-monetary outcomes.

Regions related to regret and near the striatum, namely the medial orbitofrontal cortex and rostral anterior cingulate cortex, exhibited reverse patterns of activation profiles. The medial orbitofrontal cortex has been implicated previously in studies of regret (Coricelli et al., 2005; Liu et al., 2007), while the rostral anterior cingulate has been previously implicated in emotional and error processing. Thus the rostral anterior cingulate area which is caudal to medial orbitofrontal cortex may be responsible for the emotional processes related to rejoicing (i.e., pleasure related) and suggests the possibility of a rostral-caudal gradient of different aspects of processing regret similar to that seen in the caudate for reward-prediction errors.

"Surprise" is a reflection of the ex-ante probability of a particular outcome: the lower the event's probability, the more surprising when it occurs. This network of surprise-related regions was more widespread than either the pure regret or rejoice networks. The lateral orbitofrontal cortex was the region most strongly activated by surprise. This region has more commonly been associated with aversive outcomes and losses (Hosokawa, Kato, Inoue, & Mikami, 2007; O'Doherty, Kringelbach, Rolls, Hornak, & Andrews, 2001; Rolls, 2000; Ursu & Carter, 2005). Its activation with both regret and rejoice in our study may reflect a specialization for the processing of potentially aversive outcomes, whether realized or not. Many of the surprise-related regions we observed, including the posterior cingulate, ACC, and precuneus have been linked to selective attention (Crottaz-Herbette & Menon, 2006; Hahn, Ross, & Stein, 2006; Hopfinger, Buonocore, & Mangun, 2000; Posner & Petersen, 1990; Small et al., 2003), and their activation in our study suggests a potentially augmenting effect of both regret and rejoice. In other words, the emotional response to either form of counterfactual comparison may require more attention to alternative outcomes. Without this attention, it is possible that regret and rejoice are not experienced.

REFERENCES

Abdellaoui, M. (2000). Parameter-free elicitation of utility and probability weighting functions. *Management Science*, *46*, 1497–1512.

Bell, D. E. (1982). Regret in decision-making under uncertainty. *Operations Research*, *30*, 961–981.

Bell, D. E. (1983). Risk premiums for decision regret. *Management Science*, *29*, 1156–1166.

Bentley, D. E., Derbyshire, S. W. G., Youell, P. D., & Jones, A. K. P. (2003). *Pain*, *102*, 265.

Bentley, D. E., Watson, A., Treede, R.-D., Barrtett, G., Youell, P. D., Kulkarni, B., et al. (2004). Differential effects on the laser evoked potential of selectively attending to pain localisation versus pain unpleasantness. *Clinical Neurophysiology*, *115*, 1846–1856.

Berns, G. S., Capra, C. M., Chappelow, J., Moore, S., & Noussair, C. (2008). Nonlinear neurobiological probability weighting functions for aversive outcomes. *NeuroImage*, *39*, 2047–2057.

Berns, G. S., Capra, C. M., Moore, S., & Noussair, C. (2007). A shocking new experiment: New evidence on probability weighting and common ratio violations. *Judgment and Decision-making*, *2*, 234–242.

Berns, G. S., Chappelow, J., Cekic, M., Zink, C. F., Pagnoni, G., & Martin-Skurski, M. E. (2006). Neurobiological substrates of dread. *Science*, *312*, 754–758.

Berns, G. S., McClure, S. M., Pagnoni, G., & Montague, P. R. (2001). Predictability modulates human brain response to reward. *Journal of Neuroscience*, *21*, 2793–2798.

Botvinick, M. M., Braver, T. S., Barch, D. M., Cohen, J. D., & Carter, C. S. (2001). Conflict monitoring and cognitive control. *Psychological Review*, *108*, 624–652.

Braun, M., & Muermann, A. (2004). The impact of regret on the demand for insurance. *Journal of Risk and Insurance*, *71*, 737–767.

Brooks, J., & Tracey, I. (2005). From nociception to pain perception: Imaging the spinal and supraspinal pathways. *Journal of Anatomy*, *207*, 19–33.

Camerer, C., Loewenstein, G., & Prelec, D. (2005). Neuroeconomics: How neuroscience can inform economics. *Journal of Economic Literature*, *XLIII*, 9–64.

Camille, N., Coricelli, G., Sallet, J., Pradat-Diehl, P., Duhamel, J. R., & Sirigu, A. (2004). The involvement of the orbitofrontal cortex in the experience of regret. *Science*, *304*, 1167–1170.

Caplin, A., & Leahy, J. (2001). *Quarterly Journal of Economics*, *116*, 55.

Chandrasekhar, P. V., Capra, C. M., Moore, S., Noussair, C., & Berns, G. S. (2008). Neurobiological regret and rejoice functions for aversive outcomes. *NeuroImage*, *39*(3), 1472–1484.

Cooke, A. D. J., Meyvis, T., & Schwartz, A. (2001). Avoiding future regret in purchase-timing decisions. *Journal of Consumer Research*, *27*, 447–459.

Coricelli, G., Critchley, H. D., Joffily, M., O'Doherty, J. P., Sirigu, A., & Dolan, R. J. (2005). Regret and its avoidance: A neuroimaging study of choice behavior. *Nature Neuroscience*, *8*, 1255–1262.

Craig, A. D. (2003). Pain mechanisms: Labeled lines versus convergence in central processing. *Annual Review of Neuroscience*, *26*, 1–30.

Critchley, H. D., Mathias, C. J., & Dolan, R. J. (2001). Neural activity in the human brain relating to uncertainty and arousal during anticipation. *Neuron*, *29*, 537–545.

Crottaz-Herbette, S., & Menon, V. (2006). Where and when the anterior cingulate cortex modulates attentional response: Combined fMRI and ERP evidence. *Journal of Cognitive Neuroscience*, *18*, 766–780.

Dodonova, A., & Khoroshilov, Y. (2005). *Applications of regret theory to asset pricing*. Working Paper.

Gilovich, T., Medvec, V. H., & Kahneman, D. (1998). Varieties of regret: A debate and partial resolution. *Psychological Review*, *105*, 602–605.

Glimcher, P. W. (2002). Decisions, decisions, decisions: Choosing a biological science of choice. *Neuron*, *36*, 323–332.

Glimcher, P. W., Dorris, M. C., & Bayer, H. M. (2005). Physiological utility theory and the neuroeconomics of choice. *Games and Economic Behavior*, *52*, 213–256.

Grezes, J., Frith, C. D., & Passingham, R. E. (2004). Inferring false beliefs from the actions of oneself and others: An fMRI study. *NeuroImage*, *21*, 744–750.

Hahn, B., Ross, T. J., & Stein, E. A. (2006). Neuroanatomical dissociation between bottom-up and top-down processes of visuospatial selective attention. *Neuroimage*, *32*, 842–853.

Hopfinger, J. B., Buonocore, M. H., & Mangun, G. R. (2000). The neural mechanisms of top-down attentional control. *Nature Neuroscience*, *3*, 284–291.

Hosokawa, T., Kato, K., Inoue, M., & Mikami, A. (2007). Neurons in the macaque orbitofrontal cortex code relative preference of both rewarding and aversive outcomes. *Neuroscience Research*, *57*, 434–445.

Hsu, M., Bhatt, M., Adolphs, R., Tranel, D., & Camerer, C. F. (2005). Neural systems responding to degrees of uncertainty in human decision-making. *Science*, *310*, 1680–1683.

Huettel, S. A., Stowe, C. J., Gordon, E. M., Warner, B. T., & Platt, M. L. (2006). Neural signatures of economic preferences for risk and ambiguity. *Neuron*, *49*, 765–775.

Janis, I. L., & Mann, L. (1977). *Decision-making*. New York: The Free Press.

Ji, R.-R., Kohno, T., Moore, K. A., & Woolf, C. J. (2003). Central sesitization and TLP: Do pain and memory share similar mechanism. *Trends in Neuroscience*, *26*, 696.

Kahneman, D., & Tversky, A. (1979). Prospect theory: An analysis of decision under risk. *Econometrica*, *47*, 263–291.

Kastner, S., & Pinsk, M. A. (2004). Visual attention as a multilevel selection process. *Cognitive, Affective and Behavioral Neuroscience*, *4*, 483–500.

Knutson, B., Taylor, J., Kaufman, M., Peterson, R., & Glover, G. (2005). Distributed neural representation of expected value. *Journal of Neuroscience*, *25*, 4806–4812.

Koyama, T., McHaffie, J. G., Laurienti, P. J., & Coghill, R. C. (2005). The subjective experience of pain: Where expectations become reality. *Proceedings of the National Academy of Science, USA*, *102*, 12950–12955.

LaBar, K. S., Gatenby, J. C., Gore, J. C., LeDoux, J. E., & Phelps, E. A. (1998). Human amygdala activation during conditioned fear acquisition and extinction: A mixed-trial fMRI study. *Neuron*, *20*, 937–945.

Liu, X., Powell, D. K., Wang, H., Gold, B. T., Corbly, C. R., & Joseph, J. E. (2007). Functional dissociation in frontal and striatal areas for processing of positive and negative reward information. *Journal of Neuroscience*, *27*, 4587–4597.

Loewenstein, G. (1987). Anticipation and the valuation of delayed consumption. *Economic Journal*, *97*, 666.

Lohrenz, T., McCabe, K., Camerer, C. F., & Montague, P. R. (2007). Neural signature of fictive learning signals in a sequential investment task. *Proceedings of the National Academy of Sciences of the United States of America*, *104*, 9493–9498.

Loomes, G., & Sugden, R. (1982). Regret theory: An alternative theory of rational choice under uncertainty. *The Economic Journal*, *92*, 805–824.

Loomes, G., & Sugden, R. (1987). Some implications of a more general form of regret theory. *Journal of Economic Theory*, *41*, 270–287.

McClure, S. M., Berns, G. S., & Montague, P. R. (2003). Temporal prediction errors in a passive learning task activate human striatum. *Neuron*, *38*, 339–346.

Miller, E. K., & Cohen, J. D. (2001). An integrative theory of prefrontal cortex function. *Annual Review of Neuroscience*, *24*, 167–202.

Mitchell, J. P. (2007). Activity in the right temporo-parietal junction is not selective for theory-of-mind. *Cerebral Cortex Epub ahead of print*.

Montague, P. R., King-Casas, B., & Cohen, J. D. (2006). Imaging valuation models in human choice. *Annual Review of Neuroscience*, *29*, 417–448.

Muermann, A., Mitchell, O. S., & Volkman, J. M. (2006). Regret, portfolio choice, and guarantees in defined contribution schemes. *Insurance: Mathematics and Economics*, *39*, 219–229.

Noussair, C., Robin, S., & Ruffieux, B. (2004). A comparison of hedonic rating and demand revealing auctions. *Food Quality and Preference*, *15*, 393–402.

O'Doherty, J. P., Dayan, P., Friston, K., Critchley, H., & Dolan, R. J. (2003). Temporal difference models and reward-related learning in the human brain. *Neuron*, *38*, 329–337.

O'Doherty, J., Dayan, P., Schultz, J., Deichmann, R., Friston, K., & Dolan, R. J. (2004). Dissociable roles of ventral and dorsal striatum in instrumental conditioning. *Science*, *304*, 452–454.

O'Doherty, J., Kringelbach, M. L., Rolls, E. T., Hornak, J., & Andrews, C. (2001). Abstract reward and punishment representations in the human orbitofrontal cortex. *Natural Neuroscience*, *4*, 95–102.

Pagnoni, G., Zink, C. F., Montague, P. R., & Berns, G. S. (2002). Activity in human ventral striatum locked to errors of reward prediction. *Natural Neuroscience*, *5*, 97–98.

Paulus, M. P., & Frank, L. R. (2006). Anterior cingulate activity modulates nonlinear decision weight function of uncertain prospects. *NeuroImage*, *30*, 668–677.

Petrovic, P., Petersson, K. M., Hansson, P., & Ingvar, M. (2002). A regression analysis study of the primary somatosensory cortex during pain. *NeuroImage*, *16*, 1142.

Peyron, R., Frot, M., Schneider, F., Garcia-Larrea, L., Mertens, P., Barral, F. G., Sindou, M., Laurent, B., & Mauguiere, F. (2000). Role of operculoinsular cortices in human pain processing: Converging evidence from PET, fMRI, dipole modeling, and intracerebral recordings of evoked potentials. *NeuroImage*, *17*, 1336–1346.

Phelps, E. A. (2006). Emotion and cognition, insights from studies of the human amygdala. *Annual Review of Psychology*, *57*, 27.

Platt, M. L., & Glimcher, P. W. (1999). Neural correlates of decision variables in parietal cortex. *Nature*, *400*, 233–238.

Ploghaus, A., Tracey, I., Gati, J. S., Clare, S., Menon, R. S., Matthews, P. M., & Rawlins, J. N. P. (1999). Dissociating pain from its anticipation in the human brain. *Science*, *284*, 1979–1981.

Posner, M. I., & Petersen, S. E. (1990). The attention system of the human brain. *Annual Review of Neuroscience*, *13*, 25–42.

Preuschoff, K., Bossaerts, P., & Quartz, S. R. (2006). Neural differentiation of expected reward and risk in human subcortical structures. *Neuron*, *51*, 381–390.

Raij, T. T., Numminen, J., Narvanen, S., Hiltunen, J., & Hari, R. (2005). Brain correlates of subjective reality of physically and psychologically induced pain. *Proceedings of the National Academy of Sciences, USA*, *102*, 2147.

Rolls, E. T. (2000). The orbitofrontal cortex and reward. *Cerebral Cortex*, *10*, 284–294.

Saxe, R., & Kanwisher, N. (2003). People thinking about people: The role of the temporo-parietal junction in "theory of mind". *NeuroImage*, *19*, 1835–1842.

Schultz, W., Dayan, P., & Montague, P. R. (1997). A neural substrate of prediction and reward. *Science*, *275*, 1593–1599.

Shadlen, M. N., & Newsome, W. T. (2001). Neural basis of perceptual decision in the parietal cortex (area LIP) of the rhesus monkey. *Journal of Neurophysiology*, *86*, 1916–1936.

Shulman, G. L., Astafiev, S. V., McAvoy, M. P., d'Avossa, G., & Corbetta, M. (2007). Right TPJ deactivation during visual search: Functional significance and support for a filter hypothesis. *Cerebral Cortex Epub ahead of print.*

Small, D. M., Gitelman, D. R., Gregory, M. D., Nobre, A. C., Parrish, T. B., & Mesulam, M. M. (2003). The posterior cingulate and medial prefrontal cortex mediate the anticipatory allocation of spatial attention. *Neuroimage*, *18*, 633–641.

Smith, V. (1982). Microeconomic systems as an experimental science. *American Economic Review*, *72*, 923–955.

Smith, R. D. (1996). Is regret theory an alternative basis for estimating the value of healthcare interventions? *Health Policy*, *37*, 105–115.

Sommer, M., Dohnel, K., Sodian, B., Meinhardt, J., Thoermer, C., & Hajak, G. (2007). Neural correlates of true and false belief reasoning. *NeuroImage*, *35*, 1378–1384.

Sorum, P. C., Mullet, E., Shim, J., Bonnin-Scaon, S., Chasseigne, G., & Cogneau, J. (2004). Avoidance of anticipated regret: The ordering of prostate-specific antigen tests. *Medical Decision Making*, *24*, 149–159.

Starmer, C. (2000). Developments in non-expected utility theory: The hunt for a descriptive theory of choice under risk. *Journal of Economic Literature*, *XXXVIII*, 332–382.

Tracey, I. (2005). Nociceptive processing in the human brain. *Current Opinion in Neurobiology*, *15*, 478–487.

Tsiros, M., & Mittal, V. (2000). Regret: A model of its antecedents and consequences in consumer decision-making. *Journal of Consumer Research*, *26*, 401–417.

Tversky, A., & Kahneman, D. (1992). Advances in prospect theory. Cumulative representation of uncertainty. *Journal of Risk and Uncertainty*, *5*, 297–323.

Ursu, S., & Carter, C. S. (2005). Outcome representations, counterfactual comparisons and the human orbitofrontal cortex: Implications for neuroimaging studies of decision-making. *Brain Research Cognitive Brain Research*, *23*, 51–60.

Vogt, B. A. (2005). Pain and emotion interactions in subregions of the cingulate gyrus. *Nature Reviews Neuroscience*, *6*, 533–544.

Wolfson, S., & Briggs, P. (2002). Locked into gambling: Anticipatory regret as a motivator for playing the national lottery. *Journal of Gambling Studies*, *18*, 1–17.

Wu, G., & Gonzalez, R. (1996). Curvature of the probability weighting function. *Management Science*, *42*, 1676–1690.

Yacubian, J., Glascher, J., Schroeder, K., Sommer, T., Braus, D. F., & Buchel, C. (2006). Dissociable systems for gain- and loss-related value predictions and errors of prediction in the human brain. *Journal of Neuroscience*, *26*, 9530–9537.

Zeelenberg, M. (1999). Anticipated regret, expected feedback and behavioral decision-making. *Journal of Behavioral Decision-making*, *12*, 93–106.

Zeelenberg, M., Beattie, J., van der Pligt, J., & de Vries, N. K. (1996). Consequences of regret aversion: Effects of expected feedback on risky decision-making. *Organizational Behavior and Human Decision Processes*, *65*, 148–158.

EMOTION, DECISION-MAKING AND THE BRAIN

Luke J. Chang and Alan G. Sanfey

ABSTRACT

Purpose – *Initial explorations in the burgeoning field of neuroeconomics have highlighted evidence supporting a potential dissociation between a fast automatic system and a slow deliberative controlled system. Growing research in the role of emotion in decision-making has attempted to draw parallels to the automatic system. This chapter will discuss a theoretical framework for understanding the role of emotion in decision-making and evidence supporting the underlying neural substrates.*

Design/Methodology/Approach – *This chapter applies a conceptual framework to understanding the role of emotion in decision-making, and emphasizes a distinction between expected and immediate emotions. Expected emotions refer to anticipated emotional states associated with a given decision that are never actually experienced. Immediate emotions, however, are experienced at the time of decision, and either can occur in response to a particular decision or merely as a result of a transitory fluctuation. This chapter will review research from the neuroeconomics literature that supports a neural dissociation between these two classes of emotion and also discuss a few interpretive caveats.*

Findings – *Several lines of research including regret, uncertainty, social decision-making, and moral decision-making have yielded evidence*

Neuroeconomics
Advances in Health Economics and Health Services Research, Volume 20, 31–53

ISSN: 0731-2199/doi:10.1016/S0731-2199(08)20002-6

consistent with our formulization – expected and immediate emotions may invoke dissociable neural systems.

Originality/value – *This chapter provides a more specific conceptualization of the mediating role of emotions in the decision-making process, which has important implications for understanding the interacting neural systems underlying the interface between emotion and cognition – a topic of immediate value to anyone investigating topics within the context of social-cognitive-affective-neuroscience.*

INTRODUCTION

The nascent field of neuroeconomics promises to deliver novel insights into everyday choice behavior by integrating the theories and methodologies from the diverse fields of psychology, economics, and neuroscience (Glimcher & Rustichini, 2004; Montague, King-Casas, & Cohen, 2006; Sanfey, Loewenstein, McClure, & Cohen, 2006). This approach attempts to merge economic principles, built on formal mathematical models, with measures of brain function using in vivo techniques such as single and multi-unit neuronal recordings, functional magnetic resonance imaging (fMRI), and more traditional neuropsychological methods that rely on patients with focal brain lesions. While the details of how these methods can be successfully integrated are still being developed, there have already been several interesting avenues of research (McCabe, Houser, Ryan, Smith, & Trouard, 2001; McClure, Laibson, Loewenstein, & Cohen, 2004; O'Doherty et al., 2004; O'Doherty, Hampton, & Kim, 2007; Sugrue, Corrado, & Newsome, 2005; Yechiam, Busemeyer, Stout, & Bechara, 2005), suggesting that the neuroeconomic endeavor can have a real impact in better understanding how we make choices and decisions.

One of the most promising of these directions is the notion that the brain may utilize specific subsystems when making judgments and decisions (Greene, Sommerville, Nystrom, Darley, & Cohen, 2001; McClure et al., 2004; Sanfey, Rilling, Aronson, Nystrom, & Cohen, 2003). The idea of the involvement of multiple systems in the processing of complex cognitions has a long history, dating back to the fathers of modern day psychology, including Descartes (Descartes, 1664), Wundt (Blumenthal, 1980), and James (James, 1890). This insight of William James, that decisions could be made via both automatic and controlled processes, has continued to intrigue researchers to this day. In fact, many proposed theoretical models utilize this notion of multiple systems (Chaiken & Trope, 1999; Epstein, 1994; Evans & Over, 1996; Hammond, 2000; Kahneman, 2003; Sanfey & Chang, 2008; Schneider & Shiffrin, 1977; Sloman, 1996; Stanovich & West, 2000).

Though each of these theories differs in implementational details, they all generally propose a dual-process model of decision-making, with two distinct systems that alternatively compete and cooperate to arrive at a decision (Poldrack & Packard, 2003). System 1 has consistently been described as automatic, fast, effortless, unconscious, associative, slow-learning, and emotional. System 2 can best be thought of as more controlled, slow, effortful, conscious, rule-based, fast-learning, and affectively neutral. System 1 processes are generally thought to underlie most of our more trivial decisions, where automatic responses are adaptive. System 2, which is typically more computationally demanding (Schneider & Chein, 2003), is available to monitor and potentially override System 1 when the automatic system requires more conscious control (for a more detailed review see (Sanfey & Chang, 2008). For example, when learning to drive an automobile, one's actions are largely in the control of System 2, with conscious controlled attention directed to the act of learning to operate a vehicle. With practice, many of these motor tasks become increasingly automatized under the control of System 1, which allows us to direct our attention towards conversation with passengers, listening to the radio, etc.

Standard models of decision-making have typically focused on System 2-type operations, namely the deliberative process of careful decision-making. In recent years, however, there has been a considerable effort to better specify the extent to which affective processes, such as those encompassed in System 1, can influence judgments and decisions. Traditionally, emotions have been outside the purview of decision-making researchers, and indeed emotions have often been proposed to be counterproductive to sensible decision-making. For example, we are often exhorted not to make decisions in the heat of the moment, and to cool down before making important choices. However, it is often the case that emotions may provide important signals to lead us to making more optimal decisions in certain circumstances.

Use of emotions in decision-making can have functional significance in learning what can be approached and what should be avoided (Davidson, 1995). Early work in this domain by neurologists revealed that patients who had suffered brain damage leading to impaired emotional processing often made suboptimal decisions as compared to emotionally intact controls (Bechara, Damasio, Tranel, & Damasio, 1997; Damasio, 1994). This was the first real empirical evidence suggesting that emotional processes may play a benevolent role in guiding decisions, and has since led to a growing literature on this topic. Other recent work has proposed the existence of the affect heuristic (Loewenstein, Weber, Hsee, & Welch, 2001; Slovic, Finucane, Peters, & MacGregor, 2002), by which we use the natural assessments of affective valence as the basis for judgments. These studies have largely discounted the notion that System 1 is naturally "irrational," and that System 2 provides the only set of processes capable of sensible decisions. Clearly, there is a complex exchange between these systems, and much further research will be needed before clearly defined boundaries between these systems are revealed, if indeed such boundaries exist. It is important to note at the outset that it is still largely unknown to what degree these systems are separable at the neural level. It seems very unlikely that these are two biologically distinct processes (Glimcher, Dorris, & Bayer, 2005), but evidence has shown that some degree of functional specialization may exist in the brain to distinguish the two types of processes.

The early research mentioned above used patients who had suffered brain injuries to examine the influence of emotions in decision-making. This approach is problematic for various reasons, including the heterogeneity of lesion locations, the possibility of brain damage to other areas, etc. The recent availability of brain imaging techniques that allow visualization of the normal, active human brain has allowed a wide variety of questions to be explored as to the involvement of emotions in decision-making.

The present chapter will discuss the neural underpinnings of emotion's influence on decision-making. The chapter will begin with a brief overview of how emotions are processed in the brain, highlighting key regions of interest. Next, a framework for conceptualizing emotions in the context of decision-making will be introduced. This conceptual framework, originally proposed by Loewenstein and Lerner (2003), makes an important distinction between expected and immediate emotions. The neural evidence supporting such a distinction will be evaluated using recent findings from neuroeconomic studies investigating regret, uncertainty, social decision-making, and moral decision-making. Finally, we will conclude with an integrative summary of all of the findings, noting a few interpretive caveats.

HOW THE BRAIN PROCESSES EMOTION

The study of emotion has traditionally focused on cognitive appraisals and physiological mechanisms. In recent years, however, there has been significant interest in assessing the neural response to emotional processing. One of the oldest debates in the emotion literature is whether or not the physiological responses associated with an emotional reaction precede the cognitive appraisal. William James (1884) and Carl Lange (1887) independently proposed that in response to a fearful stimulus, such as meeting a bear in the woods, the cognitive appraisal of fear will occur *after* the body has already physiologically responded to the situation. This response might take the form of a racing heart, hyperventilation, or fleeing the scene. Other theorists proposed that it was not possible to have a physiological response without the cognitive appraisal (Lazarus, 1982; Schachter & Singer, 1962). More recently, researchers have come to accept that both theories seem to be correct. The differentiation between these two responses is often referred to as either bottom–up or top–down processing. A bottom–up response is when the physiological response precedes the cognition, and a top–down response is when the cognitive appraisal leads to a physiological response.

Both of the aforementioned processes seem to have pathways in the central nervous system. For example, specific facial motor functions, like smiling, may have multiple innervations (Duchenne, 1862). Numerous cases have demonstrated that selective damage to either pathway spares the function associated with the other (Holstege, 2002; Trosch, Sze, Brass, & Waxman, 1990). Other physiological functions associated with emotion, such as respiration and heart rate, also seem to be regulated both involuntarily, via programs located in the brainstem, and voluntarily, through cortical input originating from the anterior cingulate cortex (ACC; Critchley et al., 2003; McKay, Evans, Frackowiak, & Corfield, 2003). The following section will present a brief overview of brain regions associated with emotional processing (see Fig. 1). For the purposes of this review, we will focus on negative emotions, such as fear and disgust. Investigations of this class of emotions have been considerably more extensive than studies of positive emotions. The primary reasons are that negative emotions are more straightforward to investigate in animals and can be extracted with relative ease in laboratory studies.

One emotion that has received extensive empirical investigation is fear. The experience of fear usually begins with a freezing response, a subsequent sympathetic response, and an increase in sensory perception. This allows the environment to be adequately surveyed before a fight or flight response is taken. Fear has been proposed to employ two distinct streams of processing operating in parallel. These two streams allow both a physiological response and a simultaneous cognitive appraisal (Ledoux, 1996). In the controlled

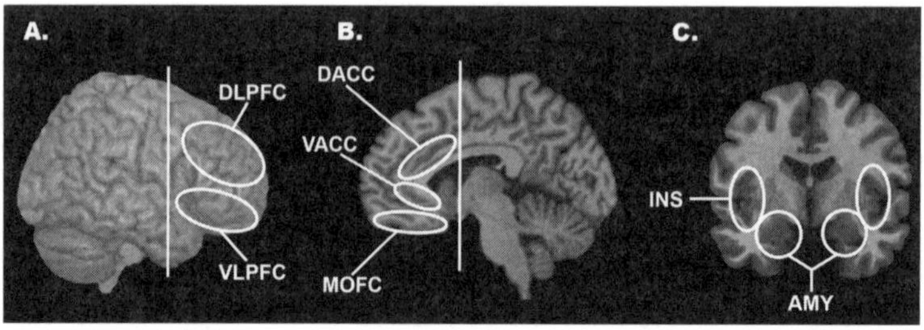

Fig. 1. Brain Areas Involved in Emotion Processing and Decision-Making. (A) The Lateral View Shows the Locations of the Dorsolateral Prefrontal Cortex (DLPFC) and Ventrolateral Prefrontal Cortex (VLPFC), Also Referred to as Lateral Orbitofrontal Cortex (LOFC). (B) The Saggital Section Shows the Locations of the Dorsal Anterior Cingulate Cortex (DACC), Ventral Anterior Cingulate Cortex (VACC), and Medial Orbitofrontal Cortex (MOFC). (C) The Coronal Section Shows the Locations of Bilateral Insular Cortex (INS) and the Bilateral Amygdalae (AMY). The Location of the Coronal Section is Indicated on the Lateral and Saggital Views by the White Vertical Line.

cortical route, information travels from the retina to the lateral geniculate nucleus of the thalamus and terminates in the contralateral primary visual cortex (Zeki, 1993). Visual information is then transmitted to the surrounding extrastriate cortex for further processing. The more controversial automatic subcortical pathway has been described as the "quick and dirty" route. It bypasses the visual cortex by traveling directly from the retina to the superior colliculus, then to the pulvinar (the posterior part of the thalamus) and amygdala, and then projecting to visual association cortex (Ledoux, 1996).

Overwhelming evidence suggests that the amygdala, a small almond shaped structure located in the medial temporal lobe (Aggleton, 1992), is essential to fear processing (Adolphs, Tranel, Damasio, & Damasio, 1994; Isenberg et al., 1999; LaBar & Cabeza, 2006; Ledoux, 1996; Morris et al., 1998; Phelps & LeDoux, 2005; Phillips, Drevets, Rauch, & Lane, 2003; Whalen et al., 1998). This makes sense from a neural framework as it is situated in a place such that it can receive higher-order inputs from multiple streams of cortical processing and signal autonomic responses in the hypothalamus to prepare the body for fight or flight.

Another negative emotion that has been reliably associated with a specific neural substrate is disgust (Calder, Lawrence, & Young, 2001; Phillips et al., 1997). Disgust is typically associated with stimuli that are revolting, inedible, or impure, and has been found to be associated with a region of the brain called the insula. The insula processes taste and smell information (Nolte, 2002; Small et al., 1999), as well as somato-visceral states of the body, such as pain, temperature, and "gut-feelings" (Craig, 2002). The insula has also been found to be associated with the experience of moral disgust (Haidt, 2001; Moll et al., 2005), autonomic arousal (Critchley, Elliott, Mathias, & Dolan, 2000), and in self-generated experiences of anger (Damasio, Grabowski, Bechara, & Damasio, 2000). Lesions to the insula can disrupt taste aversion in rats (Dunn & Everitt, 1988) and impair the recognition and experience of disgust (Calder, Keane, Manes, Antoun, & Young, 2000; Phillips et al., 1997) and other somato-sensory cravings in humans (Naqvi, Rudrauf, Damasio, & Bechara, 2007). The famous neurosurgeon Wilder Penfield found that stimulating the insula of patients during surgery led to the experience of nausea and unpleasant tastes (Penfield & Faulk, 1955). Antonio Damasio and his colleagues have proposed that the insula may be associated with the conscious experience of somatic states, and that it represents the influence of "gut-feelings" on decision-making (Bechara et al., 1997; Damasio, 1994; Naqvi et al., 2007).

The amygdala and insula have both direct and indirect reciprocal connections with regions that are associated with more cognitive functions in the prefrontal cortex (PFC). The ability to represent value and evaluate outcomes is thought to be associated with the medial orbital frontal cortex (MOFC; Gottfried, O'Doherty, & Dolan, 2003; Knutson, Adams, Fong, & Hommer, 2001; O'Doherty, Kringelbach, Rolls, Hornak, & Andrews, 2001), while the ability to override responses is associated more with lateral orbital frontal cortex (LOFC; Aron, Fletcher, Bullmore, Sahakian, & Robbins, 2003; Garavan, Ross, Murphy, Roche, & Stein, 2002). The more dorsal regions of the lateral prefrontal cortex (DLPFC) are important in maintaining and manipulating information (Baker, Frith, Frackowiak, & Dolan, 1996) and are associated with cognitive appraisals and goal maintenance (Miller & Cohen, 2001). The dorsal anterior cingulate cortex (DACC) is involved with a number of functions, including directing attention, monitoring error, and response override (Carter et al., 1998; Devinsky, Morrell, & Vogt, 1995; Miller & Cohen, 2001; Posner & Dehaene, 1994). The ventral anterior cingulate cortex (VACC) has been hypothesized to be associated with assessing the salience of emotional information and regulating emotional responses (Bush, Luu, & Posner, 2000; Devinsky et al., 1995; Drevets, 1999; Mayberg et al., 2005).

In summary, negative emotions such as fear, disgust, and anger have been reliably associated with distinct substrates of the brain, including the amygdala, insula, MOFC, and VACC. These regions process somatic states and signal physiological responses associated with arousal via the hypothalamic-pituitary axis. Likewise, they process higher-order cortical processes located in the LOFC, DACC, and DLPFC that can both up-regulate and down-regulate the emotional response. While these functions have traditionally been associated with basic emotion processing, recent evidence suggests that they may also be involved in more complex cognitive processes such as decision-making.

EMOTIONAL PROCESSES IN DECISION-MAKING

The impact of emotions on decision-making has been reviewed extensively elsewhere (Bechara, Damasio, & Damasio, 2000; Loewenstein & Lerner, 2003; Loewenstein et al., 2001; Mellers, Schwartz, & Ritov, 1997; Schwarz, 2000; Slovic et al., 2002); therefore, we will summarize here only the relevant work which has been studied in a neuroeconomic context. One useful framework for organizing the impact of affect on decision-making is to distinguish between expected and immediate emotions (Loewenstein & Lerner, 2003). Expected emotions are those that, while not experienced directly at the time of decision, are nonetheless important in the decision process itself. For example, when assessing a potentially risky investment, we may anticipate the regret we might feel should the investment fail. This anticipation of regret may in turn lead us to take the decision to avoid that financial opportunity. Immediate emotions, however, are those that are directly experienced at the time of the decision. Immediate emotions can have both direct and indirect effects on decision-making. Emotions that have direct effects can be considered "anticipatory" emotions. These emotions are experienced in anticipation of the actual decision and can include feelings of anxiety (Loewenstein et al., 2001; Slovic et al., 2002), dread (Berns et al., 2006), or excitement (Knutson, Fong, Bennett, Adams, & Hommer, 2003). Emotions that have indirect effects are referred to as "incidental" emotions. They include transient mood states that may be unrelated to the decision process, but nevertheless impact choice behavior.

Isen (2000) has shown that positive moods can lead to higher levels of risk aversion, increased reliance on heuristics, and increased efficiency in the decision-making process. Others have reported that experimentally induced incidental emotions, like sadness, can cause subjects to behave in ways that are more economically optimal, such as lessening the well-characterized endowment effect (Lerner, Small, & Loewenstein, 2004). The following sections will review the neural evidence supporting a distinction between expected and immediate emotions in the context of decision-making.

NEURAL EVIDENCE OF EXPECTED EMOTIONS

Expected emotions refer to the predicted emotional consequences associated with the result of a particular decision. These predicted emotional consequences can be positive or negative, and can therefore influence the decision accordingly. Expected emotions can be considered a top–down influence on behavior, as they are a cognitive representation of a future event, which in turn can elicit a physiological response. Previous researchers have hypothesized a dorsal/ventral distinction between the cognitive and emotional regions associated with affect (Bush et al., 2000; Lane, 2000). Candidate regions for expected emotions might include areas associated with goal maintenance and executive control (DLPFC), error or conflict monitoring (DACC), and value representation or outcome evaluation (MOFC). While there are numerous studies that have investigated the neural underpinnings of expected emotion on decision-making, we will focus on the most well studied emotion – regret.

Regret refers to the feeling that one experiences when the outcome of a decision is worse than expected. It differs from disappointment in that it is associated with a sense of personal agency (Bell, 1985; Loomes & Sugden, 1986). It was originally proposed as a way to explain behavioral violations of expected utility theory in decision-making under uncertainty, by incorporating regret minimization into the utility function (Bell, 1982; Loomes & Sugden, 1982). The experience of regret involves making a counterfactual comparison between the outcome actually experienced and an alternative outcome that was rejected (Byrne, 2002), and people generally avoid choice options that are associated with higher anticipated regret (Mellers, Schwatz, & Ritov, 1999; Zeelenberg, Beattie, van der Pligt, & de Vries, 1996). For example, one social psychology experiment found that when students were asked to exchange a lottery ticket they had personally chosen for one with better odds, the majority refused due to the anticipation of regret if their original ticket had won. Other work has demonstrated that regret is distinct from risk aversion (Zeelenberg et al., 1996), and that it can predict post-decisional affect (Mellers et al., 1999).

More recently, regret has been investigated from a neural framework using both lesion methods (Camille et al., 2004) and functional neuroimaging (Coricelli et al., 2005). Both studies utilized a task that has previously been used to investigate the influence of regret and disappointment on decision-making (Mellers et al., 1999). The task involved making a series of independent choices between two risky gambles that varied in magnitude (e.g. −\$200, −\$50, +\$50, and +\$200) and probability (e.g. 20%, 50%, and 80%). The authors elicited regret by disclosing the outcome of the alternative choice. A small actual win (e.g. \$50) compared to a large return of the un-chosen option (e.g. \$200) was hypothesized to elicit a negative emotional reaction.

Using both subjective ratings and skin conductance, Camille et al. (2004) demonstrated that healthy control subjects experienced regret when the outcome of the alternative choice was revealed, as compared to when it was not revealed. This experience of regret led subjects to adapt their behavior towards more regret-averse choices in subsequent gambles. Interestingly, patients with lesions in the orbital frontal cortex (OFC) did not generate a regret response as measured by subjective ratings or skin conductance, nor did they adapt their behavior to select more regret-averse choices in subsequent trials. The authors interpreted these findings to mean that the OFC is associated with counter-factual thinking that is crucial to the experience of regret.

In a subsequent study using fMRI, Coricelli et al. (2005) examined the brain response associated with both anticipated and experienced regret in healthy subjects. The authors parametrically manipulated experienced regret and observed an increase in activity in the MOFC, DACC, and hippocampus. This pattern of activity was distinct from outcome evaluation and experienced disappointment. Further, the authors noted that during the course of the experiment, the subjects became increasingly regret-averse.

These findings suggest that expected emotions, such as regret, can influence decision-making behavior, and are also associated with a specific neural substrate. The experience of regret seems to be associated with the MOFC, which may potentially be processing the counterfactual thinking associated with the emotion. Future research needs to experimentally tease apart exactly what aspect of regret is associated with the MOFC. Nonetheless, the behavioral evidence from the lesion patients and the neuroimaging results provides converging evidence that the MOFC is critical in the experience of this emotion, and that this in turn influences decision-making.

NEURAL EVIDENCE OF IMMEDIATE EMOTIONS

Immediate emotional reactions to a set of potential choices can also impact the decision-making process. Broadly, this has been termed the "affect heuristic" and it can occur automatically with or without conscious awareness (Slovic et al., 2002). These emotions may be associated with brain regions that automatically process information pertaining to somatic states that can lead to arousal, which in turn simultaneously signal other physiological responses and higher-order processing. These regions appear to be involved in processing of alternatives at an earlier stage as compared to expected emotions, which are more cognitive (top–down) in nature. Candidate regions involved in the processing of immediate emotions include the amygdala and insula. The following section will review evidence associated with the neural substrates of immediate emotions in a variety of domains, including uncertainty, social decision-making, and moral decision-making.

Uncertainty

Many experiments have demonstrated people's aversion to uncertainty in the context of decision-making, both in terms of the risk and the ambiguity of decision alternatives. Preliminary neural evidence supports the behavioral results that distinguish between the effects of risk and ambiguity on decision-making, and suggests that ambiguity may be associated with more negative aversive states. The neural computation of expected risk, like that of expected reward, may be localized to the ventral striatum (Fiorillo, Tobler, & Schultz, 2003). However, one study has reported a temporal dissociation, in which ventral striatal activity may be more delayed when calculating expected risk as compared to expected reward (Preuschoff, Bossaerts, & Quartz, 2006).

Ambiguity appears to be associated with even more aversive somatic states. Early conditioning studies in dogs found that unpredictable shocks lead to a state of learned helplessness (Seligman & Maier, 1967). In fear conditioning studies with humans, people are willing to withstand stronger electric shocks if they are more predictable than weaker, uncertain ones (Berns et al., 2006). Research investigating the neural substrates of ambiguity has implicated the insula, DLPFC, posterior parietal regions (Huettel, Stowe, Gordon, Warner, & Platt, 2006), amygdala and LOFC (Hsu, Bhatt, Adolphs, Tranel, & Camerer, 2005). This provides further evidence that unpredictability is associated with a negative somato-visceral state. In addition, similar to regret (Camille et al., 2004), damage to the OFC appears to lead to decreased risk and ambiguity aversion (Hsu et al., 2005).

Social Decision-Making

Immediate emotions have also been found to influence decision-making in social contexts. An economic game commonly used to study emotional processing in social situations is the Ultimatum Game (Guth, Schmittberger, & Schwarze, 1982). This game is typically played with two players – a proposer and a responder. The proposer is charged with splitting a sum of money between the two players. This split can range from fair ("We each get an equal share") to unfair ("You get nothing"). The responder must either accept or reject the offer put forth by the proposer. If the responder accepts the offer, each player is paid according to what is proposed by the proposer. If the responder rejects the offer, however, neither player receives anything. The standard game theoretic solution is for the proposer to offer the least amount of money that they believe the responder will accept. The responder should accept any offer greater than zero, on the grounds that something is better than nothing. However, many experiments have demonstrated that proposers typically offer about half of the money, and that responders reject offers of 20% of the pot or less about 50% of the time (Camerer, 2003).

Some empirical evidence has demonstrated that emotional reactions to unfairness, such as anger, underlie responder rejections (Pillutla & Murnighan, 1996; Xiao & Houser, 2005). These emotional reactions that lead to the rejection of unfair offers may be related to a fundamental evolutionary adaptive mechanism that serves to form and maintain social norms and reputation (Nowak, Page, & Sigmund, 2000).

Our group has investigated the neural systems involved in playing the ultimatum game. Sanfey et al. (2003) scanned subjects playing a one-shot ultimatum game in the role of a responder using fMRI. The subjects played with multiple human opponents and also with a computer opponent, which served as a control condition. In the comparison between unfair and fair offers, the authors observed an increase in activation in the bilateral anterior insula, DLPFC, and ACC. There was also a significant interaction in the bilateral insula between opponent type and fairness of the offer, with the activation greatest in the human unfair offers. Activity in the insula also correlated with the likelihood of rejecting an offer. Further, we found increased DLPFC activation in relation to an unfair offer, which we proposed reflects the increased cognitive demands needed to overcome the negative emotional response to an unfair offer. While this study provided a useful initial examination of how the brain makes decisions in a social context, many questions remain.

One question remaining is whether the subjects actually experienced a negative emotional reaction to unfair offers. To address this question, van 't Wout, Kahn, Sanfey, & Aleman (2006) measured electrodermal activity to assess the level of autonomic arousal experienced during the ultimatum game. Electrodermal activity has previously been found to be associated with insula activity (Critchley et al., 2000). Consistent with these findings, the authors observed increased electrodermal activity during unfair offers compared to fair offers. This activity was in turn associated with rejection of offers. Similar to the original Sanfey et al. (2003) study, this effect was specific to trials with human opponents. Subjects did not generate an electrodermal response to the computer control trials.

Another question is whether the DLPFC response to unfair offers was actually the result of maintaining a deliberative goal. To address this question, van't Wout, Kahn, Sanfey, & Aleman (2005) used repetitive transcranial magnetic stimulation (rTMS) to stimulate activity in the right DLPFC. This noninvasive technique allows for the temporary manipulation of neural activity by delivering a series of short bursts of magnetic pulses using a magnetic wand (Walsh & Pacual-Leone, 2003). The results were consistent with the prediction. Compared to sham stimulation (coil positioned but no pulse delivered), rTMS applied to the right DLPFC led to an increase in acceptances of unfair offers. This finding has recently been replicated by another group (Knoch, Pascual-Leone, Meyer, Treyer, & Fehr, 2006), though their interpretation differs somewhat.

Finally, in order to investigate the proposed role of the insula, we used simple emotional primes, namely movie clips, to elicit mood changes prior to playing the Ultimatum game. Based on the fMRI study outlined above, we hypothesized that negative emotion states would lead to increased insula activity, and thereby decrease acceptance rates of unfair offers. This is indeed what was observed, with acceptance rates while in a sad mood being significantly reduced as compared to both neutral and happy moods (Harle & Sanfey, 2007).

Recently, Koenigs and Tranel (2007) compared the performance of patients with VMPFC damage to healthy controls on the ultimatum game. They found that patients with VMPFC damage rejected more unfair offers compared to control subjects. At face value, this finding might contradict the hypothesis that patients with VMPFC damage should generate less immediate emotions to an unfair offer and therefore act in a more economically rational fashion. However, previous imaging results suggest that the emotional response to an unfair offer might be associated more with the insula (Sanfey et al., 2003). Further, there is some evidence that the

MOFC might provide inhibitory control of limbic regions such as the insula and amygdala (Critchley, Melmed, Featherstone, Mathias, & Dolan, 2001; Phelps, Delgado, Nearing, & LeDoux, 2004). Therefore, a VMPFC lesion would disinhibit the insula and lead to an increased emotional response and potentially higher rejection rates. This inability to regulate emotions is a common symptom of VMPFC damage (which typically includes the VACC) and has been well described (Bechara et al., 2000; Drevets, 2007; Rolls, Hornak, Wade, & McGrath, 1994).

Moral Decision-Making

In the domain of moral psychology, psychologists and philosophers have recently made the distinction between moral intuition and moral reasoning (Haidt, 2007). Similar to other dual-process models discussed above, moral intuition has been described as a fast, automatic emotional system. Moral reasoning has been described as more slow, deliberative, and cognitive. Greene et al. (2001) conducted a study investigating the neural correlates of moral intuition, in which subjects were presented with a number of moral dilemmas that had previously been rated as either moral-personal, moral-impersonal, or non-moral.

The authors hypothesized that moral-personal dilemmas should be the most emotionally engaging, and therefore associated with greater activity in brain regions involved with emotion processing. In support of their hypotheses, the authors observed increased activity in the MPFC, posterior cingulate cortex (PCC), and bilateral superior temporal sulci while making the moral-personal decisions. In a follow up study, the authors replicated their previous findings and observed increased activity in the DACC and DLPFC in trials where utilitarian decisions required violating personal morals, which was hypothesized to reflect increased conflict between emotional and cognitive systems. In these high emotional conflict trials, the authors also observed increased activity in the anterior insula and PCC. The authors proposed that the DLPFC is involved in making utilitarian judgments.

In support of this hypothesis, other investigators have found that patients with damage to the VMPFC endorsed more utilitarian moral judgments than either healthy controls or patients with lesions to other regions (Koenigs et al., 2007). This supports the notion that the VMPFC is necessary for generating emotional responses to moral-personal dilemmas. Patients with VMPFC lesions do not generate an emotional response to the moral-personal dilemmas and thus do not generate the conflict response described by Greene, Nystrom, Engell, Darley, and Cohen (2004). This potentially explains the increase in the endorsement of utilitarian judgments. In summary, these findings suggest that brain regions associated with emotion, such as the medial PFC, insula, and PCC, process the quick emotional responses to moral judgments, while the DLPFC may be involved in formulating more deliberative utilitarian judgments. These two systems may be arbitrated by the DACC conflict system.

DISCUSSION

The goal of neuroeconomics is to provide novel insights into processes underlying judgment and decision-making. Previous behavioral research has emphasized the importance of emotions in this process (Damasio, 1994; Loewenstein & Lerner, 2003; Loewenstein et al., 2001; Mellers et al., 1999; Slovic et al., 2002). We have attempted to present evidence that illustrates the potential neural substrates mediating emotional influences on decision-making. While the work reviewed here is preliminary in nature, there is growing evidence for a distinction between expected emotions and immediate emotions. Immediate emotions seem to be associated with more bottom–up automatic responses consistent with conceptualizations of the function of the amygdala and insula. Expected emotions, in contrast, appear to involve more top–down responses associated with regions such as the MOFC, which are important in assigning value and evaluating outcomes.

Other regions associated with higher-order cognitive functions, such as maintaining and manipulating information and goal states and response selection and control, may be linked to more dorsal PFC regions like the DLPFC and DACC (Carter et al., 2000; Miller & Cohen, 2001). Taken together, these findings suggest a neural dissociation between regions associated with automatic and controlled processing. An interesting avenue for future research would be to investigate how these systems cooperate and compete, and how this arbitration signal is generated in the brain (Daw, Niv, & Dayan, 2005). Preliminary evidence suggests that this function may be located in the DACC (Botvinick, Nystrom, Fissell, Carter, & Cohen, 1999; Carter et al., 2000), with some studies illustrating that this conflict might be observed when emotional responses contradict higher-order goal states, such as maintaining reputation, making money, or evaluating a moral dilemma (Greene et al., 2004; Sanfey et al., 2003).

In interpreting these findings, it is important to note some further caveats and limitations. First, emotion is a notoriously nebulous construct and to this day there is some disagreement about what actually constitutes an emotional state. Given the difficulty in defining this concept, it should come as no surprise that it is also difficult to measure. Emotion is typically measured using either subjective ratings or physiological measures. Unfortunately, there is conflicting evidence that these two measures are even related (for a discussion of the methods in emotion research see Coan & Allen, 2007). Additionally, a common approach within the field of neuroimaging is to observe a pattern of activation correlated with a behavioral measure, and then to use the "reverse inference" to assume that this pattern of activity necessitates the presence of this function (Poldrack, 2006). For example, repeated observation of amygdala activity in conjunction with the experience of fear does not necessarily mean that any activation of this structure *requires* that a fear response was present.

Finally, it is important to note that the theory of multiple systems remains somewhat controversial. Others have argued that "there is no neurobiological evidence that emotional and non-emotional systems are fully distinct in the architecture of the primate brain" (Glimcher et al., 2005), and indeed, the fact that all regions of the brain presumably serve multiple functions thus implies that there can never be fully dissociable emotional and cognitive regions. This criticism of the more extreme modularity view is likely true; however, the evidence discussed above does suggest that certain functions and processes may be subserved by different, probably overlapping, subsystems. Innovative multivariate statistical methods are beginning to facilitate the investigation of these systems-level networks (Damoiseaux et al., 2006; Fox et al., 2005; Greicius, Krasnow, Reiss, & Menon, 2003).

In summary, we have reviewed recent findings from the emerging field of neuroeconomics that have examined emotional influences on decision-making. These findings seem to be consistent with previous behavioral conceptualizations of emotional influences on behavior, which differentiate between expected and immediate emotions. We have also briefly discussed how emotion might fit into a dual-process framework, though it should be noted that the complex system-level dynamics of the brain most likely require a more refined and detailed theoretical framework. Nonetheless, even using this approach, we can make finer-grained distinctions between types of emotions, each of which appear to have dissociable neural substrates. Further development of this research direction, in conjunction with progress in both the theoretical and empirical understanding of emotion and techniques for better specification of neural activation, offers an exciting prospect for better understanding how our decisions are affected, for good and ill, by our emotions.

REFERENCES

Adolphs, R., Tranel, D., Damasio, H., & Damasio, A. (1994). Impaired recognition of emotion in facial expressions following bilateral damage to the human amygdala. *Nature*, *372*(6507), 669–672.

Aggleton, J. (Ed.) (1992). *The amygdala*. New York: Wiley-Liss.

Aron, A. R., Fletcher, P. C., Bullmore, E. T., Sahakian, B. J., & Robbins, T. W. (2003). Stop-signal inhibition disrupted by damage to right inferior frontal gyrus in humans. *Nature Neuroscience*, *6*(2), 115–116.

Baker, S. C., Frith, C. D., Frackowiak, R. S., & Dolan, R. J. (1996). Active representation of shape and spatial location in man. *Cerebral Cortex*, *6*(4), 612–619.

Bechara, A., Damasio, H., & Damasio, A. R. (2000). Emotion, decision making and the orbitofrontal cortex. *Cerebral Cortex*, *10*(3), 295–307.

Bechara, A., Damasio, H., Tranel, D., & Damasio, A. R. (1997). Deciding advantageously before knowing the advantageous strategy. *Science*, *275*(5304), 1293–1295.

Bell, D. E. (1982). Regret in decision making under uncertainty. *Operations Research*, *33*, 1–27.

Bell, D. E. (1985). Disappointment in decision making under uncertainty. *Operations Research*, *33*, 1–27.

Berns, G. S., Chappelow, J., Cekic, M., Zink, C. F., Pagnoni, G., & Martin-Skurski, M. E. (2006). Neurobiological substrates of dread. *Science*, *312*(5774), 754–758.

Blumenthal, A. (1980). A Wundt primer: The operating characteristics of consciousness. In: R. Rieber & D. Robinson (Eds), *Wilhelm Wundt in historical perspective* (pp. 121–144). New York: Plenum.

Botvinick, M., Nystrom, L. E., Fissell, K., Carter, C. S., & Cohen, J. D. (1999). Conflict monitoring versus selection-for-action in anterior cingulate cortex. *Nature*, *402*(6758), 179–181.

Bush, G., Luu, P., & Posner, M. I. (2000). Cognitive and emotional influences in anterior cingulate cortex. *Trends in Cognitive Sciences*, *4*(6), 215–222.

Byrne, R. M. (2002). Mental models and counterfactual thoughts about what might have been. *Trends in Cognitive Sciences*, *6*(10), 426–431.

Calder, A. J., Keane, J., Manes, F., Antoun, N., & Young, A. W. (2000). Impaired recognition and experience of disgust following brain injury. *Nature Neuroscience*, *3*(11), 1077–1078.

Calder, A. J., Lawrence, A. D., & Young, A. W. (2001). Neuropsychology of fear and loathing. *Nature Reviews Neuroscience*, *2*(5), 352–363.

Camerer, C. F. (2003). Dictator, ultimatum, and trust games. In: C. F. Camerer (Ed.), *Behavioral game theory* (pp. 43–116). New York: Russell Sage Foundation.

Camille, N., Coricelli, G., Sallet, J., Pradat-Diehl, P., Duhamel, J. R., & Sirigu, A. (2004). The involvement of the orbitofrontal cortex in the experience of regret. *Science*, *304*(5674), 1167–1170.

Carter, C. S., Braver, T. S., Barch, D. M., Botvinick, M. M., Noll, D., & Cohen, J. D. (1998). Anterior cingulate cortex, error detection, and the online monitoring of performance. *Science*, *280*(5364), 747–749.

Carter, C. S., Macdonald, A. M., Botvinick, M., Ross, L. L., Stenger, V. A., Noll, D., & Cohen, J. D. (2000). Parsing executive processes: Strategic vs. evaluative functions of the anterior cingulate cortex. *Proceedings of the National Academy of Sciences of the United States of America*, *97*(4), 1944–1948.

Chaiken, S., & Trope, Y. (1999). *Dual process theories in social psychology*. New York: The Guilford Press.

Coan, J. A., & Allen, J. B. (Eds). (2007). *Handbook of emotion elicitation and assessment*. New York, NY: Oxford University Press.

Coricelli, G., Critchley, H. D., Joffily, M., O'Doherty, J. P., Sirigu, A., & Dolan, R. J. (2005). Regret and its avoidance: A neuroimaging study of choice behavior. *Nature Neuroscience*, *8*(9), 1255–1262.

Craig, A. D. (2002). How do you feel? Interoception: The sense of the physiological condition of the body. *Nature Reviews Neuroscience*, *3*(8), 655–666.

Critchley, H. D., Elliott, R., Mathias, C. J., & Dolan, R. J. (2000). Neural activity relating to generation and representation of galvanic skin conductance responses: A functional magnetic resonance imaging study. *Journal of Neuroscience*, *20*(8), 3033–3040.

Critchley, H. D., Mathias, C. J., Josephs, O., O'Doherty, J., Zanini, S., Dewar, B. K., Cipolotti, L., Shallice, T., & Dolan, R. J. (2003). Human cingulate cortex and autonomic control: Converging neuroimaging and clinical evidence. *Brain*, *126*(Pt 10), 2139–2152.

Critchley, H. D., Melmed, R. N., Featherstone, E., Mathias, C. J., & Dolan, R. J. (2001). Brain activity during biofeedback relaxation: A functional neuroimaging investigation. *Brain*, *124*(Pt 5), 1003–1012.

Damasio, A. R. (1994). *Descartes' error: Emotion, reason, and the human brain*. New York: Penguin Putnam.

Damasio, A. R., Grabowski, T. J., Bechara, A., Damasio, H., Ponto, L. L., Parvizi, J., & Hichwa, R. D. (2000). Subcortical and cortical brain activity during the feeling of self-generated emotions. *Nature Neuroscience*, *3*, 1049–1056.

Damoiseaux, J. S., Rombouts, S. A., Barkhof, F., Scheltens, P., Stam, C. J., Smith, S. M., & Beckmann, C. F. (2006). Consistent resting-state networks across healthy subjects. *PNAS*, *103*(37), 13848–13853.

Davidson, R. J. (1995). Cerebral asymmetry, emotion, and affective style. In: R. J. Davidson & K. Hughdal (Eds), *Brain asymmetry* (pp. 361–387). Cambridge: MIT Press.

Daw, N. D., Niv, Y., & Dayan, P. (2005). Uncertainty-based competition between prefrontal and dorsolateral striatal systems for behavioral control. *Nature Neuroscience*, *8*(12), 1704–1711.

Descartes, R. (1664). *L'Homme (Treatise on Man)*. (T. S. Hall, Trans.). Cambridge, MA: Harvard University Press.

Devinsky, O., Morrell, M. J., & Vogt, B. A. (1995). Contributions of anterior cingulate cortex to behaviour. *Brain*, *118*(Pt 1), 279–306.

Drevets, W. C. (1999). Prefrontal cortical-amygdalar metabolism in major depression. *Annals of the New York Academy of Sciences*, *877*, 614–637.

Drevets, W. C. (2007). Orbitofrontal cortex function and structure in depression. *Annals of the New York Academy of Sciences*.

Duchenne, G. B. A. (1862). *Mecanisme de la Physionomie Humaine, ou Analyse Electro-Physiologique de l'Expression des Passions Applicble a la Practique des Arts Plastiques.* Paris: J.B. Balliere.

Dunn, L. T., & Everitt, B. J. (1988). Double dissociations of the effects of amygdala and insular cortex lesions on conditioned taste aversion, passive avoidance, and neophobia in the rat using the excitotoxin ibotenic acid. *Behavioral Neuroscience, 102*(1), 3–23.

Epstein, S. (1994). Integration of the cognitive and the psychodynamic unconscious. *American Psychologist, 49*(8), 709–724.

Evans, J. S. B. T., & Over, D. E. (1996). *Rationality and reasoning*. Hove, East Sussex, UK: Psychology Press.

Fiorillo, C. D., Tobler, P. N., & Schultz, W. (2003). Discrete coding of reward probability and uncertainty by dopamine neurons. *Science, 299*(5614), 1898–1902.

Fox, M. D., Snyder, A. Z., Vincent, J. L., Corbetta, M., Van Essen, D. C., & Raichle, M. E. (2005). The human brain is intrinsically organized into dynamic, anticorrelated functional networks. *Proceedings of the National Academy of Sciences of the United States of America, 102*(27), 9673–9678.

Garavan, H., Ross, T. J., Murphy, K., Roche, R. A., & Stein, E. A. (2002). Dissociable executive functions in the dynamic control of behavior: Inhibition, error detection, and correction. *Neuroimage, 17*(4), 1820–1829.

Glimcher, P. W., Dorris, M. C., & Bayer, H. M. (2005). Physiological utility theory and the neuroeconomics of choice. *Games and Economic Behavior, 52*(2), 213–256.

Glimcher, P. W., & Rustichini, A. (2004). Neuroeconomics: The consilience of brain and decision. *Science, 306*(5695), 447–452.

Gottfried, J. A., O'Doherty, J., & Dolan, R. J. (2003). Encoding predictive reward value in human amygdala and orbitofrontal cortex. *Science, 301*(5636), 1104–1107.

Greene, J. D., Nystrom, L. E., Engell, A. D., Darley, J. M., & Cohen, J. D. (2004). The neural bases of cognitive conflict and control in moral judgment. *Neuron, 44*(2), 389–400.

Greene, J. D., Sommerville, R. B., Nystrom, L. E., Darley, J. M., & Cohen, J. D. (2001). An fMRI investigation of emotional engagement in moral judgment. *Science, 293*(5537), 2105–2108.

Greicius, M. D., Krasnow, B., Reiss, A. L., & Menon, V. (2003). Functional connectivity in the resting brain: A network analysis of the default mode hypothesis. *Proceedings of the National Academy of Sciences of the United States of America, 100*(1), 253–258.

Guth, W., Schmittberger, R., & Schwarze, B. (1982). An experimental analysis of ultimatum bargaining. *Journal of Economic Behavior and Organization, 3*, 367.

Haidt, J. (2001). The emotional dog and its rational tail: A social intuitionist approach to moral judgment. *Psychological Review, 108*(4), 814–834.

Haidt, J. (2007). The new synthesis in moral psychology. *Science, 316*(5827), 998–1002.

Hammond, K. R. (2000). *Judgment under stress.* New York: Oxford University Press.

Harle, K., & Sanfey, A. G. (2007). Incidental sadness biases social economic decisions in the ultimatum game. *Emotion, 7*(4), 876–881.

Holstege, G. (2002). Emotional innervation of facial musculature. *Movement Disorders, 17*(Suppl 2), S12–S16.

Hsu, M., Bhatt, M., Adolphs, R., Tranel, D., & Camerer, C. F. (2005). Neural systems responding to degrees of uncertainty in human decision-making. *Science, 310*(5754), 1680–1683.

Huettel, S. A., Stowe, C. J., Gordon, E. M., Warner, B. T., & Platt, M. L. (2006). Neural signatures of economic preferences for risk and ambiguity. *Neuron, 49*(5), 765–775.

Isen, A. M. (2000). Positive affect and decision making. In: M. Lewis & J. M. Haviland-Jones (Eds), *Handbook of emotions* (pp. 417–435). New York: Guilford Press.

Isenberg, N., Silbersweig, D., Engelien, A., Emmerich, S., Malavade, K., Beattie, B., Leon, A. C., & Stern, E. (1999). Linguistic threat activates the human amygdala. *Proceedings of the National Academy of Sciences of the United States of America*, *96*(18), 10456–10459.

James, W. (1884). What is an emotion?. *Mind*, *9*, 188–205.

James, W. (1890). *The principles of psychology*. New York: Henry Holt and Co.

Kahneman, D. (2003). A perspective on judgment and choice: Mapping bounded rationality. *American Psychologist*, *58*(9), 697–720.

Knoch, D., Pascual-Leone, A., Meyer, K., Treyer, V., & Fehr, E. (2006). Diminishing reciprocal fairness by disrupting the right prefrontal cortex. *Science*, *314*(5800), 829–832.

Knutson, B., Adams, C. M., Fong, G. W., & Hommer, D. (2001). Anticipation of increasing monetary reward selectively recruits nucleus accumbens. *Journal of Neuroscience*, *21*(16), RC159.

Knutson, B., Fong, G. W., Bennett, S. M., Adams, C. M., & Hommer, D. (2003). A region of mesial prefrontal cortex tracks monetarily rewarding outcomes: Characterization with rapid event-related fMRI. *Neuroimage*, *18*(2), 263–272.

Koenigs, M., & Tranel, D. (2007). Irrational economic decision-making after ventromedial prefrontal damage: Evidence from the Ultimatum Game. *Journal of Neuroscience*, *27*(4), 951–956.

Koenigs, M., Young, L., Adolphs, R., Tranel, D., Cushman, F., Hauser, M., & Damasio, A. (2007). Damage to the prefrontal cortex increases utilitarian moral judgements. *Nature*, *446*(7138), 908–911.

LaBar, K. S., & Cabeza, R. (2006). Cognitive neuroscience of emotional memory. *Nature Reviews Neuroscience*, *7*(1), 54–64.

Lane, R. D. (2000). Neural correlates of conscious emotional experience. In: R. D. Lane & L. Nadel (Eds), *Cognitive neuroscience of emotion* (pp. 345–370). New York: Oxford University Press.

Lange, C. S. (1887). Ueber Gemuthsbewegungen, *3*, 8.

Lazarus, R. S. (1982). Thoughts on the relations between emotion and cognition. *American Psychologist*, *37*(9), 1019–1024.

Ledoux, J. (1996). *The emotional brain*. New York: Simon & Schuster.

Lerner, J. S., Small, D. A., & Loewenstein, G. (2004). Heart strings and purse strings: Carryover effects of emotions on economic decisions. *Psychological Science*, *15*(5), 337–341.

Loewenstein, G., & Lerner, J. S. (2003). The role of affect in decision making. In: R. J. Davidson, K. R. Scherer & H. H. Goldsmith (Eds), *Handbook of affective sciences*. New York, NY: Oxford University Press.

Loewenstein, G. F., Weber, E. U., Hsee, C. K., & Welch, N. (2001). Risk as feelings. *Psychological Bulletin*, *127*(2), 267–286.

Loomes, G., & Sugden, R. (1982). Regret theory: An alternative of rational choice under uncertainty. *Economic Journal*, *92*, 805–824.

Loomes, G., & Sugden, R. (1986). Disappointment and dynamic consistency in choice under uncertainty. *Review of Economic Studies*, *53*, 271–282.

Mayberg, H. S., Lozano, A. M., Voon, V., McNeely, H. E., Seminowicz, D., Hamani, C., Schwalb, J. M., & Kennedy, S. H. (2005). Deep brain stimulation for treatment-resistant depression. *Neuron*, *45*(5), 651–660.

McCabe, K., Houser, D., Ryan, L., Smith, V., & Trouard, T. (2001). A functional imaging study of cooperation in two-person reciprocal exchange. *Proceedings of the National Academy of Sciences of the United States of America*, *98*(20), 11832–11835.

McClure, S. M., Laibson, D. I., Loewenstein, G., & Cohen, J. D. (2004). Separate neural systems value immediate and delayed monetary rewards. *Science*, *306*(5695), 503–507.

McKay, L. C., Evans, K. C., Frackowiak, R. S., & Corfield, D. R. (2003). Neural correlates of voluntary breathing in humans. *Journal of Applied Physiology*, *95*(3), 1170–1178.

Mellers, B., Schwartz, A., & Ritov, I. (1997). Elation and disappointment: Emotional responses to risky options. *Psychological Science*, *8*, 423–429.

Mellers, B., Schwatz, A., & Ritov, I. (1999). Emotion-based choice. *Journal of Experimental Psychology*, *128*(3), 332–345.

Miller, E. K., & Cohen, J. D. (2001). An integrative theory of prefrontal cortex function. *Annual Review of Neuroscience*, *24*, 167–202.

Moll, J., de Oliveira-Souza, R., Moll, F. T., Ignacio, F. A., Bramati, I. E., Caparelli-Daquer, E. M., & Eslinger, P. J. (2005). The moral affiliations of disgust: A functional MRI study. *Cognitive and Behavioral Neurology*, *18*(1), 68–78.

Montague, P. R., King-Casas, B., & Cohen, J. D. (2006). Imaging valuation models in human choice. *Annual Review of Neuroscience*, *29*, 417–448.

Morris, J. S., Friston, K. J., Buchel, C., Frith, C. D., Young, A. W., Calder, A. J., & Dolan, R. J. (1998). A neuromodulatory role for the human amygdala in processing emotional facial expressions. *Brain*, *121*(Pt 1), 47–57.

Naqvi, N. H., Rudrauf, D., Damasio, H., & Bechara, A. (2007). Damage to the insula disrupts addiction to cigarette smoking. *Science*, *315*(5811), 531–534.

Nolte, J. (2002). *The human brain: An introduction to its functional anatomy*. St. Louis, MO: Mosby.

Nowak, M. A., Page, K. M., & Sigmund, K. (2000). Fairness versus reason in the ultimatum game. *Science*, *289*(5485), 1773–1775.

O'Doherty, J., Dayan, P., Schultz, J., Deichmann, R., Friston, K., & Dolan, R. J. (2004). Dissociable roles of ventral and dorsal striatum in instrumental conditioning. *Science*, *304*(5669), 452–454.

O'Doherty, J., Kringelbach, M. L., Rolls, E. T., Hornak, J., & Andrews, C. (2001). Abstract reward and punishment representations in the human orbitofrontal cortex. *Nature Neuroscience*, *4*(1), 95–102.

O'Doherty, J. P., Hampton, A., & Kim, H. (2007). Model-based fMRI and its application to reward learning and decision making. *Annals of the New York Academy of Sciences*, *1104*, 35–53.

Penfield, W., & Faulk, M. E., Jr. (1955). The insula; further observations on its function. *Brain*, *78*(4), 445–470.

Phelps, E. A., Delgado, M. R., Nearing, K. I., & LeDoux, J. E. (2004). Extinction learning in humans: Role of the amygdala and vmPFC. *Neuron*, *43*(6), 897–905.

Phelps, E. A., & LeDoux, J. E. (2005). Contributions of the amygdala to emotion processing: From animal models to human behavior. *Neuron*, *48*(2), 175–187.

Phillips, M. L., Drevets, W. C., Rauch, S. L., & Lane, R. (2003). Neurobiology of emotion perception I: The neural basis of normal emotion perception. *Biological Psychiatry*, *54*(5), 504–514.

Phillips, M. L., Young, A. W., Senior, C., Brammer, M., Andrew, C., Calder, A. J., Bullmore, E. T., Perrett, D. I., Rowland, D., & Williams, S. C. (1997). A specific neural substrate for perceiving facial expressions of disgust. *Nature*, *389*(6650), 495–498.

Pillutla, M. M., & Murnighan, J. K. (1996). Unfairness, anger, and spite: Emotional rejection of ultimatum offers. *Organizational Behavior and Human Decision Processes*, *68*, 208.

Poldrack, R. A. (2006). Can cognitive processes be inferred from neuroimaging data? *Trends in Cognitive Sciences*, *10*(2), 59–63.

Poldrack, R. A., & Packard, M. G. (2003). Competition among multiple memory systems: Converging evidence from animal and human brain studies. *Neuropsychologia*, *41*(3), 245–251.

Posner, M. I., & Dehaene, S. (1994). Attentional networks. *Trends in Neurosciences*, *17*(2), 75–79.

Preuschoff, K., Bossaerts, P., & Quartz, S. R. (2006). Neural differentiation of expected reward and risk in human subcortical structures. *Neuron*, *51*(3), 381–390.

Rolls, E. T., Hornak, J., Wade, D., & McGrath, J. (1994). Emotion-related learning in patients with social and emotional changes associated with frontal lobe damage. *Journal of Neurology, Neurosurgery, and Psychiatry*, *57*(12), 1518–1524.

Sanfey, A. G., & Chang, L. J. (2008). Multiple systems in decision-making. In: W. T. Tucker, S. Ferson, A. Finkel, T. F. Long, D. Slavin & P. Wright (Eds.), *Strategies for risk communication: Evolution, evidence, experience*. New York: Annals of the New York Academy of Sciences.

Sanfey, A. G., Loewenstein, G., McClure, S. M., & Cohen, J. D. (2006). Neuroeconomics: Cross-currents in research on decision-making. *Trends in Cognitive Sciences*, *10*(3), 108–116.

Sanfey, A. G., Rilling, J. K., Aronson, J. A., Nystrom, L. E., & Cohen, J. D. (2003). The neural basis of economic decision-making in the Ultimatum Game. *Science*, *300*(5626), 1755–1758.

Schachter, S., & Singer, J. E. (1962). Cognitive, social, and physiological determinants of emotional state. *Psychological Review*, *69*, 379–399.

Schneider, W., & Chein, J. M. (2003). Controlled & automatic processing: Behavior, theory, and biological mechanisms. *Cognitive Science*, *27*, 525–559.

Schneider, W., & Shiffrin, R. M. (1977). Controlled and automatic human information processing: I. detection, search, attention. *Psychological Review*, *84*(1), 1–66.

Schwarz, N. (2000). Emotion, cognition, and decision-making. *Cognition and Emotion*, *14*(4), 433–440.

Seligman, M. E., & Maier, S. F. (1967). Failure to escape traumatic shock. *Journal of Experimental Psychology*, *74*(1), 1–9.

Sloman, S. (1996). The empirical case for two systems of reasoning. *Psychological Bulletin*, *119*(1), 3–22.

Slovic, P., Finucane, M. L., Peters, E., & MacGregor, D. G. (2002). The affect heuristic. In: T. Gilovich, D. Griffin & D. Kahneman (Eds), *Heuristics and biases* (pp. 397–420). New York: Cambridge University Press.

Small, D. M., Zald, D. H., Jones-Gotman, M., Zatorre, R. J., Pardo, J. V., Frey, S., & Petrides, M. (1999). Human cortical gustatory areas: A review of functional neuroimaging data. *Neuroreport*, *10*(1), 7–14.

Stanovich, K. E., & West, R. F. (2000). Individual differences in reasoning: Implications for the rationality debate? *Behavioral and Brain Functions*, *23*, 645–726.

Sugrue, L. P., Corrado, G. S., & Newsome, W. T. (2005). Choosing the greater of two goods: Neural currencies for valuation and decision making. *Nature Reviews Neuroscience*, *6*(5), 363–375.

Trosch, R. M., Sze, G., Brass, L. M., & Waxman, S. G. (1990). Emotional facial paresis with striatocapsular infarction. *Journal of the Neurological Sciences*, *98*(2–3), 195–201.

van't Wout, M., Kahn, R. S., Sanfey, A. G., & Aleman, A. (2005). Repetitive transcranial magnetic stimulation over the right dorsolateral prefrontal cortex affects strategic decision-making. *Cognitive Neuroscience and Neuropsychology*, *16*(16), 1849–1852.

van't Wout, M., Kahn, R. S., Sanfey, A. G., & Aleman, A. (2006). Affective state and decision-making in the Ultimatum Game. *Experimental Brain Research*, *169*(4), 564–568.

Walsh, V., & Pacual-Leone, A. (2003). *Transcranial magnetic stimulation: A neuro-chronometrics of mind.* Cambridge, MA: MIT Press.

Whalen, P. J., Rauch, S. L., Etcoff, N. L., McInerney, S. C., Lee, M. B., & Jenike, M. A. (1998). Masked presentations of emotional facial expressions modulate amygdala activity without explicit knowledge. *Journal of Neuroscience*, *18*(1), 411–418.

Xiao, E., & Houser, D. (2005). Emotion expression in human punishment behavior. *Proceedings of the National Academy of Sciences of the United States of America*, *102*(20), 7398–7401.

Yechiam, E., Busemeyer, J. R., Stout, J. C., & Bechara, A. (2005). Using cognitive models to map relations between neuropsychological disorders and human decision-making deficits. *Psychological Science*, *16*(12), 973–978.

Zeelenberg, M., Beattie, J., van der Pligt, J., & de Vries, N. (1996). Consequences of regret aversion: Effects of expected feedback on risky decision making. *Organizational Behavior and Human Decision Processes*, *65*, 148–158.

Zeki, S. (1993). *A vision of the brain.* London: Blackwell.

ANXIETY AND DECISION-MAKING: TOWARD A NEUROECONOMICS PERSPECTIVE

Andrei C. Miu, Mircea Miclea and Daniel Houser

ABSTRACT

Purpose – *This chapter focuses on individual differences in anxiety, by reviewing its neurobiology, cognitive effects, with an emphasis on decision-making, and recent developments in neuroeconomics.*

Methodology – *A review and discussion of anxiety and decision-making research.*

Practical implications – *This chapter argues that by making the step from emotional states to individual differences in emotion, neuroeconomics can extend its neurobiological roots and outreach its current clinical relevance.*

Value of chapter – *This chapter contributes to the literature on individual differences in emotion and their effects on decision-making, which is increasingly important in mainstream behavioral economics and neuroeconomics.*

Neuroeconomics
Advances in Health Economics and Health Services Research, Volume 20, 55–84

ISSN: 0731-2199/doi:10.1016/S0731-2199(08)20003-8

INTRODUCTION

Different people facing the same problem often make different decisions that seem difficult to reconcile with standard expected utility theory. Particularly when the problem involves a high degree of uncertainty and risk, human decision-making often deviates from economic models of rational behavior. Tversky and Kahneman explained this phenomenon with their groundbreaking identification of heuristics that systematically bias decision-making (Tversky & Kahneman, 1974). This paradigm shift set the stage for a boom in behavioral economics, along with a systematic interest in individual differences in decision-making.

Behavioral economics, and more recently, neuroeconomics, have subsequently become more interested in emotion and the individual differences related to emotion. In this respect, behavioral economics parallels cognitive psychology, which previously separated emotion from cognitive processes (Neisser, 1967), but now extensively studies emotion and cognition interactions in mainstream science (for review, see Dalgleish & Power, 1999; Damasio, 2000; Dolan, 2002). Similarly, behavioral economics has become more receptive to the potential role of emotion in adaptive decision-making. As a result, it no longer adheres to the earlier view that people behave more rationally to the extent that they can free themselves of emotion.

Originally, neither psychologists nor economists fully appreciated the idea that emotions could have a positive role in decision-making. They exemplified the representiveness heuristic in scientific thinking by considering only those emotions (e.g., social anxiety) that subjectively stood out, essentially because they interfered with cognition. The reason for this is that traditional methods of measuring emotion relied mostly on evaluative reports. In fact, psychological research only recently began to dominantly view emotions as multidimensional subjective, behavioral, and psychological responses. The change occurred in part due to the realization that: (a) emotions reflect states of activation in two complementary appetitive and defensive motivational systems, and (b) these systems may have evolved independently of a link to a developed language system. Both insights contributed to the ensuing shift from subjective reports to behavioral and physiological measures of emotions (for review, see Bradley & Lang, 2007). These theoretical and methodological changes in studying emotions stemmed from multidisciplinary efforts bridging psychology, physiology, and neuroscience. Such collaborative efforts were instrumental in helping scholars to understand the effects of emotional responses.

Emotional responses can be associated with psychophysiological signals that sometimes exert a sub-conscious influence on decision-making. The somatic marker hypothesis developed this neuropsychological perspective. The theory was based on the discovery of skin conductance increases, typically associated with emotional arousal, which anticipated advantageous choices in a decision-making task simulating uncertainty and risk (Bechara, Damasio, Damasio, & Anderson, 1994). This finding was striking because the somatic markers predicted advantageous choices, even before participants knew the strategy that could maximize their long-term gain. Since first articulated (Damasio, Tranel, & Damasio, 1991), the association between decision-making deficits in what became known as the Iowa Gambling Task, and the absence of anticipatory skin conductance increases in patients with lesions in the ventromedial prefrontal cortex, has stimulated tremendous research in the neuropsychology of emotion and decision (for review, see Bechara, Damasio, & Damasio, 2000).

Accumulating evidence on the somatic marker hypothesis and other theories of emotion and cognition in neuropsychology have drawn the attention of scholars in psychology, neuroscience, and economics to the role of emotion in decision-making. Ideas such as J.A. Gray's reinforcement sensitivity theory (for review, see Gray & McNaughton, 2003) have generated interest in individual differences related to emotion. Studies of the neurobiological basis of emotion, decision, and individual differences have appeared in the developing field of neuroeconomics. Such studies often use non-invasive electrophysiological and functional neuroimaging procedures to draw inferences with respect to brain activity in healthy humans (see, e.g., McCabe, 2003; Camerer, Loewenstein, & Prelec, 2005; Sanfey, Loewenstein, McClure, & Cohen, 2006; Loewenstein, Rick, & Cohen, 2008).

In this chapter, we provide a neuroeconomics perspective on the relationship between a particular individual difference, state/trait anxiety, and decision-making. Further, we discuss the dysregulation of this relationship in anxiety and affective disorders. Affective states are passing emotional experiences or moods, whereas affective traits (e.g., trait anxiety, trait optimism, trait rumination; see Scheier, Carver, & Bridges, 1994; Sharot, Riccardi, Raio, & Phelps, 2007; Trapnell & Campbell, 1999; Ray et al., 2005) are chronic dispositions towards such experiences (Gasper & Clore, 1998). This chapter outlines how the investigation of individual differences related to emotion, such as trait anxiety, has begun to factor into the current understanding of emotion's role in decision-making. We focus on trait anxiety for the reason that it is significantly genetic in nature and is relevant to the risk of anxiety and affective disorders in its impact on the brain and behavior. Using this focus, we implicitly argue that by making the step from emotional states to affective traits or individual differences in emotion, neuroeconomics can extend its neurobiological roots and outreach its current clinical relevance. The same view has also been defended in other complementary reviews (Rahman, Sahakia, Cardinal, Rogers, & Robbins, 2001; Paulus, 2007).

NEUROBIOLOGY OF ANXIETY

Some people, when asked to make predictions about their future, will tend to overestimate the risk of personally relevant negative events (e.g., being diagnosed with cancer sometime later in life). Consequently, avoiding these perceived risks will drive their behavior. We chose to focus here on the trait of anxiety because this affective trait has a strong biological determination, is relatively stable during life, and has been shown to influence cognition, behavior, health, and underlying brain activity. In our view, this trait is one whose study is currently at the frontier of the psychobiology of personality.

A personality trait implies a generalized and enduring predisposition to react to many situations in a relatively consistent manner (Allport, 1937). Early factor analyses of behavioral tendencies first distinguished anxiety from stress. Scholars originally viewed anxiety as being caused by frustration of one's values (Cattell & Scheier, 1958). Stress, however, was thought to be triggered when the demands of a situation exceeded one's biological, psychological, or social resources (for review, see Lazarus, 1993). Later work coined this distinction, defining state anxiety as an emotion characterized by a subjective feeling of tension, cognitions involving fear and worry, increased autonomic activation, and sometimes specific behaviors such as verbal incoherence, immobility, or tremor (Spielberger, 1966; Endler & Kocovski, 2001; see Kowalski, 2000). Nonetheless, this definition sometimes fails to clearly differentiate state anxiety from other emotions like fear. State anxiety can be further distinguished from these other emotions based on cognitive appraisal, behavior, or neurobiological underpinnings. For instance, fear is the response to an identifiable threat; it involves behaviors like active avoidance, and is supported by neural circuits in which the medial temporal lobe's amygdala serves an important function. Anxiety, however, is the response to an unidentifiable threat or anticipated danger. As such, it involves active exploration for avoiding risk or active avoidance, and is implemented through septo-hippocampal neural circuits (Lazarus, 1982; Blanchard & Blanchard, 1990; Gray & McNaughton,

2000/2003; LeDoux, 2000). These dissociations have played a major part in the development of the so-called ethoexperimental approach to emotions (for review, see Blanchard, Griebel, & Blanchard, 2001; Rodgers, Cao, Dalvi, & Holmes, 1997), which has provided insightful perspectives into the pathogenesis of anxiety disorders (Mineka & Zinbarg, 2006; Miclea, 2001). The reader who is unfamiliar with the functional neuroanatomy of emotion and cognition is referred to Fig. 1.

Cattell and Scheier were among the first to describe anxiety as a function of both states and traits. Trait anxiety refers to one's sensitivity to threat, and high trait anxiety denotes an increased predisposition to display state anxiety toward even mild or ambiguous threat. Both state and trait anxieties are multimensional constructs, with at least two facets of trait – cognitive worry and autonomic-emotional – and four facets of state: social evaluation, physical danger, ambiguousness, and daily routines (Endler & Kocovski, 2001). Self-report measures of both global (Spielberger, 1983) and multimensional anxiety (Endler, Edwards, & Vitelli, 1991) have thus been created

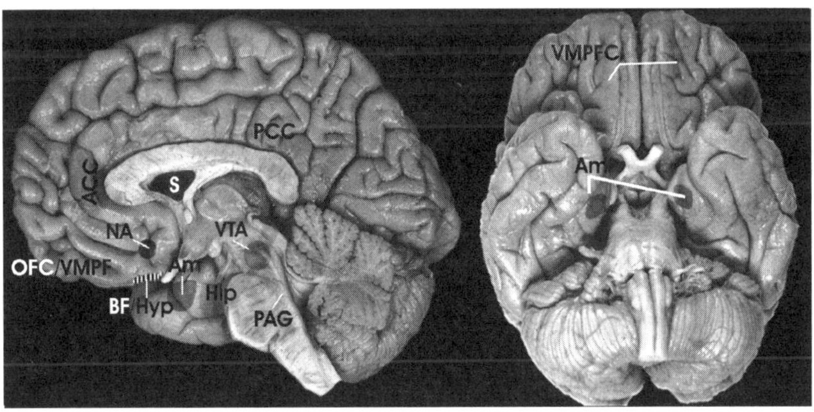

Fig. 1. The Brain Structures Starring in Studies of Emotion and Cognition Include the Subcortical (i.e., Since They Lie Beneath the Underlying Cortex, Most are Shown Here in Phantom Views) Amygdala (Am), the Nucleus Accumbens (NA), the Basal Forebrain and Hypothalamus (BF/Hyp), as Well as Areas Associated with the Ventral Tegmental Area (VTA), the Hippocampus (Hip), the Periaquaeductal Grey (PAG), and the Septum (S); and, Cortically, the Orbitofrontal/Ventromedial Prefrontal Cortex (OFC/VMPFC), the Anterior (ACC) and Posterior Cingulate Cortex (PCC). For Analyses of the Involvement of These Structures in Emotion and Cognition, See Pessoa (2008) and Phan, Wager, Taylor, and Liberzon (2002).

and corroborated with cognitive, behavioral (e.g., increased attention to aversive stimuli, augmented startle), biochemical (e.g., salivary cortisol), psychophysiological (e.g., skin conductance, cardiovascular activity, face electromyogram), and functional imaging correlates (e.g., activation of the amygdala) of anxiety (for reviews, see Cacioppo, Tassinary, & Berntson, 2007; Andreassi, 2000; Davidson, Scherer, & Goldsmith, 2003).

Our dispositional tendency toward state anxiety (i.e., trait anxiety, which is conceptually and psychometrically related to harm avoidance, neuroticism, and pessimism) is partially determined genetically, as indicated by behavioral and molecular genetics and imaging genomics approaches. A twin study indicated that state anxiety is largely mediated by non-shared environmental factors with minimal genetic effects, in contrast to trait anxiety, which shows substantial genetic effects (Lau, Eley, & Stevenson, 2006). Over 30% of the variance in trait anxiety can be explained by additive genetic factors, and 15% can be explained by shared environment. It is noteworthy that trait anxiety displays a much higher level of genetic determination than do medical disorders such as Parkinson's disease or breast cancer (for review, see Plomin, Owen, & McGuffin, 1994).

According to the study of Lau et al. (2006) threats from individual experience (e.g., physical or social threat, school and academic difficulties, peer relationship difficulties) would need to interact with genetic and familial vulnerability factors (e.g., dysfunctional family relationships, neighborhood conditions, parents' socioeconomic status) to produce an anxious phenotype.

Indeed, at least two likely genetic candidates have been identified, both of which are related to brain serotonin metabolism. Scholars have linked high trait anxiety scores with one or two copies of the short variant of a polymorphism (5-HTTLPR, 17q11, where LPR comes from gene-*linked polymorphic region*) identified in the regulatory region of the serotonin transporter (5-HTT) gene (e.g., Lesch et al., 1996; Osher, Hamer, & Benjamin, 2000), which reduces the transcriptional efficiency of the 5-HTT gene promoter and consequently the expression of 5-HTT and the serotonin reuptake.

In neuroimaging studies, the 5-HTTLPR genotype has been associated with increased amygdala activity, reduced gray matter volume in perigenual cingulate cortex and amygdala, and reduced functional coupling between these two neural structures during the processing of emotional faces (e.g., Hariri et al., 2002; Pezawas et al., 2005). These imaging genomics studies suggest that a key aspect of dispositional anxiety is the reduced control over extinction of negative affect, or, in psychological terms, low emotional resilience (see Davidson, 2004). One or two copies of 5-HTTLPR may also influence autonomic reactivity to stress (e.g., heart rate variability during exposure to CO_2), although in a less predictable manner (see Schmidt et al., 2000).

If trait anxiety is indeed a risk marker of anxiety and affective disorders, as has often been claimed (for review, see Bienvenu & Brandes, 2005), one would expect anxiety and 5-HTTLPR to have identified an endophenotype of these disorders. Endophenotypes refer to neurophysiological, biochemical, endocrinological, neuroanatomical, cognitive, or neuropsychological patterns of signs that are more closely related to the biological processes giving rise to psychiatric illness than to diagnostic categories (for review, see Gottesman & Gould, 2003; Flint & Munafò, 2007). Indeed, patients with social phobia, generalized anxiety disorder, panic disorder, or bulimia, who are heterozygous or homozygous for 5-HTTLPR (this genetic variant influences phenotype in a dominant-recessive manner) display increased state anxiety and activation of the amygdala in a public speaking condition (Furmark et al., 2004; Hariri et al., 2005), as well as reduced response to serotonin reuptake inhibitors (Stein, Seedat, & Gelernter, 2006; Perna, Favaron, Di Bella, Bussi, & Bellodi, 2005; Monteleone et al., 2005). Trait anxiety can thus be considered an indicator of risk for initial and comorbid anxiety and depression. Likewise, 5-HTTLPR, as well as other candidate genes contributing to the genetic variance of trait anxiety, can likely help identify endophenotypes of anxiety and affective disorders for which more targeted medication and psychotherapy can be designed.

However, one must consider that 5-HTTLPR only contributes up to 10% of the genetic variance of trait anxiety (Lesch et al., 1996; for review, see Munafo, Brown, & Hariri, 2008). Another part of trait anxiety's genetic variance can be attributed to a low expressing polymorphism in the promoter region of the monoamine oxidase A (MAO-A uVNTR, where VNTR comes from *variable number of tandem repeat located upstream*) gene, an enzyme involved in the catabolism of monoaminergic neurotransmitters such as serotonin, norepinephrine, epinephrine, and dopamine. The male carriers of this genetic variant of MAO-A showed increased harm avoidance (i.e., trait anxiety) and reduced reward dependence, in addition to both dysregulated amygdala activity and stronger functional coupling between the amygdala and the ventromedial prefrontal cortex (Buckholtz et al., 2008). This MAO-A genotype has also been associated with reduced amygdala and supragenual cingulate volumes, hyperreactive amygdala and hippocampus during retrieval of negative emotional memories, and reduced supragenual cingulate activation during cognitive inhibition tasks (see Meyer-Lindenberger, 2006).

Notably, both the 5-HTTLPR and the MAO-A uVNTR genetic variants influence amygdala activation, which is essential to emotional evaluation. Likewise, both variants affect cingulate regulatory circuitry for extinction of negative emotions. These shared attributes may indicate that these structures are at the heart of the neural substrates of anxiety. Other genetic candidates (e.g., polymorphisms in the catechol O-methyltransferase gene; see Stein, Fallin, Schork, & Gelernter, 2005) may also contribute to genetic variance of trait anxiety.

Given the fact that trait anxiety is substantially genetic in nature, one would expect it to be associated with differences in brain structure and function. Indeed, an early magnetic resonance spectroscopy study indicated that trait anxiety is associated with higher concentrations of the excitatory neurotransmitter precursor N-acetyl aspartate in the orbitofrontal cortex (Grachev & Apkarian, 2000). Subsequent neuroimaging work supported the view that trait anxiety is associated with structural and functional differences in the neural structures related to emotion and emotion regulation, particularly in the temporal and frontal lobe.

For instance, a recent magnetic resonance imaging study showed that both women and men with high trait anxiety display reduced volume of the right hippocampus; however, only the women have also reduced volume of the left anterior prefrontal cortex (Yamasue et al., 2008). Dispositional anxiety has also been negatively correlated with resting regional cerebral blood flow in the left parahippocampal gyrus and orbitoinsular junction, as well as other regions in the frontal, temporal, and parietal cortex (Sugiura et al., 2000). During a state of anticipatory anxiety, the levels of oxyhemoglobin, which indicates a local rise in energy demands, increased more in the right than in the left medial prefrontal cortex. This increase was positively correlated with dispositional anxiety (Morinaga et al., 2007).

Finally, functional magnetic resonance imaging studies indicated that activity in frontal and medial temporal lobe structures also varies as a function of dispositional anxiety in cognitive tasks. Dispositional anxiety was correlated with anterior cingulate response to emotionally positive stimuli (Canli, Amin, Haas, Omura, & Constable, 2004; for discussion, see Hamann & Harenski, 2004). Also, trait anxiety predicted activation of the basolateral amygdala to subliminally processed fearful faces (Etkin et al., 2004). Several studies using psychophysiological measures of autonomic activity during rest or emotion generally supported the view that there are also functional autonomic differences (e.g., potentiated startle reflex and increased heart rate during speech anticipation in social anxiety) related to trait anxiety (Cornwell, Johnson, Berardi, & Grillon, 2006; Gonzalez-Bono et al., 2002; see also Mauss, Wilhelm, & Gross, 2003).

COGNITIVE EFFECTS OF ANXIETY

Some early studies indicated that high trait anxiety is associated with reduced accuracy and increased time on analogical reasoning tasks (Mandler & Sarason, 1952; Siegman, 1956; Mayer, 1977). Subsequent research showed that if the same type of task was administered in a state of stress, high trait anxiety participants still made a high number of errors, but they also spent significantly less time on the task compared to low trait anxiety participants (Leon & Revelle, 1985). These results highlighted the possibility that the effects of trait anxiety on cognition may develop more during state anxiety than emotionally neutral states. This possibility was supported using other cognitive tasks (see Williams, Mathews, & MacLeod, 1996).

Some authors have gone further to suggest that the cognitive differences associated with trait anxiety are mediated by state anxiety. This idea was supported by studies showing that participants who tend to react extremely negatively to perceived stress displayed greater anxiety toward a simple laboratory visit (Shackman et al., 2006). However, many studies have controlled for state anxiety and still reported specific associations between trait anxiety and cognitive and physiological effects (e.g., Cornwell et al., 2006; Paulus, Feinstein, Simmons, & Stein, 2004). It is nonetheless recommendable to control for state anxiety immediately before or after the experiment. The ideal method of control is self-report questionnaires coupled with physiological measures.

Researchers began to study the cognitive effects of anxiety more systematically in order to test the predictions of Gordon Bower's network model of emotion and cognition (for review, see MacLeod & Rutherford, 1992). According to Bower's theory, human associative memory is organized as a network in which information is stored in connecting nodes (Anderson & Bower, 1973). Within this network, nodes corresponding to each emotional state are connected to other nodes storing affectively congruent information. Thus, when someone experiences an emotional state, the corresponding node becomes activated and automatically activates its connecting nodes. This process biases the cognitive system toward further favoring the processing of stimuli that are congruent with the current emotional state.

Aaron Beck developed a similar theory; however, in contrast to Bower, who viewed emotional information-processing biases as dependent on mood and thus transitory, Beck argued that these biases, or schemas, tend to be intraindividually stable. He further maintained that the biases relate to dispositions toward clinical depression or anxiety (Beck, 1976). The possibility that affective traits like trait anxiety could bias information processing throughout attention, reasoning, and memory has been very appealing. This prospect is particularly interesting from a clinical perspective developed around Beck and others who argued for the involvement of cognitive and personality variables in the pathogenesis of mental and psychosomatic disorders (for review, see Mathews & MacLeod, 2005; Coles & Heimberg, 2002; Miclea, 2006). For instance, much research has dealt with high trait anxiety as a vulnerability factor for generalized anxiety disorder (for review, see Eysenck, 1997).

Numerous studies on the cognitive effects of anxiety followed this line of reasoning. They endorsed the idea that, from a functional perspective, one can view anxiety as part of a defense mechanism against potential dangers: at the cognitive level, it facilitates the cognitive anticipation and detection of danger, and at the behavioral level it mobilizes resources for the situation when the perceived danger proves real (Keltner & Gross, 1999; Calvo, Avero, Castillo, & Miguel-Tobal, 2003). In order to detect early indications of potential dangers and prepare appropriate defensive responses, trait anxiety could bias the cognitive system in at least three ways, affecting: (a) attention, by favoring the detection of potentially threatening relative to emotionally neutral stimuli; (b) interpretation, by favoring the interpretation of ambiguous stimuli as potentially threatening; and (c) memory, by favoring the recall of information related to potential threats.

In fact, emotion's interference with attentional processing is higher in high trait anxiety participants, particularly in conditions where the perceived state anxiety is high (Mogg, Mathews, Bird, & Macgregor-Morris, 1990; MacLeod & Rutherford, 1992; see also Mogg, Bradley, Williams, & Mathews, 1993). Researchers generally study emotion's interference with attention by using variants of the emotional Stroop task. This task requires participants to name the color of the presented words while ignoring the emotionally salient meaning of some of those words. The attentional bias in anxiety has been attributed to the increased tendency of high trait anxiety participants to attend to even mild aversive stimuli, or to show a higher resistance to disengaging from the processing of these stimuli (e.g., Yiend & Mathews, 2001; MacLeod & Rutherford, 1992; Koster, Crombez, Verschuere, & Houwer, 2006; Fox, 1993; Mogg et al., 2000).

Regarding memory biases in anxiety, several early studies (e.g., Reidy & Richards, 1997a, 1997b) reported that high trait anxiety participants recalled more threatening words in explicit memory tasks, or that trait anxiety was only correlated with implicit memory for threat information (Harrison & Turpin, 2003). These studies were unable to discriminate between subclinical anxiety (e.g., over average trait anxiety scores of healthy volunteers in self-report questionnaires) and generalized anxiety disorder (Mathews, Mogg, May, & Eysenck, 1989). However, subsequent studies found little or no enhancement of memory associated with high trait anxiety (Richards & French, 1991; Reidy, 2004; Oldenburg, Lundh, & Kivistö, 2002).

More recent studies have drawn attention to the fact that emotion has both enhancing *and* impairing effects on memory. This latter effect refers to the reduced recall of neutral stimuli that are temporally associated with an emotional event, in comparison to other neutral stimuli. High trait anxiety is associated with an increased impairing effect of emotion on explicit memory (Miu, Heilman, Opre, & Miclea, 2005). This finding may significantly contribute to changing the direction of the currently equivocal view of trait anxiety's effects on memory. In contrast to the study of memory biases in anxiety, persuasive evidence has indicated that high trait anxiety participants tend to interpret ambiguous information in a self-relevant, negative manner (e.g., Brendle & Wenzel, 2004; Burke & Mathews, 1992).

The recent attentional control theory (Eysenck, Derakshan, Santos, & Calvo, 2007) concerns the assumption that the effects of anxiety on attention are key to understanding how anxiety influences cognitive performance. The theory posits that state anxiety decreases attentional control by impairing goal-directed attention and increasing the extent to which attentional information processing is driven by stimuli. This would indicate an impairment in the selection of cues which may be relevant to the goal. Thus, the cognitive system would be left at the will of perceptually or emotionally salient stimuli. In high trait anxiety, the cognitive system would be biased toward increased distraction by stimuli related to threat. Unless compensatory strategies (e.g, enhanced effort, increased use of processing resources) are used, state anxiety would increasingly impair cognitive efficiency (i.e., the relationship between quality of task performance and the effort spent) and efficacy. Given that state anxiety has been associated with reduced inhibition of prepotent responses and reduced task-switching capacity, its effect on cognitive efficiency might be chiefly mediated by two central executive functions that involve attentional control: inhibition and shifting. The final section of this chapter will explore the neuroeconomical support for this theory.

ANXIETY AND DECISION-MAKING

Janis and Mann (1977) first distinguished between vigilant and hypervigilant decision-making patterns. Vigilant decision-making is an ideal pattern of decision-making in predictable and controllable situations. It involves systematic information search, thorough consideration of all available alternatives, allocation of sufficient time to the evaluation of alternatives, and close reexamination and review of data before making a decision. In contrast, hypervigilant decision-making is characterized by a non-systematic or selective information search, limited consideration of alternatives, rapid evaluation of data, and selection of a solution without extensive review or reappraisal. This kind of decision-making, although originally acknowledged as saving time and effort, was nonetheless viewed as a defective coping pattern that interrupted the cognitive processes required for optimal decision-making. Stress tended to increase the use of hypervigilant decision-making and the frequency of errors in logical analogy tasks (Baradell & Klein, 1993; Keinan, 1987). Subsequent work emphasized that hypervigilant decision-making is an attempt to maintain a reasonable balance between task demand and effort. Consequently, it is adaptive in highly demanding tasks.

Using a computer simulation of navy radar monitoring and classification, administered in either a normal or high-stress condition (i.e., auditory distraction, task load, and time pressure), researchers showed that under both conditions, people using hypervigilant decision-making displayed a greater number of accurate target identifications than people using a vigilant strategy. This result occurred notwithstanding the fact that hypervigilant decision-makers deviated more frequently from a fixed sequence in scanning information and checked or reviewed data less frequently before making a decision (Johnston, Driskell, & Salas, 1997). However, stress tended to impair decision-making irrespective of the decision-making strategy, showing that although hypervigilant decision-making may be adaptive in more demanding situations, it may still be susceptible to the effects of high stress (Johnston, Driskell, & Salas, 1997).

The above study and others like it highlighted the possibility that since anxiety and other negative emotions (e.g., fear, anger, sadness, disgust; see Raghunathan & Pham, 1999; Lerner & Keltner, 2000; Fessler,

Pillsworth, & Flamson, 2004) are characterized by an increased sense of vulnerability, they may be associated with pessimistic risk appraisal and risk-aversive decision-making, if not hypervigilant decision-making *per se*. Risk is usually defined as the probability, size, or so-called subjective "negative utility" of a potential loss (Vlek & Stallen, 1980). Early studies associated positive effect with lower estimates of negative events (Johnson & Tversky, 1983), or higher negative utility for losses (Isen, Nygren, & Ashby, 1988). However, by the end of the 1990s, no study had reported estimates of probability and utility together; this data was necessary for grasping a more complete picture of the relationship between affect and risk (Stöber, 1997).

One of the first empirical studies on anxiety and risk in healthy volunteers used a task in which participants had to choose between different lotteries. The study found that low trait anxiety participants focused on the probability to win, whereas high trait anxiety participants focused on the size of the possible loss (Gaul, 1977). Another study argued that state anxiety specifically influences only the risk estimates related to the source to which state anxiety is attributed (e.g., an exam); trait anxiety, on the other hand, is associated with a global effect on risk estimates of self-relevant events (Butler & Mathews, 1987; see also Eisenberg, Baron, & Seligman, 1996).

Butler and Mathews' study compared risk estimates made one month before an examination with risk estimates made one day before an examination. They found that at the second measurement, when state anxiety was high, participants gave higher estimates only of those negative events related to the forthcoming exam. However, if the same participants were grouped for their trait anxiety, those with higher scores estimated higher probabilities for all self-relevant negative events. In another study, Stöber (1997) used a musical induction procedure and a risk evaluation task in which participants had to estimate both the probability and the utility of the events described in several texts. Stöber reported that high trait anxiety participants, in comparison to low trait anxiety participants, estimated larger probabilities and negative utilities when the events were negative and smaller probabilities and utilities when the events were positive. He concluded that the results imply that high trait anxiety subjects seem to consider bad luck as more plausible and good luck as less plausible. This could be interpreted as a general pessimistic bias in the trait-anxious individuals' perception of risk and chance (Stöber, 1997).

Trait anxiety is associated not only with increased risk estimates, but also with behavioral risk avoidance. Trait anxiety correlated with risk avoidance in both self-report questionnaires (i.e., Risk-Taking Behaviors Scale; Weber,

Blais, & Betz, 2002; see Maner & Schmidt, 2006) and behavioral tasks (i.e., Balloon Analog Risk Task; Lejuez et al., 2002; see Maner et al., 2007). Briefly, Balloon Analog Risk Task is a computer-based measure of risk-taking, in which participants can earn financial rewards by pumping balloons presented on a screen; different balloons have variable explosion points, and once a balloon explodes, the money deposited for pumping that balloon is lost. Risk-taking is defined in terms of mean pumps per unexploded balloon. Although anxiety is associated with risk avoidance in this task, dispositionally anxious persons may not avoid risks in all decision-making situations. When dispositionally anxious participants were forced to choose between a sure contract and a risky contract, involving either achieving a gain or avoiding a loss, they avoided risks when they could achieve a gain; however, they seemed to take more risks compared to non-anxious participants when they had to avoid suffering a loss (Lauriola & Levin, 2001). These results resemble those previously reported by Kahneman and Tversky (1984), who were first to find that participants show risk aversion in the domain of gains and risk-seeking in the domain of losses. Dispositional anxiety can thus be a predictor of individual susceptibility to this framing effect.

Using the Ultimatum Game, we also provided evidence that personality interacts with motivation to elicit different patterns of behavior (for review, see Revelle, 1993). The Ultimatum Game involves sharing a sum of money between a proposer and a responder; the proposer decides how to share the money between him/herself and the responder, and the responder decides whether to accept or reject the offer made by the proposer (Güth, Schmittberger, & Schwarze, 1982). The rule of this economic game is that if the responder accepts the offer, the money is split accordingly, but if the responder rejects the offer, neither player receives anything. Offers are generally categorized as fair (i.e., 50/50 offers on average), unfair (i.e., the proposer keeps more than 70% of the sum for him/herself), or hyperfair (i.e., the proposer keeps less than 30% of the sum for him/herself). Using an Ultimatum Game, we observed that different conditions motivated extreme dispositional anxiety proposers to reduce the risk of having their offer rejected by making more generous offers to the responder (Raghunathan and Pham's low risk/low reward mode). Dispositionally anxious individuals tend to be cooperators rather than free riders or conditional cooperators in bargaining (see Kurzban & Houser, 2001); nonetheless, low trait anxiety proposers were more likely to display a tendency toward a low risk/low reward mode of behavior when they had to avoid a loss in a modified Ultimatum Game. In contrast, high trait anxiety proposers were more likely to display a tendency toward this mode of behavior when the size of the pie increased in a repeated Ultimatum Game (Heilman, Miu, Opre, & Houser, 2006). This result supports the possibility that dispositional anxiety interacts with motivation in bargaining behavior.

What are the mechanisms of pessimistic risk appraisal and increased risk aversion in anxiety? One such mechanism is related to the tendency of high trait anxiety individuals to rely more on the emotions (i.e., negative emotions like state anxiety) that are congruent with their dispositional tendency. High trait anxiety is associated with attributing negative feelings to stable and general sources (i.e., internal attribution), whereas low trait anxiety is associated with attributing negative feelings to transitory and contextual sources (i.e., external attribution) (Abramson, Metalsky, & Alloy, 1989). The "affect-as-information" approach states that affective cues influence judgments when such cues are experienced as providing relevant information (Clore, 1992; Schwarz & Clore, 1983; see also Loewenstein & O'Donoghue, 2004; Slovic, Finucane, Peters, & MacGregor, 2007).

In keeping with this approach, Gasper and Clore (1998) confirmed that high trait anxiety participants estimated higher risks of negative events, especially when the events were self-relevant (e.g., having something stolen, doing something embarrassing). They further showed that they were able to reduce the risk estimates of low trait anxiety participants simply by reminding the participants that their state anxiety, originally attributed to the upcoming exam, might instead be attributable to an irrelevant source. This tactic, however, was unable to reduce the risk estimates of high trait anxiety participants. These results consequently demonstrate that attribution manipulations more consistently reduce emotion's influence on judgment when the emotion is incongruent with one's affective traits (Gasper & Clore, 1998).

Similarly, when attribution of state anxiety was not manipulated, and students were asked to predict the upcoming results of a test, anxiety correlated with less optimistic predictions. This was not the case when participants were induced to attribute their anxiety to an external cause (i.e., the cup of decaffeinated coffee they had all drank before making the predictions; see Shepperd, Grace, Cole, & Klein, 2005). The authors of this latter study emphasized that anxiety's adaptive function is to alert people that more circumspect predictions are in order. This alert may help prepare the cognitive system for coping with a potentially negative outcome.

Based on the proven tendency of high trait anxiety individuals to choose a negative interpretation for ambiguous stimuli (for review, see Eysenck, 1997), Bensi and Giusberti hypothesized that this trait would be associated with reduced tolerance to uncertainty and a "jump-to-conclusions" style of decision-making (Bensi & Giusberti, 2007). High trait anxiety participants asked for significantly less evidence to make a decision in a formal probabilistic task (i.e., Bead Task; see Garety, Hemsley, & Wessely, 1991). They also gathered a lesser amount of data before answering in a hypothetical real-life decision-making situation (i.e., Scenario Task; see Bensi & Giusberti, 2007). Even when participants were free to ask for the amount of evidence they needed to decide whether a coin was genuine or forged, based on a series of coin tosses, the high trait anxiety participants needed significantly fewer tosses in order to decide.

Another hypothesis testing task reached the same result (i.e., Card Task; see Young & Bentall, 1995). In that test task, not only did high trait anxiety participants need fewer feedback cards to decide, but they also provided fewer correct answers (Bensi & Giusberti, 2007). Given that anxious individuals experience uncertainty more stressfully, their implicit goal, rather than solving the task correctly, may instead be to reduce uncertainty and eliminate the discomfort of ambiguity by providing the first acceptable conclusion.

Several distinctions might be kept in mind in regarding risk aversion in anxiety. One such distinction is between occasional and frequent risk-taking, corroborated with the domain of risk-taking (e.g., substance use, behavior on the road, sexual relations, deviant behavior). Among these domains of risk-taking, negative affectivity, to which high trait anxiety individuals are prone, specifically predicted only frequent risk-taking in the domain of substance use (Desrichard & Denarie, 2005). Attitudes (e.g., attitudes toward traffic safety; see Ulleberg & Rundmo, 2003), situational factors framing the decision (e.g., level of exposure to risk or protective factors for a disease; see Lauriola, Russo, Lucidi, Violani, & Levin, 2005), and coping (e.g., establishing one's own priorities and goals; see Hall, 1972; O'Hare & Tamburri, 1986) might also be important mediators of the effects of dispositional anxiety on risk-taking in traffic behavior, health decisions, and career decision-making.

Another mechanism underlying the pessimistic risk appraisal and increased risk avoidance associated with high trait anxiety is related to the availability heuristic. This heuristic refers to the observation that judgments regarding the likelihood of certain events are biased by the ease with which past occurrences of similar events can be accessed from memory (Tversky & Kahneman, 1974). Yet another mechanism may be related to the increased elaboration of threat-related schemata in memory (Butler & Mathews, 1987). Kverno (2000) tested these two mechanisms in a memory task.

The task required participants selected for trait anxiety either to estimate the frequency, or freely recall the neutral and physically threatening words that had been presented several times during acquisition. Kverno predicted that high trait anxiety would estimate greater frequencies for threatening words compared to low trait anxiety, but would show similar rates of recall. The results indicated that high trait anxiety participants indeed estimated significantly larger frequencies for threatening, but not neutral words, in comparison to low trait anxiety participants. This effect was not confounded by a better recognition of threatening words. Although participants generally recalled threatening words better than neutral words, there were no differences between trait anxiety groups.

ANXIETY IN NEUROECONOMICS

Considering the effects of dispositional anxiety on brain, emotion, and cognition, one can hypothesize that this trait is associated with different physiological correlates and neural substrates of emotion in decision-making. Decision-making involves complex computational interactions: for instance, between response selection, response conflict, reward processing, and attentional control. Not surprisingly, such interactions are supported by activation in a distributed network of neural structures. These structures include the orbitofrontal and dorsolateral prefrontal cortex, the insular cortex and the anterior cingulate cortex in the frontal lobe, the precuneus and the bilateral superior parietal lobules in the parietal cortex, the thalamus, and the caudate (Krain, Wilson, Arbuckle, Castellanos, & Milham, 2006b). As recognized, studying the differences associated with anxiety in the activity of these neural networks would contribute to our growing appreciation of personality as a predictor of brain responses to cognitive demands (e.g., Kumari, ffytche, Williams, & Gray, 2004; Canli et al., 2004; Etkin et al., 2004); likewise, it would contribute to our understanding of the neural substrates engaged in the preferential processing of aversive stimuli and their involvement in the pathogenesis of anxiety and affective disorders (e.g., Ernst & Paulus, 2005; Paulus, 2007). Since researchers have only recently begun to systematically examine these issues, the rest of this chapter reviews the studies published to date and also outlines some outstanding issues for future studies.

The "risk-as-feelings" and somatic marker hypotheses highlighted the role of affect experienced at the moment of decision-making. They have consequently offered a good framework for understanding why dispositional anxiety is associated with impaired decision-making (for reviews, see Loewenstein, Weber, Hsee, & Welch, 2001; Bechara et al., 2000). We have reviewed evidence that dispositional anxiety can modulate the genesis and quality of emotions, as well as their neural and physiological underpinnings. By way of emotion, dispositional anxiety could have significant effects on decision-making, by reducing information-processing efficiency (i.e., the effort that is necessary to maintain quality of performance) and even efficacy, when compensatory strategies are not successful (see Eysenck et al., 2007). Based on the analysis of cognitive biases in anxiety, researchers have predicted that decision-making is likely to be influenced by anxiety in two stages: (a) the assessment and formation of preferences among possible options, and (b) the experience or evaluation of outcomes (see Ernst & Paulus, 2005).

Dispositional anxiety may be associated with hyperarousal or increased interoception (i.e., homeostatic sensing of the internal state of the body), as well as increased top-down modulation of interoceptive signals through biased attention and interpretation. Accordingly, anxious individuals may show "an altered pattern of aversive somatic markers during the assessment stage of decision-making […], as well as during the experience of outcome […]" (Ernst & Paulus, 2005, p. 602). We recently used an Iowa Gambling Task and psychophysiological correlates of emotional response to find this exact pattern in participants selected for extreme trait anxiety (Miu, Heilman, & Houser, 2008). Iowa Gambling Task simulates real-life decision-making in the way it factors uncertainty of premises and outcomes, as well as reward and punishment (Bechara et al., 1994). It measures the degree to which individuals learn to choose small immediate gains associated in the long term with smaller losses, over large immediate gains associated in the long term with larger losses.

High trait anxiety was associated with a pattern of increased anticipatory skin conductance increases prior to advantageous trials, increased heart rate deceleration to punishment, and impaired decision-making. These results clearly indicate that high trait anxiety is associated with defective modulation of somatic signals, coupled with disrupted discrimination of advantageous and disadvantageous choices in decision-making tasks involving learning from emotional cues. However, considering that previous psychophysiological studies did not always replicate hyperarousal in high trait anxiety (e.g., Mauss et al., 2003), it seems reasonable to assume that the increased impairing effect of negative emotions on decision-making in anxious individuals might be the combined result of hyperarousal and increased top-down modulation (e.g, increased attention to autonomic bodily processes) of bottom-up interoceptive afferents (Paulus, 2007). Indeed, anxiety scores correlate with interoceptive accuracy, subjective negative emotional experience, and activity in the right anterior insular/opercular cortex during a heartbeat detection condition. This result points to the cortical region as a neural mechanism for the increased awareness of visceral responses during negative emotional states in high trait anxiety (Critchley, Wiens, Rotshtein, Ohman, & Dolan, 2004).

The biases toward increased risk aversion and reduced tolerance to uncertainty have been associated with anxiety and might be reflected by neural activity in brain areas related to uncertainty and risk processing (e.g., Fukui, Murai, Fukuyama, Hayashi, & Hanakawa, 2005; Critchley, Mathias, & Dolan, 2001; Breiter, Aharon, Kahneman, Dale, & Shizgal, 2001). A recent meta-analysis suggested that risk and ambiguity in decision-making illustrate affective "hot" and cognitive "cool" processes. The analysis found that the neural substrates of risk and ambiguity can be functionally dissociated: the probability of activation in the orbitofrontal cortex, the middle frontal gyrus, the bilateral superior parietal regions, and the left inferior parietal regions was higher in conditions when risk predominated, whereas the probability of activation in the dorsolateral prefrontal cortex, the cingulate gyrus, the subcallosal portion of the anterior cingulate, the precuneus, and the left inferior parietal regions was higher when ambiguity predominated (Krain et al., 2006b).

Although risk and ambiguity can be dissociated based on their neural substrates, decision-making under ambiguity cannot be considered more complex than risky decision-making (see Huettel, Stowe, Gordon, Warner, & Platt, 2006). Moreover, risk involving potential losses or gains may be further dissociated. A recent neuropsychological study indicated that patients with amygdala lesions displayed impaired decision-making under risk of potential gains, but not losses. In contrast, patients with damage to the ventromedial prefrontal cortex showed alterations in both types of risky decision-making (Weller, Levin, Shiv, & Bechara, 2007). The results of a functional neuroimaging study seem to support this view. The tendency to be risk-averse in decisions framed by gains, and risk-seeking in decisions framed by losses was correlated with amygdala activity. The reverse pattern, however, was correlated with activity in the anterior cingulate cortex (De Martino, Kumaran, Seymour, & Dolan, 2006; for discussion see Kahneman & Frederick, 2007).

Researchers previously associated dispositional anxiety with increased susceptibility to this framing effect, and thus, reduced rationality (Lauriola & Levin, 2001). Considering that reduced susceptibility to the gain/loss framing effects was correlated with enhanced activity in the ventromedial prefrontal cortex, one would expect that high trait anxiety individuals had increased amygdala activity correlated with reduced activity in these frontal areas. Future functional neuroimaging studies might investigate this possibility. It would also be interesting to verify how centrally acting drugs would change the high amygdala-low frontal activity potentially involved in the increased susceptibility of high trait anxiety to framing effects. Two good candidates for a psychopharmalogical study of susceptibility to framing effects in anxiety would be: (a) the GABA-ergic agonist lorazepam, which is known to reduce risk-taking in a dose-dependent manner (Arce, Miller, Feinstein, Stein, & Paulus, 2006), and (b) the beta-adrenergic antagonist propranolol, which reduces the impact of emotion on memory (Cahill, Prins, Weber, & McGaugh, 1994).

A landmark neuroimaging study, which brought trait anxiety closer to the attention of neuroeconomists, showed that high and low trait anxiety healthy volunteers had similar behavioral performance in a two-choice prediction task at three different error rates. High trait anxiety participants, however, had higher activations in the anterior cingulate and medial prefrontal specifically in the low-error-rate condition (Paulus et al., 2004). This result seems to support the hypothesis that trait anxiety is sometimes associated with reduced cognitive efficiency. Activity in the anterior cingulate has also been associated with intolerance to uncertainty in decision-making. This may suggest that this activity is also involved in reduced decision-making efficiency in high trait anxiety.

Intolerance to uncertainty, viewed as an affective trait, has been positively correlated with anterior cingulate activity during decision-making in healthy adolescents, but not adults. Research suggests that these findings may point to a developmental mechanism involved in the pathogenesis of generalized anxiety disorder (Krain et al., 2006a). Across two groups of healthy adolescents and age-matched patients with generalized anxiety disorder, intolerance to uncertainty indeed correlated positively with activity in the bilateral amygdala, medial frontal gyrus, anterior cingulate cortex, and other more posterior brain regions (Krain et al., 2008). Intolerance to uncertainty identified a subgroup of patients which activated frontal and limbic regions (see Krain et al., 2008) in response to uncertainty in decision-making. In contrast, patients with lower scores on this trait responded to uncertainty by deactivating the same regions.

According to Ernst and Paulus (2005), anxiety may also influence the experience or evaluation of outcomes. Neuropsychological evidence gathered around the reinforcement sensitivity theory (Gray & McNaughton, 2000/2003) has compellingly argued that trait anxiety is associated with higher sensitivity to punishment. The theory maintains that this higher sensitivity is functionally attributable to a behavioral inhibition system implemented by the septo-hippocampal system (i.e., all those structures which receive direct inhibitory GABA-ergic input from the medial septal area, such as hippocampus proper, dentate gyrus, the entorhinal cortex, the subicular area, the posterior cingulate cortex). According to the theory, the behavioral inhibition system mainly mediates the detection of conflicts between concurrently active goals. When conflict is detected, it increases the valence of affectively negative stimuli and associations until a behavioral solution in favor of approach or avoidance is attained (for review, see Corr, 2004).

The reinforcement sensitivity theory is largely based on data from experimental neuropsychology; that is, animal studies of septo-hippocampal lesions and the effects of barbiturates, ethanol, and anxiolytics. We used this theory to hypothesize that high trait anxiety would be associated with increased somatic markers to punishment in an Iowa Gambling Task. This prediction was supported by the higher cardiac deceleration associated with punishment in high trait anxiety (Miu et al., 2008). Future neuroimaging studies will investigate the effect of the differential sensitivity to reinforcements associated with trait anxiety on decision-making.

In conclusion, studies on trait anxiety and other individual differences related to emotion have started to show their potential of contributing to the understanding of the role of emotion in decision-making. Studies of individual differences in emotion and their effects on decision-making might serve as a platform for extending the neurobiological roots and widen the clinical perspective of neuroeconomics. Future neuroeconomic studies might go beyond mapping brain activity associated with emotion and decision-making, to manipulating brain activity through methods such as transcranial magnetic stimulation (for review, see Hallett, 2007) or psychopharmacological interventions, ideally coupled with neuroimaging. In addition, neuroeconomists might increase their efforts of formalizing the results of neuroimaging studies and integrate them in mainstream economic thinking (e.g., physiological utility; Glimcher, Dorris, & Bayer, 2005). In much the same way neuroscience and artificial intelligence stimulated the development of the information-processing approach in cognitive psychology in the late 1950s, neuroecomics should nowadays catalyze efforts to diversify paradigms of decision-making measurement that are long overdue in psychology. Finally, neuroeconomics might also more closely follow current trends in mainstream cognitive neuroscience (e.g., imaging genomics). These are only several ways neuroeconomics might increase its impact on fundamental and applied biomedical and socioeconomic thinking.

REFERENCES

Abramson, L. Y., Metalsky, F. I., & Alloy, L. B. (1989). Hopelessness depression: A theory based subtype of depression. *Psychological Review*, *96*(2), 358–372.

Allport, G. W. (1937). *Personality*. New York: Holt.

Anderson, J., & Bower, G. (1973). *Human associative memory*. Washington, DC: Winston.

Andreassi, J. L. (2000). *Psychophysiology: Human behavior and physiological response* (3rd ed.). Hillsdale, NJ: Lawrence Erlbaum Associates.

Arce, E., Miller, D. A., Feinstein, J. S., Stein, M. B., & Paulus, M. P. (2006). Lorazepam dose-dependently decreases risk-taking related activation in limbic areas. *Psychopharmacology (Berlin)*, *189*(1), 105–116.

Baradell, J., & Klein, K. W. (1993). The relationship of life stress and body consciousness to hypervigilant decision making. *Journal of Personality and Social Psychology*, *64*, 267–273.

Bechara, A., Damasio, A. R., Damasio, H., & Anderson, S. W. (1994). Insensitivity to future consequences following damage to human prefrontal cortex. *Cognition*, *50*(1–3), 7–15.

Bechara, A., Damasio, H., & Damasio, A. R. (2000). Emotion, decision making and the orbitofrontal cortex. *Cerebral Cortex*, *10*(3), 295–307.

Beck, A. T. (1976). *Cognitive therapy and the emotional disorders*. New York: Meridian.

Bensi, L., & Giusberti, F. (2007). Trait anxiety and reasoning under uncertainty. *Personality and Individual Differences*, *43*(4), 827–838.

Bienvenu, O. J., & Brandes, M. (2005). The interface of personality traits and anxiety disorders. *Primary Psychiatry*, *12*(3), 35–39.

Blanchard, D. C., & Blanchard, R. J. (1990). Behavioral correlates of chronic dominance–subordination relationships of male rats in a seminatural situation. *Neuroscience and Biobehavioral Review*, *14*(4), 455–462.

Blanchard, D. C., Griebel, G., & Blanchard, R. J. (2001). Mouse defensive behaviors: Pharmacological and behavioral assays for anxiety and panic. *Neuroscience and Biobehavioral Review*, *25*(3), 205–218.

Bradley, M. M., & Lang, P. J. (2007). Emotion and motivation. In: J. T. Cacioppo, L. G. Tassinary & G. G. Berntson (Eds), *Handbook of psychophysiology*. New York: Cambridge University Press.

Breiter, H. C., Aharon, I., Kahneman, D., Dale, A., & Shizgal, P. (2001). Functional imaging of neural responses to expectancy and experience of monetary gains and losses. *Neuron*, *30*(2), 619–639.

Brendle, J. R., & Wenzel, A. (2004). Differentiating between memory and interpretation biases in socially anxious and nonanxious individuals. *Behavior Research and Therapy*, *42*(2), 155–171.

Buckholtz, J. W., Callicott, J. H., Kolachana, B., Hariri, A. R., Goldberg, T. E., Genderson, M., Egan, M. F., Mattay, V. S., Weinberger, D. R., & Meyer-Lindenberg, A. (2008). Genetic variation in MAOA modulates ventromedial prefrontal circuitry mediating individual differences in human personality. *Molecular Psychiatry*, *13*(3), 313–324.

Burke, M., & Mathews, A. (1992). Autobiographical memory and clinical anxiety. *Cognition and Emotion*, *6*, 23–35.

Butler, G., & Mathews, A. (1987). Anticipatory anxiety and risk perception. *Cognitive Research and Therapy*, *11*, 551–565.

Cacioppo, J. T., Tassinary, L. G., & Berntson, G. G. (2007). *Handbook of psychophysiology* (3rd ed.). Cambridge, UK: Cambridge University Press.

Cahill, L., Prins, B., Weber, M., & McGaugh, J. L. (1994). Beta-adrenergic activation and memory for emotional events. *Nature*, *371*(6499), 702–704.

Calvo, M. G., Avero, P., Castillo, M. D., & Miguel-Tobal, J. J. (2003). Multidimensional anxiety and content-specificity effects in preferential processing of threat. *European Psychologist*, *8*(4), 252–265.

Camerer, C. F., Loewenstein, G. F., & Prelec, D. (2005). Neuroeconomics: How neuroscience can inform economics. *Journal of Economic Literature*, *43*, 9–64.

Canli, T., Amin, Z., Haas, B., Omura, K., & Constable, R. T. (2004). A double dissociation between mood states and personality traits in the anterior cingulate. *Behavioral Neuroscience*, *118*(5), 897–904.

Cattell, R. B., & Scheier, I. H. (1958). The nature of anxiety: A review of thirteen multivariate analyses comprising 814 variables. *Psychological Reports*, *4*, 351–388.

Clore, G. L. (1992). Cognitive phenomenology: Feelings and the construction of judgment. In: L. L. Martin & A. Tesser (Eds), *The construction of social judgments* (pp. 133–163). Hillsdale, NJ: Erlbaum.

Coles, M. E., & Heimberg, R. G. (2002). Memory biases in the anxiety disorders: Current status. *Clinical Psychological Review*, *22*(4), 587–627.

Cornwell, B. R., Johnson, L., Berardi, L., & Grillon, C. (2006). Anticipation of public speaking in virtual reality reveals a relationship between trait social anxiety and startle reactivity. *Biological Psychiatry*, *59*(7), 664–666.

Corr, P. J. (2004). Reinforcement sensitivity theory and personality. *Neuroscience and Biobehavioral Review*, *28*(3), 317–332.

Critchley, H. D., Mathias, C. J., & Dolan, R. J. (2001). Neural activity in the human brain relating to uncertainty and arousal during anticipation. *Neuron*, *29*(2), 537–545.

Critchley, H. D., Wiens, S., Rotshtein, P., Ohman, A., & Dolan, R. J. (2004). Neural systems supporting interoceptive awareness. *Nature Neuroscience*, *7*(2), 189–195.

Dalgleish, T., & Power, M. (1999). *Handbook of cognition and emotion*. New York: Wiley.

Damasio, A. R. (2000). A second chance for emotion. In: R. Lane & L. Nadel (Eds), *Cognitive neuroscience of emotion* (pp. 12–23). New York: Oxford University Press.

Damasio, A. R., Tranel, D., & Damasio, H. (1991). Somatic markers and the guidance of behaviour: Theory and preliminary testing. In: H. S. Levin, H. M. Eisenberg & A. L. Benton (Eds), *Frontal lobe function and dysfunction*. New York: Oxford University Press.

Davidson, R., Scherer, K., & Goldsmith, H. H. (2003). *Handbook of affective sciences*. London: Oxford University Press.

Davidson, R. J. (2004). Well-being and affective style: Neural substrates and biobehavioural correlates. *Philosophical Transactions of the Royal Society of London Series B, Biological Sciences*, *359*(1449), 1395–1411.

De Martino, B., Kumaran, D., Seymour, B., & Dolan, R. J. (2006). Frames, biases, and rational decision-making in the human brain. *Science*, *313*(5787), 684–687.

Desrichard, O., & Denarie, V. (2005). Sensation seeking and negative affectivity as predictors of risky behaviors: A distinction between occasional versus frequent risk-taking. *Addictive Behaviors*, *30*(7), 1449–1453.

Dolan, R. J. (2002). Emotion, cognition, and behavior. *Science*, *298*(5596), 1191–1194.

Eisenberg, A. E., Baron, J., & Seligman, M. E. P. (1996). *Individual differences in risk aversion and anxiety* (Downloaded on January 9. Available at http://www.sas.upenn.edu/~baron/amyold.html).

Endler, N. S., Edwards, J., & Vitelli, R. (1991). *Test manual for the Endler Multidimensional Anxiety Scales (EMAS)*. Los Angeles: Western Psychological Services.

Endler, N. S., & Kocovski, N. L. (2001). State and trait anxiety revisited. *Journal of Anxiety Disorder*, *15*(3), 231–245.

Ernst, M., & Paulus, M. P. (2005). Neurobiology of decision making: A selective review from a neurocognitive and clinical perspective. *Biological Psychiatry*, *58*(8), 597–604.

Etkin, A., Klemenhagen, K. C., Dudman, J. T., Rogan, M. T., Hen, R., Kandel, E. R., & Hirsch, J. (2004). Individual differences in trait anxiety predict the response of the basolateral amygdala to unconsciously processed fearful faces. *Neuron*, *44*(6), 1043–1055.

Eysenck, M. W. (1997). *Anxiety and cognition: A unified theory*. Hove: Psychology Press.

Eysenck, M. W., Derakshan, N., Santos, R., & Calvo, M. G. (2007). Anxiety and cognitive performance: Attentional control theory. *Emotion*, *7*(2), 336–353.

Fessler, D. M. T., Pillsworth, E. G., & Flamson, T. J. (2004). Angry men and disgusted women: An evolutionary approach to the influence of emotions on risk taking. *Organizational Behavior and Human Decision Processes*, *95*, 107–123.

Flint, J., & Munafo, M. R. (2007). The endophenotype concept in psychiatric genetics. *Psychological Medicine*, *37*(2), 163–180.

Fox, E. (1993). Attentional bias in anxiety: Selective or not? *Behavior Research and Therapy*, *31*(5), 487–493.

Fukui, H., Murai, T., Fukuyama, H., Hayashi, T., & Hanakawa, T. (2005). Functional activity related to risk anticipation during performance of the Iowa Gambling Task. *Neuroimage*, *24*(1), 253–259.

Furmark, T., Tillfors, M., Garpenstrand, H., Marteinsdottir, I., Langstrom, B., Oreland, L., & Fredrikson, M. (2004). Serotonin transporter polymorphism related to amygdala excitability and symptom severity in patients with social phobia. *Neuroscience Letters*, *362*(3), 189–192.

Garety, P. A., Hemsley, D. R., & Wessely, S. (1991). Reasoning in deluded schizophrenic and paranoid patients. Biases in performance on a probabilistic inference task. *Journal of Nervous and Mental Disease*, *179*(4), 194–201.

Gasper, K., & Clore, G. L. (1998). The persistent use of negative affect by anxious individuals to estimate risk. *Journal of Personality and Social Psychology*, *74*(5), 1350–1363.

Gaul, M. (1977). Influences of anxiety level on evaluation of dimensional importance in risky tasks. *Polish Psychological Bulletin*, *8*, 165–170.

Glimcher, P. W., Dorris, M. C., & Bayer, H. M. (2005). Physiological utility theory and the neuroeconomics of choice. *Games and Economic Behavior*, *52*(2), 213–256.

Gonzalez-Bono, E., Moya-Albiol, L., Salvador, A., Carrillo, E., Ricarte, J., & Gomez-Amor, J. (2002). Anticipatory autonomic response to a public speaking task in women: The role of trait anxiety. *Biological Psychology*, *60*(1), 37–49.

Gottesman, I. I., & Gould, T. D. (2003). The endophenotype concept in psychiatry: Etymology and strategic intentions. *American Journal of Psychiatry*, *160*(4), 636–645.

Grachev, I. D., & Apkarian, A. V. (2000). Anxiety in healthy humans is associated with orbital frontal chemistry. *Molecular Psychiatry*, *5*(5), 482–488.

Gray, J. A., & McNaughton, N. (2000/2003). *The neuropsychology of anxiety: An enquiry into the functions of the septo-hippocampal system* (2nd ed.). Oxford: Oxford University Press.

Gray, J. A., & McNaughton, N. (2003). *The neuropsychology of anxiety*. New York, NY: Oxford University Press.

Güth, W., Schmittberger, R., & Schwarze, B. (1982). An experimental analysis of ultimatum bargaining. *Journal of Economic Behavior and Organization*, *3*(4), 367–388.

Hall, D. T. (1972). A model of coping with role conflict: The role behavior of college educated women. *Administrative Science Quarterly*, *17*(4), 471–486.

Hallett, M. (2007). Transcranial magnetic stimulation: A primer. *Neuron*, *55*(2), 187–199.

Hamann, S., & Harenski, C. L. (2004). Exploring the brain's interface between personality, mood, and emotion: Theoretical comment on Canli et al. (2004). *Behavioral Neuroscience*, *118*(5), 1134–1136.

Hariri, A. R., Drabant, E. M., Munoz, K. E., Kolachana, B. S., Mattay, V. S., Egan, M. F., & Weinberger, D. R. (2005). A susceptibility gene for affective disorders and the response of the human amygdala. *Archives of General Psychiatry*, *62*(2), 146–152.

Hariri, A. R., Mattay, V. S., Tessitore, A., Kolachana, B., Fera, F., Goldman, D., Egan, M. F., & Weinberger, D. R. (2002). Serotonin transporter genetic variation and the response of the human amygdala. *Science*, *297*(5580), 400–403.

Harrison, L. K., & Turpin, G. (2003). Implicit memory bias and trait anxiety: A psychophysiological analysis. *Biological Psychology*, *62*(2), 97–114.

Heilman, R. M., Miu, A. C., Opre, A., & Houser, D. (2006). The thrills of decision-making: Trait anxiety, neuroticism and sensation seeking in ultimatum game and Iowa gambling task. Paper presented at the IAREP-SABE Conference on Behavioural Economics & Economic Psychology, Paris, Franta.

Huettel, S. A., Stowe, C. J., Gordon, E. M., Warner, B. T., & Platt, M. L. (2006). Neural signatures of economic preferences for risk and ambiguity. *Neuron*, *49*(5), 765–775.

Isen, A. M., Nygren, T. E., & Ashby, F. G. (1988). Influence of positive affect on the subjective utility of gains and losses: It is just not worth the risk. *Journal of Personality and Social Psychology*, *55*(5), 710–717.

Janis, I., & Mann, L. (1977). *Decision making: A psychological analysis of conflict, choice, and commitment*. New York: The Free Press.

Johnson, E. J., & Tversky, A. (1983). Affect, generalization, and the perception of risk. *Journal of Personality and Social Psychology*, *45*(1), 20–31.

Johnston, J. H., Driskell, J. E., & Salas, E. (1997). Vigilant and hypervigilant decision making. *Journal of Applied Psychology*, *82*(4), 614–622.

Kahneman, D., & Frederick, S. (2007). Frames and brains: Elicitation and control of response tendencies. *Trends in Cognitive Sciences*, *11*(2), 45–46.

Kahneman, D., & Tversky, A. (1984). Choices, values and frames. *American Psychologist*, *39*, 341–350.

Keinan, G. (1987). Decision making under stress: Scanning of alternatives under controllable and uncontrollable threats. *Journal of Personality and Social Psychology*, *52*(3), 639–644.

Keltner, D., & Gross, J. J. (1999). Functional accounts of emotions. *Cognition and Emotion*, *13*(5), 467–480.

Koster, E. H. W., Crombez, G., Verschuere, B., & De Houwer, J. (2006). Attention to threat in anxiety-prone individuals: Mechanisms underlying attentional bias. *Cognitive Therapy and Research*, *30*, 635–643.

Kowalski, R. M. (2000). Anxiety. In: A. E. Kazdin (Ed.), *Encyclopedia of psychology*. Washington: APA.

Krain, A. L., Gotimer, K., Hefton, S., Ernst, M., Castellanos, F. X., Pine, D. S., Milham, M. P. (2008). A functional magnetic resonance imaging investigation of uncertainty in adolescents with anxiety disorders. *Biological Psychiatry*, *63*(6), 563–568.

Krain, A. L., Hefton, S., Pine, D. S., Ernst, M., Castellanos, F. X., Klein, R. G., & Milham, M. P. (2006a). An fMRI examination of developmental differences in the neural correlates of uncertainty and decision-making. *Journal of Child Psychology and Psychiatry*, *47*(10), 1023–1030.

Krain, A. L., Wilson, A. M., Arbuckle, R., Castellanos, F. X., & Milham, M. P. (2006b). Distinct neural mechanisms of risk and ambiguity: A meta-analysis of decision-making. *Neuroimage*, *32*(1), 477–484.

Kumari, V., ffytche, D. H., Williams, S. C., & Gray, J. A. (2004). Personality predicts brain responses to cognitive demands. *Journal of Neurosciences*, *24*(47), 10636–10641.

Kurzban, R., & Houser, D. (2001). Individual differences and cooperation in a circular public goods game. *European Journal of Personality*, *15*, S37–S52.

Kverno, S. (2000). Trait anxiety influences on judgments of frequency and recall. *Personality and Individual Differences*, *29*(3), 395–404.

Lau, J. Y., Eley, T. C., & Stevenson, J. (2006). Examining the state-trait anxiety relationship: A behavioural genetic approach. *Journal of Abnormal Child Psychology*, *34*(1), 19–27.

Lauriola, M., & Levin, I. P. (2001). Personality traits and risky decision making in a controlled experimental task: An exploratory study. *Personality and Individual Differences*, *31*, 215–226.

Lauriola, M., Russo, P. M., Lucidi, F., Violani, C., & Levin, I. P. (2005). The role of personality in positively and negatively framed risky health decisions. *Personality and Individual Differences*, *38*, 45–59.

Lazarus, R. S. (1982). Thoughts on the relation between emotion and cognition. *American Psychologist*, *37*(9), 1019–1024.

Lazarus, R. S. (1993). From psychological stress to the emotions: A history of changing outlooks. *Annual Review of Psychology*, *44*, 1–21.

LeDoux, J. E. (2000). Emotion circuits in the brain. *Annual Review of Neuroscience*, *23*, 155–184.

Lejuez, C. W., Read, J. P., Kahler, C. W., Richards, J. B., Ramsey, S. E., Stuart, G. L., Strong, D. R., & Brown, R. A. (2002). Evaluation of a behavioral measure of risk taking: The Balloon Analogue Risk Task (BART). *Journal of Experimental Psychology. Applied*, *8*(2), 75–84.

Leon, M. R., & Revelle, W. (1985). Effects of anxiety on analogical reasoning: A test of three theoretical models. *Journal of Personality and Social Psychology*, *49*(5), 1302–1315.

Lerner, J. S., & Keltner, D. (2000). Beyond valence: Toward a model of emotion-specific influences on judgement and choice. *Cognition and Emotion*, *14*(4), 473–493.

Lesch, K. P., Bengel, D., Heils, A., Sabol, S. Z., Greenberg, B. D., Petri, S., et al. (1996). Association of anxiety-related traits with a polymorphism in the serotonin transporter gene regulatory region. *Science*, *274*(5292), 1527–1531.

Loewenstein, G., Rick, S., & Cohen, J. D. (2008). Neuroeconomics. *Annual Reviews of Psychology*, *59*, 647–672.

Loewenstein, G. F., & O'Donoghue, T. (2004, May). *Animal spirits: Affective and deliberative processes in economic behavior* (Downloaded on January 9. Available at http://cbdr.cmu.edu/seminar/Loewenstein.pdf).

Loewenstein, G. F., Weber, E. U., Hsee, C. K., & Welch, E. S. (2001). Risk as feelings. *Psychological Bulletin, 127*, 267–286.

MacLeod, C., & Rutherford, E. M. (1992). Anxiety and the selective processing of emotional information: Mediating roles of awareness, trait and state variables, and personal relevance of stimulus materials. *Behavior Research and Therapy, 30*(5), 479–491.

Mandler, G., & Sarason, S. B. (1952). A study of anxiety and learning. *Journal of Abnormal Psychology, 47*(2), 166–173.

Maner, J. K., Richey, J. A., Cromer, K., Mallott, M., Lejuez, C. W., Joiner, T. E., & Schmidt, N. B. (2007). Dispositional anxiety and risk-avoidant decision-making. *Personality and Individual Differences, 42*, 665–675.

Maner, J. K., & Schmidt, N. B. (2006). The role of risk avoidance in anxiety. *Behavior Therapy, 37*(2), 181–189.

Mathews, A., & MacLeod, C. (2005). Cognitive vulnerability to emotional disorders. *Annual Review of Clinical Psychology, 1*, 167–195.

Mathews, A., Mogg, K., May, J., & Eysenck, M. (1989). Implicit and explicit memory bias in anxiety. *Journal of Abnormal Psychology, 98*(3), 236–240.

Mauss, I. B., Wilhelm, F. H., & Gross, J. J. (2003). Autonomic recovery and habituation in social anxiety. *Psychophysiology, 40*(4), 648–653.

Mayer, R. E. (1977). Problem-solving performance with task overload: Effects of self-pacing and trait anxiety. *Bulletin of Psychonomic Society, 9*, 283–286.

McCabe, K. (2003). Neuroeconomics. In: L. Nadel (Ed.), *Encyclopedia of cognitive science* (Vol. 3, pp. 294–298). New York: Macmillan Publishers Ltd.

Meyer-Lindenberger, A. (2006). Functional imaging genetics of neural circuits for social cognition. Paper presented at the Second International Imaging Genetics Conference, UC Irvine, CA.

Miclea, M. (2001). Defense mechanisms. Some lessons from cognitive neurosciences and ethoexperimental studies. In: O. Benga & M. Miclea (Eds), *Development and cognition* (pp. 173–193). Cluj-Napoca: Presa Universitara Clujeana [Cluj University Press].

Miclea, M. (2006). *Anxiety. Current perspectives* (Special Issue of *Cognition, Brain, Behavior*, the Official Journal of the Romanian Association for Cognitive Science). Cluj-Napoca: Romanian Association for Cognitive Science Press.

Mineka, S., & Zinbarg, R. (2006). A contemporary learning theory perspective on the etiology of anxiety disorders: It's not what you thought it was. *American Psychologist, 61*(1), 10–26.

Miu, A. C., Heilman, R. M., & Houser, D. (2008). Anxiety impairs decision-making: Psychophysiological evidence from an Iowa Gambling Task. *Biological Psychology, 77*(3), 353–358.

Miu, A. C., Heilman, R. M., Opre, A., & Miclea, M. (2005). Emotion-induced retrograde amnesia and trait anxiety. *Journal of Experimental Psychology. Learning, Memory, and Cognition, 31*(6), 1250–1257.

Mogg, K., Bradley, B. P., Dixon, C., Fischer, S., Twelftree, H., & McWilliams, A. (2000). Trait anxiety, defensiveness and selective processing of threat: An investigation using two measures of attentional bias. *Personality and Individual Differences, 28*, 1063–1077.

Mogg, K., Bradley, B. P., Williams, R., & Mathews, A. (1993). Subliminal processing of emotional information in anxiety and depression. *Journal of Abnormal Psychology, 102*(2), 304–311.

Mogg, K., Mathews, A., Bird, C., & Macgregor-Morris, R. (1990). Effects of stress and anxiety on the processing of threat stimuli. *Journal of Personality and Social Psychology*, *59*(6), 1230–1237.

Monteleone, P., Santonastaso, P., Tortorella, A., Favaro, A., Fabrazzo, M., Castaldo, E., Caregaro, L., Fuschino, A., & Maj, M. (2005). Serotonin transporter polymorphism and potential response to SSRIs in bulimia nervosa. *Molecular Psychiatry*, *10*(8), 716–718.

Morinaga, K., Akiyoshi, J., Matsushita, H., Ichioka, S., Tanaka, Y., Tsuru, J., & Hanada, H. (2007). Anticipatory anxiety-induced changes in human lateral prefrontal cortex activity. *Biological Psychology*, *74*(1), 34–38.

Munafo, M. R., Brown, S. M., & Hariri, A. R. (2008). Serotonin transporter (5-HTTLPR) genotype and amygdala activation: A meta-analysis. *Biological Psychiatry*, *63*(9), 852–857.

Neisser, U. (1967). *Cognitive psychology*. Englewood Cliffs, NJ: Prentice-Hall.

O'Hare, M. O., & Tamburri, E. (1986). Coping as a moderator of the relation between anxiety and career decision making. *Journal of Counseling Psychology*, *33*, 255–264.

Oldenburg, C., Lundh, L. G., & Kivistö, P. (2002). Explicit and implicit memory, trait anxiety, and repressive coping style. *Personality and Individual Differences*, *32*, 107–119.

Osher, Y., Hamer, D., & Benjamin, J. (2000). Association and linkage of anxiety-related traits with a functional polymorphism of the serotonin transporter gene regulatory region in Israeli sibling pairs. *Molecular Psychiatry*, *5*(2), 216–219.

Paulus, M. P. (2007). Decision-making dysfunctions in psychiatry – Altered homeostatic processing? *Science*, *318*(5850), 602–606.

Paulus, M. P., Feinstein, J. S., Simmons, A., & Stein, M. B. (2004). Anterior cingulate activation in high trait anxious subjects is related to altered error processing during decision making. *Biological Psychiatry*, *55*(12), 1179–1187.

Perna, G., Favaron, E., Di Bella, D., Bussi, R., & Bellodi, L. (2005). Antipanic efficacy of paroxetine and polymorphism within the promoter of the serotonin transporter gene. *Neuropsychopharmacology*, *30*(12), 2230–2235.

Pessoa, L. (2008). On the relationship between emotion and cognition. *Nature Reviews in Neuroscience*, *9*(2), 148–158.

Pezawas, L., Meyer-Lindenberg, A., Drabant, E. M., Verchinski, B. A., Munoz, K. E., Kolachana, B. S., Egan, M. F., Mattay, V. S., Hariri, A. R., & Weinberger, D. R. (2005). 5-HTTLPR polymorphism impacts human cingulate-amygdala interactions: A genetic susceptibility mechanism for depression. *Nature Neuroscience*, *8*(6), 828–834.

Phan, K. L., Wager, T., Taylor, S. F., & Liberzon, I. (2002). Functional neuroanatomy of emotion: A meta-analysis of emotion activation studies in PET and fMRI. *Neuroimage*, *16*(2), 331–348.

Plomin, R., Owen, M. J., & McGuffin, P. (1994). The genetic basis of complex human behaviors. *Science*, *264*(5166), 1733–1739.

Raghunathan, R., & Pham, M. T. (1999). All negative moods are not equal: Motivational influences of anxiety and sadness on decision-making. *Organizational Behavior and Human Decision Processes*, *79*(1), 56–77.

Rahman, S., Sahakia, B., Cardinal, R., Rogers, R., & Robbins, T. (2001). Decision making and neuropsychiatry. *Trends in Cognitive Sciences*, *5*(6), 271–277.

Ray, R. D., Ochsner, K. N., Cooper, J. C., Robertson, E. R., Gabrieli, J. D., & Gross, J. J. (2005). Individual differences in trait rumination and the neural systems supporting cognitive reappraisal. *Cognitive, Affective and Behavioral Neuroscience*, *5*(2), 156–168.

Reidy, J. (2004). Trait anxiety, trait depression, worry, and memory. *Behavior Research and Therapy*, *42*(8), 937–948.

Reidy, J., & Richards, A. (1997). Anxiety and memory: A recall bias for threatening words in high anxiety. *Behavior Research and Therapy*, *35*(6), 531–542.

Revelle, W. (1993). Individual differences in personality and motivation: Non-cognitive determinants of cognitive performance. In: A. Baddeley & L. Weiskrantz (Eds), *Attention: Selection, awareness and control. A tribute to Donald Broadbent* (pp. 346–373). Oxford: Oxford University Press.

Richards, A., & French, C. C. (1991). Effects of encoding and anxiety on implicit and explicit memory performance. *Personality and Individual Differences*, *12*, 131–139.

Rodgers, R. J., Cao, B. J., Dalvi, A., & Holmes, A. (1997). Animal models of anxiety: An ethological perspective. *Brazilian Journal of Medical and Biological Research*, *30*(3), 289–304.

Sanfey, A. G., Loewenstein, G., McClure, S. M., & Cohen, J. D. (2006). Neuroeconomics: Cross-currents in research on decision-making. *Trends in Cognitive Sciences*, *10*(3), 108–116.

Scheier, M. F., Carver, C. S., & Bridges, M. W. (1994). Distinguishing optimism from neuroticism (and trait anxiety, self-mastery, and self-esteem): A reevaluation of the Life Orientation Test. *Journal of Personality and Social Psychology*, *67*(6), 1063–1078.

Schmidt, N. B., Storey, J., Greenberg, B. D., Santiago, H. T., Li, Q., & Murphy, D. L. (2000). Evaluating gene x psychological risk factor effects in the pathogenesis of anxiety: A new model approach. *Journal of Abnormal Psychology*, *109*(2), 308–320.

Schwarz, N., & Clore, G. L. (1983). Mood, misattribution, and judgments of well-being: Informative and directive functions of affective states. *Journal of Personality and Social Psychology*, *45*, 513–523.

Shackman, A. J., Sarinopoulos, I., Maxwell, J. S., Pizzagalli, D. A., Lavric, A., & Davidson, R. J. (2006). Anxiety selectively disrupts visuospatial working memory. *Emotion*, *6*(1), 40–61.

Sharot, T., Riccardi, A. M., Raio, C. M., & Phelps, E. A. (2007). Neural mechanisms mediating optimism bias. *Nature*, *450*(7166), 102–105.

Shepperd, J. A., Grace, J., Cole, L. J., & Klein, C. (2005). Anxiety and outcome predictions. *Personality and Social Psychology Bulletin*, *31*(2), 267–275.

Siegman, A. W. (1956). The effect of manifest anxiety on a concept formation task, a nondirected learning task and on timed and untimed intelligence tests. *Journal of Consulting Psychology*, *20*(3), 176–178.

Slovic, P., Finucane, M. L., Peters, E., & MacGregor, D. G. (2007). The affect heuristic. *European Journal of Operational Research*, *177*, 1333–1352.

Spielberger, C. D. (1983). *Manual for the State-Trait Anxiety Inventory*. Palo Alto: Consulting Psychologists Press.

Spielberger, C. S. (1966). *Anxiety and behaviour*. New York: Academic Press.

Stein, M. B., Fallin, M. D., Schork, N. J., & Gelernter, J. (2005). COMT polymorphisms and anxiety-related personality traits. *Neuropsychopharmacology*, *30*(11), 2092–2102.

Stein, M. B., Seedat, S., & Gelernter, J. (2006). Serotonin transporter gene promoter polymorphism predicts SSRI response in generalized social anxiety disorder. *Psychopharmacology (Berlin)*, *187*(1), 68–72.

Stöber, J. (1997). Trait anxiety and pessimistic appraisal of risk and chance. *Personality and Individual Differences*, *22*, 465–476.

Sugiura, M., Kawashima, R., Nakagawa, M., Okada, K., Sato, T., Goto, R., Sato, K., Ono, S., Schormann, T., Zilles, K., & Fukuda, H. (2000). Correlation between human personality and neural activity in cerebral cortex. *Neuroimage*, *11*(5 Pt 1), 541–546.

Trapnell, P. D., & Campbell, J. D. (1999). Private self-consciousness and the five-factor model of personality: Distinguishing rumination from reflection. *Journal of Personality and Social Psychology*, *76*(2), 284–304.

Tversky, A., & Kahneman, D. (1974). Judgment under uncertainty: Heuristics and biases. *Science*, *185*(4157), 1124–1131.

Ulleberg, P., & Rundmo, T. (2003). Personality, attitudes and risk perception as predictors of risky driving behaviour among young drivers. *Safety Science*, *41*(5), 427–443.

Vlek, C., & Stallen, P. J. (1980). Rational and personal aspects of risk. *Acta Psychologica*, *45*(1–3), 273–300.

Weber, E. U., Blais, A.-R., & Betz, N. (2002). A domain-specific risk-attitude scale: Measuring risk perceptions and risk behaviors. *Journal of Behavioral Decision Making*, *15*, 263–290.

Weller, J. A., Levin, I. P., Shiv, B., & Bechara, A. (2007). Neural correlates of adaptive decision making for risky gains and losses. *Psychological Science*, *18*(11), 958–964.

Williams, J. M., Mathews, A., & MacLeod, C. (1996). The emotional Stroop task and psychopathology. *Psychological Bulletin*, *120*(1), 3–24.

Yamasue, H., Abe, O., Suga, M., Yamada, H., Rogers, M. A., Aoki, S., Kato, N., & Kasai, K. (2008). Sex-linked neuroanatomical basis of human altruistic cooperativeness. *Cerebral Cortex*, *18*(10), 2331–2340.

Yiend, J., & Mathews, A. (2001). Anxiety and attention to threatening pictures. *Quarterly Journal of Experimental Psychology A*, *54*(3), 665–681.

Young, H. F., & Bentall, R. P. (1995). Hypothesis testing in patients with persecutory delusions: Comparison with depressed and normal subjects. *British Journal of Clinical Psychology*, *34*(Pt 3), 353–369.

THE POTENTIAL ROLE OF REGRET IN THE PHYSICIAN–PATIENT RELATIONSHIP: INSIGHTS FROM NEUROECONOMICS

Giorgio Coricelli

ABSTRACT

Purpose – *The aim of the chapter is to show how two important facts of physicians' behavior, (i) their tendency to "create" the demand for medical practices, and (ii) their delay and reluctance in using new treatments and therapies, can be explained with the lens of the neuroeconomics research on the neural and behavioral basis of regret.*

Methodology – *This chapter adopts a neuroeconomics perspective on decision-making, asking how the brain represents values and generates emotional states, which consequently influence choices. In the line of recent work on emotion-based decision-making, we expect to be able to characterize the brain areas underlying the studied processes and to specify the functional relationship between rational decision-making and the emotional influences that modulate these decisional processes.*

Originality – *Neurobiological approaches can contribute significantly to a better understanding of the cognitive and emotional underpinnings of*

Neuroeconomics
Advances in Health Economics and Health Services Research, Volume 20, 85–97

ISSN: 0731-2199/doi:10.1016/S0731-2199(08)20004-X

medical decision-making, from how physicians might evaluate and anticipate the effect of alternative therapies, to how patients might anticipate future consequences of their health choice. This can explain some features of the doctor–patient relationship which are not consistent with simple maximization models.

Findings – *Our findings suggest that physicians' behavior can be often explained by regret avoidance. Likewise, they suggest that physicians play as actual agents when they make medical decisions that will affect the future well-being of their patients.*

Research limitations – *We limited our analysis to the potential role of anticipated regret; therefore, this chapter neglects many important factors of the health sector.*

1. INTRODUCTION

The introduction of neuroscience tools, coupled with increasing evidence on the importance of emotional and social states in economic decision-making, is opening new perspectives in the field of neuroeconomics (Camerer, 2003; McCabe, 2003; Glimcher & Rustichini, 2004; Rustichini, 2005). In this chapter we adopt a neuroeconomics approach on decision-making in the health sector. We propose new hypotheses based on the relationship between cognitive and emotional component during medical decision-making.

Our analysis relies on the study of the behavioral and the neural basis of the emotion of regret and its role in complex decision-making processes, such as those involved in health care decisions.

Two important questions regarding physician–patient interaction can be better understood using the lens of neuroeconomics. Specifically, why do physicians tend to induce the demand for medical practices, and why are they reluctant to introduce new treatments and new therapies? We propose that a possible explanation of these contradictory facts can be found in the role of anticipated regret in the decisions made by the patients and the physicians. We present here a formal model of regret-averse physician behavior and (analogical) evidence from recent neuroeconomics studies that support this possible explanation.

The chapter is organized as follows: the second and third sections briefly describe the psychological and economic theories of regret. The final sections present the theoretical model and the neuroeconomics evidence related to the doctor–patient interaction.

2. THE PSYCHOLOGY OF PERSONAL RESPONSIBILITY

The feeling of responsibility for the consequence of our choices has an important role in decision-making (Zeelenberg & Beattie, 1997). This is particularly true when our choice might affect the well-being of others. On one hand, we tend to compare factual or imaginative alternatives, engaging in a mental process called counterfactual (Lewis, 1973; Roese & Olson, 1995; Byrne, 2002). On the other hand, we often "prefer not to know" the outcome of the option that we have rejected, if only for the fact that it might be better than the outcome of our choice (Kahneman & Tversky, 1982). Counterfactuals amplify (Kahneman & Miller, 1986) and in some cases even generate emotional responses (Mellers, Ritov, & Schwartz, 1999; Zeelenberg & van Dijk, 2004).

Humans use strategies to avoid intense negative emotions, and can anticipate the effects of future thinking about "how I would have been better if I had chosen differently." This thinking determines the feeling of regret. Regret is a cognitive-based emotion characterized by the feeling of responsibility for the negative outcome of our choice (Gilovich & Melvec, 1994). Disappointment is the emotion related to an unexpected negative outcome independent of the responsibility component (Bell, 1985; Loomes & Sugden, 1986). Anticipation of regret induces changes in behavioral strategies (Ritov, 1996) and characterizes the learning process in decision-making (Zeelenberg, Beattie, van der Pligt, & de Vries, 1996). Regret results from a decision made and the possibility to compare the obtained outcome with better outcomes of rejected alternatives.

Norm theory by Kahneman and Miller (1986) suggests that the norms used in outcome evaluation are evaluated after the outcome occurs. Kahneman and Miller suggest that the norm is an appropriate context point of reference, used in the evaluation processes. This theoretical concept postulates that an outcome automatically evokes alternatives for comparison, in terms of what could/might have been. The recruited alternative plays as a point of reference for the comparison. The norms of "what might have happened if I had chosen differently" evoke a strong affective reaction, namely regret.

3. ECONOMIC MODELS OF REGRET

Classical economic models of regret suggest (Bell, 1982; Loomes & Sugden, 1982) that incorporating regret into the utility function might reconcile the utility theory with observed behavior (Allais paradox types of behavior) in decision-making under uncertainty. The main point is that many violations of the axioms of von Neumann and Morgenstern (1944) expected utility theory might be explained by the anticipated regret; thus, a decision-maker might incur in a suboptimal choice in order to avoid future regrettable situations. Monetary assets and a measure of regret are incorporated in a multiattribute utility function. Bell emphasizes the decision aspect of regret. Thus, regret arises from a decision and "is measured as the difference in value between the received assets and the highest level of assets produced by other alternatives (cf. Bell, 1982)." Bell gives this formal definition of the multiattribute utility function:

$$U(x, y) = v(x) + f(v(x) - v(y))$$

where x indicates the final asset x and y is the foregone asset. The utility is a function of the asset value ($v(x)$) and of the regret ($v(x) - v(y)$). These two terms are additive. f is decreasingly concave in the case of regret aversion.

Loomes and Sugden (1982) considered anticipated regret as rational, and regret theory as an "alternative theory of rational choice under uncertainty." They introduced the concept of choiceless utility. Choiceless utility is the utility derived from a certain consequence (outcome) without having chosen. Loomes and Sugden focused on two main points of regret theory: first, the fact that regret is commonly experienced; and, second, that people try to anticipate and avoid the experience of future regret.

Anticipated regret is based on considering choosing an alternative and simultaneously rejecting other alternatives. The type of feedback information is indeed crucial to determining the emotional response, and the decisional process is influenced by the knowledge about the future feedback available.

4. THE ROLE OF REGRET IN THE PHYSICIAN–PATIENT INTERACTION

Feedback information about the success or the failure of different therapies and medical practices is increasingly accessible (there are thousands of web pages dedicated to medical information,[1] informative brochures offered by national and international health care organizations, medical information offered by the media in terms of news, health product updates, and chat forums) to both physicians and patients. Thus, the choice of a therapy and the simultaneous rejection of other practices represent a scenario where the likelihood of future regret might arise.

Here, we show how two important facts of physicians' behavior can be explained with the lens of the neuroeconomics research on the neural and behavioral basis of regret. First (Fact 1), physicians tend to "create" the demand for medical practices; and, second (Fact 2), they are often slow and sometimes reluctant in using new treatments and therapies.

There are several possible explanations for the first fact (Newhouse, 1970; Feldstein, 1970; Evans, 1974). For instance, Evans (1974) modeled the physician–patient interaction as a game of asymmetric information, in which physicians would prescribe excessive (over the optimal level from the patients' perspective) medical treatments with the only purpose of maximizing their own income. Models of this type underestimate the uncertainty effect and the moral (Arrow, 1963) and reputational considerations that characterize physicians' choice behavior.

We can reasonably assume that even fully opportunistic physicians would not profit from the negative consequences of their choice in terms of reduction of well-being of their patients (which would negatively affect physicians' reputations, careers, and self esteem). We suggest that they might offer more than the optimal level of medical practices in order to avoid possible regret for "not having done enough." The action–inaction effect is an important factor related to the psychology of regret. As shown in Gilovich and Medvec (1994–1995), inaction generates more long-term regret than action. In this specific case, the physician would prescribe more practices than the ones presumably needed in order to avoid the regret of not having done enough for the patient's health. Another important consideration in this context is the fact that patients tend to negatively evaluate (wrongly assuming that the quantity of the offered practices is perfectly correlated with the effort and the skills of their physicians; see Tversky & Kahneman, 1973) physicians that do not prescribe enough medical products according to the patient's perspective. This is often more than what patients really need. In this sense, over-offering is a strategy that matches both the physician and the patient's regret avoidance behavior.

The second fact, the reluctance of physicians to prescribe innovative and more risky medical practices, is highly related to the uncertainty on the efficacy of novel products. Uncertainty on the efficacy of different treatments is a main component of medical choices. Models that consider the uncertainty in the productivity of medical practices better explain physicians' behavior than models based merely on the asymmetric information between physicians and patients and the resulting moral hazard from the physicians' side.

From a different perspective, we can actually consider the asymmetric information, in terms of physicians' (compared to patients) better knowledge of possible consequences of different medical products, as more important for explaining the reluctance of offering new products (Fact 2) than the tendency to create their own demand (Fact 1). In this sense, "knowing that you know more" might induce a higher sense of responsibility. In this chapter we argue that the uncertainty in the efficacy of novel medical products and therapies affects the physician's behavior, inducing regret avoidance choices, such as avoiding practices that might be extremely risky for the patients' health.

Put in these terms, there is an analogy between the physicians' behavior described by Facts 1 and 2, and the behavior of investors during the choice of their pension plan. Both agents, the physicians and the investors, "hedge away from the extremes" in order to minimize their future regret. The "extremes" for the investors are to invest all in the risk-free assets (bonds) or all in the risky assets (stocks). The investors that try to avoid regret would choose a riskier portfolio if the equity premium is low, and a more moderate portfolio if the equity premium is high, compared to the behavior of a risk-averse investor. In other words, the regret-averse investor will hold a positive amount of stocks even if the equity premium is close to zero, and will always hold a positive amount of bonds even though the equity premium is quite large. Similarly, following our interpretation, regret-averse physicians will offer more than optimal levels of standard practices (Fact 1) and at the same time they will be reluctant to offer innovative practices (Fact 2). However, a purely risk-averse physician will offer less-standard practices to avoid the risk of prescribing products that might be dangerous for the patients (e.g., allergy reactions), and he/she will offer a higher level of innovative (low risk) practices compared to a regret-averse physician.

4.1. Formal Model of Regret-Averse Physician Behavior

Formally, we can describe a physician's choice between combinations of levels of standard and innovative therapies, following the model of Muermann, Mitchell, and Volkman (2006) on portfolio selection. We call γ the proportion of standard therapies chosen by the physician. The objective of the physician is to maximize the patient's health level h. The standard therapies give a deterministic return (in terms of health level), while the innovative therapies give a stochastic return. Ex ante, a regret-averse physician would choose the level of γ that maximizes the following equation (adapted from Maccheroni, Marinacci, & Rustichini, 2006):

$$E[u(h_\gamma) - k\rho(u(\max\ H) - u(h_\gamma))]$$

where, $\rho(u(\max\ H) - u(h_\gamma))$ is the regret term, measured as the difference between the ex-post optimal level of health (max H) and the final level given the choice of $\gamma(h_\gamma)$, with $\rho' > 0$ and $\rho'' > 0$ for regret aversion; k indicates the relative importance of anticipating regret with respect to the mere risk avoidance behavior (described by a $u' > 0$ and $u'' < 0$). Thus, if the physician does not anticipate regret, $k = 0$, he/she will behave as a risk-averse expected utility maximizer.

This model predicts different patterns of behavior according to the level of k. If $k > 0$, thus the physician tries to avoid future regret, he/she will choose to prescribe respectively a larger level of standard practices and less innovative therapies, compared with a risk-averse physician (see Proposition 2 in Muermann et al., 2005).

Behavioral data from Mellers et al. (1999), Camille et al. (2004), and Coricelli et al. (2005) show that anticipated regret is the main determinant of subjects' choice behavior in situations where the subjects know, prior to making a decision, that they will get information about the outcomes of the rejected alternatives (complete feedback). Risk aversion prevails, however, in situations where the feedback on the foregone alternative is not provided (partial feedback). These findings suggest the empirical plausibility of a $k > 0$, and of its theoretical predictions (i.e., excessive standard practices and reduced level of innovative therapies).

4.2. What Might Happen in the Brain of a Regret-Averse Physician?

As we mentioned above, the explanation of the Facts 1 and 2 in terms of physicians' regret avoidance behavior is analogous to the interpretation of the investors' behavior of "hedging away from the extremes" in a pension plan. Given this interpretation, we can conclude that the physicians play as actual agents when they take a medical decision that will affect the future well-being of their patients. The results from a brain imaging study (Coricelli et al., 2005[2]) showed that physiological responses (heart rate) and brain activity are modulated as a function of whether the subject is involved in an actual choice (that is, whether the subject is agent) or is following a computer program choice (where choice is computer-selected, meaning the subject had no agency). Brain structures (many portions of the prefrontal cortex) usually involved in decision-making, and specifically involved in regret processing (orbitofrontal cortex,[3] anterior cingulated cortex and hippocampus) activated only when the subjects were agents. The influence of personal responsibility on the processing of the outcomes was evident in contrasting outcome-related activity for choose trials (where the subject selected which gamble to "play") with follow trials (where "choice," i.e., follow, was computer-selected) (Fig. 1 The effect of agency). Thus, outcome evaluation is influenced by the level of responsibility in the process of choice (agency) and by the available information regarding alternative outcomes (complete or partial feedback).

The explanation of Facts 1 and 2 in terms of anticipated regret supports the hypothesis that physicians might play as "perfect agents" during choices that might affect the future health of the patients. Thus, we could expect the physicians' brain activity during medical decision-making to look like the neuronal activity related to agency (i.e., when a subject is taking a decision that will affect his future well-being). We expect a "transfer" between patient and physician in terms of actual emotional and cognitive processes. Indeed, just "following" patients' directions would not induce the feeling and the anticipation of regret (see Fig. 1), and therefore would not explain the coexistence of Facts 1 and 2.

5. SUMMARY AND CONCLUSIONS

This chapter uses recent findings from neuroeconomics on the neural and theoretical basis of the emotion of regret to explain behavioral facts observed in physician–patients interactions. Regret is an emotion associated with a decision that turns out badly. It is usually elicited by a comparison (counterfactual) between the outcome of choice and the better outcome of rejected alternatives. In the context of medical decision-making, the feedback on the efficacy of different medical practices is almost unavoidable; thus, the prospect of future regret is always present. The behavioral impact of regret is expressed by the fact that people often try to avoid the likelihood of future regret even when this conflicts with the prescription of decision based upon rational choice.

Here we suggest, with the support of neuroeconomics findings, that regret aversion is a good predictor of physicians' behavior. The studies on the neural basis of regret show the involvement of a brain circuitry (orbitofrontal cortex, anterior cingulate, and temporal areas) in the experience and in the anticipation of this cognitive-based emotion. The orbitofrontal cortex is found to play an important role during the entire process of decision-making

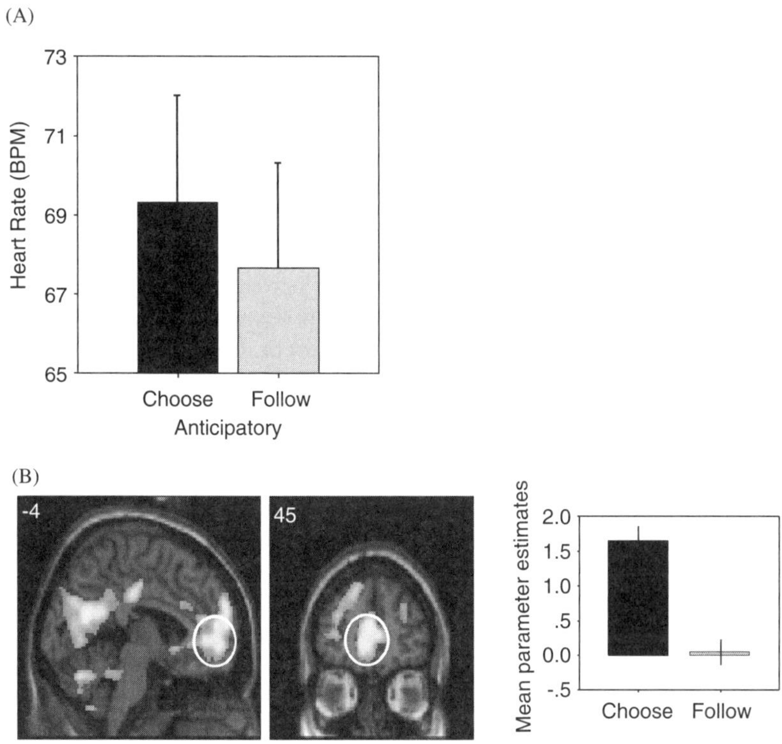

Fig. 1. The Responsibility (Agency) Effect. In Coricelli et al. (2005) Subjects Participated in the Regret Gambling Task. Regret Was Induced by Providing Information Regarding the Outcome of the Unchosen Gamble (Complete Feedback Condition). Half of the Trials Were "Choose" Trials, Where the Subject Had a Choice; the Other Half Were "Follow" Trials, Where the Subjects Were Informed That the Computer Would Randomly Choose One of the Two Gambles. The Follow Trials Were Introduced in Order to Remove Any Feeling of Responsibility. (A) During Task Performance, Subjects' Physiological Responses (Heart Rate) Were Significantly Higher in "Choose" Trials Than in "Follow" Trials ($P = .001$). (B) Irrespective of Whether the Subject Experienced Financial Gain or Loss on a Particular Trial, Responsibility for Selecting the Initial Gamble Influenced the Pattern of Outcome-Related Brain Activity. Notably, Initial Selection between the Gambles (in Contrast to "Following" the Computer-Selected Gamble) Was Associated with Enhancement of Activity in Themedial Prefrontal Cortex (Including Genual Cingulate, Paracingulate, and Mediodorsal Prefrontal Cortices) and the Primary Visual and Anterior Superior Temporal (STG) Cortices. In Contrast, Following Computer-Selected Choices Was Associated with Relative Enhancement of Activity in Thalamus, Supplementary Motor (SMA) and Bilateral Superior Parietal Cortices. This Pattern is Similar to That Observed During Passive Anticipation (Nagai, Critchley, Featherstone, Trimble, & Dolan, 2004). The Agency Effect Was Significant Only for Choose Trials Where the Subject Was Responsible for the Choice, i.e., When the Subject (Rather Than the Computer) Selected between Two Gambles. Group Data (Thresholded at $P<0.001$, Uncorrected) Is Plotted on Sagittal and Coronal Sections of a Normalized Canonical Template Brain. In the Right Panel We Plot the Average Parameter Estimates ($\pm$s.e.m.) for Relative Difference in BOLD Activity at Outcome in Choose and Follow Trials.

in contexts where regret might arise. This particular portion of the prefrontal cortex integrates cognitive and emotional components of decision-making. Results from a recent neuroimaging study (Coricelli et al., 2005) demonstrate how the activity of the regret circuitry is found only when the experimental subject is actually an agent, meaning that he/she is actually taking a decision. It is not activated when the subject is merely following the choice of another agent (the patient). We use this result to suggest that physicians actually play as agent when they are taking decisions that might primarily have consequences for the future of their patients. With this interpretation, we can reconcile apparently contradictory facts of the physicians' behavior, such as their tendency to offer more than the optimal level of standard practices and less than the optimal level of innovative therapies. Thus, we suggest that these less-than-rational medical choices are made in order to avoid the prospect of future regret.

Many important factors of the health sector, such as the effect of different institutions and the health insurance system (Arrow, 1963; Cutler & Reber, 1998), have been neglected in this chapter. We limited our analysis to a single and specific factor (anticipated regret) that we suggest (see also Thaler, 1980) might explain some features of the doctor–patient relationship which are not consistent with simple maximization models.

NOTES

1. For instance, these are the top ten most useful websites listed (in alphabetical order) by the Medical Library Association: Cancer.gov, Centers for Disease Control and Prevention (CDC), familydoctor.org, healthfinder, HIV InSite, Kidshealth, Mayo Clinic, MEDEM: an information partnership of medical societies, MEDLINEplus, and NOAH: New York Online Access to Health.

2. Coricelli et al. (2005) measured brain activity using functional magnetic resonance imaging (fMRI) while subjects selected between two gambles wherein regret was induced by providing information about the outcome of the unchosen gamble. Increasing regret enhanced activity in the medial orbitofrontal region, the dorsal anterior cingulate cortex, and hippocampus. Both, the dorsal portion of the cingulate cortex and the hippocampal activities reveal an underlying cognitive-based declarative process of regret. The portion of the anterior cingulate which was activated in our task during regret has been identified (meta-analysis) to be a purely cognitive area. And the observed hippocampus activity suggests the presence of a declarative memory activity (the lesson to remember is: "in the future pay more attention at the consequences of your choice").

3. The orbitofrontal cortex represents the relative values of different rewards (Rolls, 1999; Rolls, 2000; Breiter, Ahron, Kahneman, Dale, & Shizgal, 2001; O'Doherty, Krigelbach, Rolls, Hornak, & Andrews, 2001; Dreher, Kohn, & Berman, 2006), and

the subjective pleasantness of reinforcers (primary reinforcers, such as food, sex; and secondary, abstract reinforcers, such as money). Neurons in this region of the brain encode the relative values of different choice alternatives (Padoa-Schioppa & Assad, 2006). Tremblay and Schultz (1999) demonstrated how OFC neurons fire when the relatively preferred available reward, between pairs of rewards, is delivered, thus "revealing" the monkey preferences. Corroborating results come from a more recent study (Padoa-Schioppa & Assad, 2006), where monkey is asked to choose between combinations of amounts of different rewards. Also in this case, the OFC neurons fire according to the monkey's preference structure and actual choices. This activity of the OFC corresponds to a high-level representational function of the values of external stimuli.

ACKNOWLEDGMENTS

I gratefully acknowledge financial support from the Human Frontier Science Program (HFSP, RGP 56/2005, "Decision making and strategies in the brain: a multidisciplinary approach for understanding social behaviour"), ANR (Agence Nationale de la Recherche), and PAT (Provincia Autonoma di Trento).

REFERENCES

Arrow, K. J. (1963). Uncertainty and the welfare economics of medical care. *The American Economic Review*, *53*, 941–973.

Bell, D. E. (1982). Regret in decision-making under uncertainty. *Operations Research*, *30*, 961–981.

Bell, D. E. (1985). Disappointment in decision-making under uncertainty. *Operations Research*, *33*, 1–27.

Breiter, H. C., Ahron, I., Kahneman, D., Dale, A., & Shizgal, P. (2001). Functional imaging of neural responses to expectancy and experience of monetary gains and losses. *Neuron*, *30*, 619–639.

Byrne, R. M. J. (2002). Mental models and counterfactual thoughts about what might have been. *Trends Cognitive Science*, *6*, 426–431.

Camerer, C. F. (2003). Psychology and economics. Strategizing in the brain. *Science*, *300*, 1673–1675.

Camille, N., Coricelli, G., Sallet, J., Pradat, P., Duhamel, J. R., & Sirigu, A. (2004). The involvement of the orbitofrontal cortex in the experience of regret. *Science*, *304*, 1167–1170.

Coricelli, G., Critchley, H. D., Joffily, M., O'Doherty, J. D., Sirigu, A., & Dolan, R. J. (2005). Regret and its Avoidance: A Neuroimaging Study of Choice Behavior. *Nature Neuroscience*, *8*, 1255–1262.

Cutler, D. M., & Reber, S. J. (1998). Paying for health insurance: The trade-off between competition and adverse selection. *Quarterly Journal of Economics*, *113*, 433–466.

Dreher, J. C., Kohn, P., & Berman, K. F. (2006). Neural coding of distinct statistical properties of reward information in humans. *Cerebral Cortex*, *16*, 561–573.

Evans, R. G. (1974). Supplier-induced demand: Some empirical evidence and implications. In: M. Perlman (Ed.), *The Economics of Health and Medical Care*. New York: Wiley.

Feldstein, M. S. (1970). The rising price of physicians' services. *Review of Economics and Statistics*, *51*, 121–133.

Gilovich, T., & Medvec, V. H. (1995). The experience of regret: What, when, and why. *Psychological Review*, *102*, 379–395.

Gilovich, T., & Melvec, V. H. (1994). The temporal pattern to the experience of regret. *Journal of Personality and Social Psychology*, *67*, 357–365.

Glimcher, P. W., & Rustichini, A. (2004). Neuroeconomics: The consilience of brain and decision. *Science*, *306*, 447–452.

Kahneman, D., & Miller, D. (1986). Norm theory: Comparing reality to its alternatives. *Psychological Review*, *93*, 136–153.

Kahneman, D., & Tversky, A. (1982). The psychology of preferences. *Scientific American*, *246*, 160–173.

Lewis, D. (1973). *Counterfactuals*. Cambridge, MA: Harvard University Press.

Loomes, G., & Sugden, R. (1982). Regret theory: An alternative theory of rational choice under uncertainty. *Economic Journal*, *92*, 805–824.

Loomes, G., & Sugden, R. (1986). Disappointment and dynamic inconsistency in choice under uncertainty. *Review of Economic Studies*, *53*, 271–282.

Maccheroni, F., Marinacci, M., & Rustichini, A. (2006). Social decision theory. Bocconi University, Milano, Italy.

McCabe, K. A. (2003). Neuroeconomics. In: L. Nadel (Ed.), *Encyclopedia of cognitive science* (Vol. 3, pp. 294–298). Publishing Group, Macmillan Publishers Ltd.

Mellers, B., Ritov, I., & Schwartz, A. (1999). Emotion-based choice. *Journal of Experimental Psychology: General*, *3*, 332–345.

Muermann, A., Mitchell, O. S., & Volkman J. M. (2006). Regret, portfolio choice, and guarantees in defined contribution schemes. *Insurance: Mathematics and Economics*, *39*, 219–229.

Nagai, Y., Critchley, H. D., Featherstone, E., Trimble, M. R., & Dolan, R. J. (2004). Activity in ventromedial prefrontal cortex covaries with sympathetic skin conductance level: A physiological account of a "default mode" of brain function. *Neuroimage*, *22*, 243–251.

Newhouse, J. P. (1970). A model of physician pricing. *Southern Economics Journal*, *37*, 174–183.

O'Doherty, J., Krigelbach, M. L., Rolls, E. T., Hornak, J., & Andrews, C. (2001). Abstract reward and punishment representations in the human orbitofrontal cortex. *Nature Neuroscience*, *4*, 95–102.

Padoa-Schioppa, C., & Assad, J. A. (2006). Neurons in the orbitofrontal cortex encode economic value. *Nature*, *441*, 223–226.

Ritov, I. (1996). Probabilities of regret: Anticipation of uncertainty resolution in choice. *Organizational Behavior and Human Decision Processes*, *66*, 228–236.

Roese, N. J., & Olson, J. M. (1995). *What might have been: The social psychology of counterfactual thinking*. Mahwah, NJ: Erlbaum.

Rolls, E. T. (1999). *The brain and emotion*. New York: Oxford University Press.

Rolls, E. T. (2000). The orbitofrontal cortex and reward. *Cerebral Cortex*, *10*, 284–294.

Rustichini, A. (2005). Neuroscience. Emotion and reason in making decisions. *Science*, *310*, 1624–1625.

Thaler, R. (1980). Toward a positive theory of consumer choice. *Journal of Economic Behavior and Organization*, *1*, 39–60.

Tremblay, L., & Schultz, W. (1999). Relative reward preference in primate orbitofrontal cortex. *Nature*, *398*, 704–708.

Tversky, A., & Kahneman, D. (1973). Availability: A heuristic for judging frequency and probability. *Cognitive Psychology*, *5*, 207–232.

von Neumann, J., & Morgenstern, O. (1944). *Theory of games and economic behavior*. Princeton, NJ: Princeton University Press.

Zeelenberg, M., & Beattie, J. (1997). Consequences of regret aversion: Additional evidence for effects of feedback on decision-making. *Organizational Behavior and Human Decision Processes*, *72*, 63–78.

Zeelenberg, M., Beattie, J., van der Pligt, J., & de Vries, N. K. (1996). Consequences of regret aversion: Effects of expected feedback on risky decision-making. *Organizational Behavior and Human Decision Processes*, *65*, 148–158.

Zeelenberg, M., & van Dijk, E. (2004). On the comparative nature of the emotion regret. In: D. Mandel, D. Hilton & P. Catelani (Eds), *The Psychology of Counterfactual Thinking*. Routledge: London.

HOW PRIMATES (INCLUDING US!) RESPOND TO INEQUITY

Sarah F. Brosnan

ABSTRACT

Purpose – *Responding negatively to inequity is not a uniquely human trait. Some of our closest evolutionary ancestors respond negatively when treated less well than a conspecific. Comparative work between humans and other primates can help elucidate the evolutionary underpinnings of humans' social preferences.*

Methodology/approach – *Results from studies of nonhuman primates, in particular chimpanzees and capuchin monkeys, are presented in comparison to human results that have been collected during economic game studies in humans, such as in the Ultimatum Game or Impunity Game.*

Findings – *Among nonhuman primates, a frequent behavioral reaction to inequity is to refuse to continue the interaction. While in some cases this response appears to be caused by the inequitable distribution, in others, it seems to be caused by another individual's inequitable behavior. While these reactions are similar to those of humans, this reaction does not appear to be a sense of fairness in the way that we think of it in humans. Neither nonhuman primate species alters their behavior when they are the benefited individual, and in an experimental situation, chimpanzees do not alter their behavior to obtain food for their partner as well as for themselves.*

Neuroeconomics
Advances in Health Economics and Health Services Research, Volume 20, 99–124

ISSN: 0731-2199/doi:10.1016/S0731-2199(08)20005-1

Originality/value of the chapter – *Although there are differences between human and nonhuman primate responses, such studies allow us to better understand the evolution of our own responses to inequity. Given the strong behavioral reactions that even monkeys show to inequitable treatment, it is not surprising that humans are concerned with equity. Such comparisons increase understanding of issues such as healthcare disparities in humans.*

Imagine this situation. Your department chair walks in to the conference room for a meeting with you and a colleague. She's promised to bring the coffee and, without further ado, gives your colleague a *venti* cappuccino from Starbucks and you a fifty-cent cup of lukewarm instant from the vending machine. How do you feel? Does it make a difference if your cheaper coffee tastes fine, or if you actually prefer regular coffee to cappuccino? Probably not – you would still feel slighted.

In fact, you would probably be uncomfortable even if you were the one who got the cappuccino. You might offer to share it with your unlucky colleague, equalizing the outcome (if not the process). You might suggest that your colleague get a cappuccino at the next meeting, equalizing the process and, over the long term, the outcome. You might justify to yourself why you actually deserved the better drink – after all, yours was the funded grant. This is a phenomenon that psychologists refer to as a psychological leveling mechanism. This will result in equity (from your perspective), although not equality. If you fail to notice the inequity, you are an unusual human indeed.

What if you replace the characters in this scenario with another species, and the cappuccinos with foods that this species happens to really like? This is precisely what my colleagues and I have been studying in monkeys and apes. By studying the reactions of nonhuman primates to situations similar to this, I attempt to understand both the situations that will evoke an inequity response and the evolution of these reactions. In so doing, we may learn ways in which to restructure our own institutions and behaviors to better accommodate humans' evolved propensities.

In this chapter, I first discuss why it is useful to investigate human behavior by examining these behaviors in nonhuman species. Following this, I lay out a framework for the evolution of inequity responses, to help us predict which behaviors we might expect to see in other species. I then discuss work that I and others have done to investigate responses to inequity in nonhuman primates (hereafter, primates) and place their behaviors in the context of this evolutionary framework. I end with a summary of what we know, and how it relates to human behavior, specifically in the context of health and healthcare decisions.

BEHAVIORAL PHYLOGENY

Studying monkeys and apes to learn about human decision-making may seem like a stretch. What could a chimpanzee possibly tell us that is relevant to ourselves? A lot, it turns out. Studying nonhuman primates, our closest evolutionary relatives, tells us a great deal about how and why we behave in the ways that we do. Moreover, primates offer an added advantage in that we typically know their full social history and often have more control over the experimental environment. Nonhuman species are also unencumbered with complex cultural institutions, such as religious organizations, schools, and governments, so their responses are likely to indicate what primates have evolved to do, rather than what they have learned to do.[1] By studying how nonhuman primates make decisions, we learn the basis of human decision-making and can begin to tease apart what is evolved and what is the result of our extensive culture.

Comparative studies rely on the similarities and differences between either closely related species, or species that may or may not be very closely related, but share similar environments. To address the first possibility, there might be a close evolutionary link between the species in question. This means that the behavior first evolved to increase the fitness of an ancestor to *both* species in question, then was maintained through evolutionary time to be present in both species. This is termed homology. As an example, both blue jays and hummingbirds have wings; the reason is that they both evolved from a common avian ancestor that had wings, and that trait has existed continually in the lines that subsequently led to both blue jays and hummingbirds. Humans are primates, so our closest evolutionary ancestors in the animal kingdom are monkeys and apes. Within the primates, we are most closely related to apes (chimpanzees, bonobos, gorillas, and orangutans), followed by Old World monkeys, New World Monkeys (including capuchin monkeys, a species discussed in detail later), and prosimians. Thus like the birds' wings, shared characteristics in the Order[2] *Primates* may be homologous, or shared by common descent, throughout the Order.

However, that is not the only way that species can share traits. Convergent traits are those which evolved in two or more distantly linked species because similar environmental pressures favored the evolution of the same trait. This is termed homoplasy. Back to the example of wings: both blue jays and bats have wings, but the common ancestor to both did not have wings, nor do many intervening species between the two. Rather, both blue jays and bats (or, specifically, an ancestor to each, which lived since the two species split) experienced the appropriate series of mutations to allow wing development, concurrent with facing environmental pressures which favored this development. This is the second way in which comparisons may be relevant. If a nonhuman species faced similar pressures to those humans faced, we would expect similar (if not identical) traits to evolve.

Although these examples are for physical traits, this analysis can be done with behaviors as well. A technique known as behavioral phylogeny allows comparisons to be made between different species to extrapolate the likelihood of common descent for any behavior (Boehm, 1999; Preuschoft & van Hooff, 1995; Wrangham & Peterson, 1996). In this chapter, I will discuss comparisons between decision-making strategies in humans, chimpanzees, and capuchin monkeys. All three species share behaviors such as cooperation and food sharing, which implicates convergence. However, chimpanzees are, along with the bonobo, our closest living ancestors. This implicates similarities as being due to homology, or shared descent.

Note, however, that even if these species do share some traits in common with us, they may manifest slightly differently among the species. Some might have developed to a greater degree, or different environmental pressures may have altered the expression of a trait. Thus, it is important to establish beforehand what we are looking for, and why we might expect to see it. In the next section, I briefly summarize how a response to inequity might have evolved, and what behaviors we might expect to see in nonhuman primates.

THE EVOLUTION OF INEQUITY

Few would disagree that humans have a sense of fairness. We respond badly when we are treated unfairly. We give more than the minimum required in experimental games (Henrich et al., 2001) and we frequently punish in situations in which another individual behaves non-cooperatively (Fehr & Rockenbach, 2003; Kahneman, Knetsch, & Thaler, 1986; Zizzo & Oswald, 2001). To varying degrees, these inequity-averse responses are seen across a wide variety of cultures (Henrich et al., 2001) and vary significantly depending upon the quality of the relationship between the individuals involved (Clark & Grote, 2003). They have recently been linked to emotional, as well as rational, processes, both at the level of behavior and at the level of neural activity (Frank, 1988, 2001; Sanfey, Rilling, Aronson, Nystrom, & Cohen, 2003).

Inequity occurs when one individual receives a payoff or outcome that is in some dimension inferior to that which was expected *based on another's outcome* (Brosnan, 2006b; Hatfield, Walster, & Berscheid, 1978). Often, equity is equated with equality, although an outcome may be equitable and not equal (or equal and not equitable). Moreover, inequity must be differentiated from 'greed,' or wanting more for its own sake rather than because another individual got more. That is, a reaction to inequity must be based on a comparison of one's payoffs with those of another, and hence is inherently social.

It is unlikely that a behavior as complex as responding to inequity arose de novo. Instead, it probably developed over time through a series of stages that were each beneficial to the performer in their own right, ultimately resulting in the sort of complex understanding of inequity and fairness that we see in humans. Thus, while other species may or may not show behaviors that are identical to those of humans, the behaviors they do exhibit are likely to be steps in the same evolutionary process. Obviously, we expect to see more similarities in species that are more closely related (such as chimpanzees and humans) than other species (such as capuchin monkeys or non-primate species and humans).

I have previously proposed four distinct steps in the evolution of the inequity response as we see it in humans (Brosnan, 2006a, 2006b; Brosnan & de Waal, 2004a). The first is an ability to notice when rewards differ between individuals. While this seems obvious from a human perspective, it is not at all certain in other species. This requires an individual to step outside of its self-involved life and pay attention to another individual – outside of any context in which the other individual is directly affecting them (e.g., not during a fight, a sexual encounter, etc). Moreover, it requires fairly advanced cognition to compare one's own rewards with those of another. However, it is likely that this ability arose in a different context than inequity. Many species (primate and non-primate) socially learn, meaning that they acquire information or techniques from watching other individuals' actions or outcomes. This is often more efficient than acquiring information through individual experience. Any individual that learns socially must pay attention to other individuals' rewards. Since many primate species are known to socially learn, including the species we will discuss, chimpanzees and capuchin monkeys, (Brosnan & de Waal, 2004b; Custance, Whiten, & Fredman, 1999; McGrew, 2004; Whiten, 1998) we can assume that they possess the capability to compare their rewards to those of another.

A second step is to react negatively to discrepancies in rewards between oneself and another. Essentially, this requires individuals to not only notice the outcomes of another (step 1), but to react negatively to this difference. In fact, this alone may provide a fitness benefit. If this negative response to inequity caused individuals to seek new partners, by chance their next encounter may be more equitable, hence increasing fitness. For instance, both capuchins and chimpanzees cooperatively hunt, and share the prey after the kill (Boesch, 1994; Rose, 1997). If one individual in a partnership consistently receives little or no meat after the hunt, hunting with another partner might increase their meat consumption (and fitness) if the new partner shares more generously. In fact, if one's current partner is particularly stingy, then almost any move will be fitness-enhancing. Note that for this to work, individuals need not intentionally seek out better sharers, nor do they need to understand their motives for switching partners. The outcome will yield a fitness benefit to any individual who is inclined to 'shop around' for a better partner when in a blatantly inequitable relationship.

The third step is to take deliberate action to rectify inequity. This behavior, which is seen in humans, involves paying a cost of some sort to reduce the relative level of inequity between oneself and another. This strong dislike of inequity is referred to in behavioral economics as 'disadvantageous inequity aversion' (Fehr & Schmidt, 1999). In experimental games, individuals will pay to reduce others' earnings (Fehr & Gachter, 2002; Fehr & Rockenbach, 2003; Kahneman et al., 1986; Zizzo & Oswald, 2001), although other factors, such as culture (Henrich et al., 2001), anonymity (Bolton & Zwick, 1995), entitlement (Hoffman, McCabe, Shachat, & Smith, 1994), a taste for egalitarianism (Dawes, Fowler, Johnson, McElreath, & Smirnov, 2007), and the availability of an emotional outlet (Xiao & Houser, 2005) clearly play a role as well. This is the most complex of the reactions against disadvantageous inequity. The reason is that it requires an understanding of how one's actions will alter the outcome of the partner, and requires some ability to inhibit, since punishment in this sense requires giving up an immediate reward. Nonhuman primates can inhibit their behavior, even in the face of an immediate reward (Beran, 2002; Evans & Westergaard, 2006). They also show a basic understanding of how their actions will be perceived by others (Hare, Call, Agnetta, & Tomasello, 2000). Thus, the psychological building blocks are in place for this sort of behavior in nonhuman primates.

The fourth and final step in the evolution of inequity responses is a response against overcompensation (Hatfield et al., 1978). In this situation, individuals are uncomfortable that another individual receives less than they do – think back to the introductory example and imagine you were the individual who got the cappuccino while your colleague got the instant coffee. This response can be activated when the advantaged party is both the self or a third party (Andreoni, Brown, & Vesterlund, 2002). Rectification usually takes the form of psychological leveling mechanisms (e.g., derogation, justification for receipt of the superior reward), or, more practically, material compensation. This response is driven by what has been termed, in economics, 'advantageous inequity aversion' (Fehr & Schmidt, 1999).

While it is easy to intuit the fitness benefits which accrue based on a response to inequity against the self, (steps 1–3), there are also fitness benefits to responding negatively to overcompensation. These benefits are not immediate material gain, but rather stem from a long-term commitment which generates rewards in the future. By materially rectifying inequity, one is sending a very powerful message about one's interactions with others. This information – that you are a person who looks out for others' interests and lives by a standard of equity – is given to anyone who witnesses the act, and to those whom they tell. Because rectifying overcompensation requires sacrifice, it is difficult to fake and as such is a very effective commitment device (Frank, 1988). Thus, a small sacrifice now leads to great benefits in the future. Note that for a negative response to overcompensation to be most effective, witnesses to the act need to be able to pass this information on to others who did not witness it. This is accomplished primarily through language, so if these responses have primarily evolved as commitment devices, we would expect to see weaker responses in nonhuman species, which lack communication as sophisticated as that of humans.

There is some disagreement as to the strength of aversion to overcompensation in humans. While it is often found that people prefer equity to any sort of inequity, advantageous inequity is typically preferred to disadvantageous inequity (Lowenstein, Thompson, & Bazerman, 1989). Moreover, sometimes inequity (which favors the in group) is even preferred (Diekmann, Samuels, Ross, & Bazerman, 1997). Furthermore, people tend to rectify inequity through psychological balancing mechanisms rather than material compensation (Hatfield et al., 1978) and, given the opportunity, will usually choose to ignore information that could lead to a more fair outcome at a cost to the self (Dana, Weber, & Kuang, 2003).

I assume that these steps evolved more or less in the order presented, since they build upon each other, although some variation from this is possible. Note that all four of these stages need to be developed in order to consider the response a sense of 'fairness' or justice in the sense that we mean it in humans (Brosnan, 2006b). Particularly if a reaction to overcompensation is missing, the response is a one-sided, self-centered response that is focused purely on the individual. This is not the same as the human goal, which holds justice or fairness to all as an ideal to be striven for. Generally among humans there is an appeal to an objective level of fairness or justice, almost a platonic ideal, which is the standard by which actions are to be judged. I do not mean to imply there is one such standard – there certainly is not, and each person's standard may shift with the circumstances – but there is a relating of current events to a separate, 'objective,' standard removed from the current situation. Since it is difficult or impossible to determine a nonhuman's ideals, in these studies we examine purely behavior, not motivation. In studies on inequity in nonhumans, the goal, then, is to determine situations in which the primates show evidence of one of these stages, and determine a potential evolutionary trajectory from comparisons between these species.

In my own work, I have investigated how two species of nonhuman primates, capuchin monkeys (*Cebus apella*) and chimpanzees (*Pan troglodytes*), respond to inequity (Brosnan & de Waal, 2003a; Brosnan, Schiff, & de Waal, 2005). Both species show characteristics which imply that they expect equity in their day-to-day lives; they do not take objects from one another's possession, and they share food and work together to obtain rewards that must be divided amongst themselves (Boesch, 1994; Brosnan & de Waal, 2002; de Waal & Berger, 2000; de Waal & Brosnan, 2006; de Waal & Davis, 2002; Mendres & de Waal, 2000). Below I briefly summarize a number of these studies and try to place them in the context of the framework delineated earlier.

DO NONHUMAN PRIMATES RESPOND NEGATIVELY TO INEQUITY?

The earliest work on inequity in nonhuman primates simply established the presence of distributional inequity in two species, capuchin monkeys and chimpanzees (Brosnan & de Waal, 2003a; Brosnan et al., 2005). In initial tests, my colleague Frans de Waal and I tested subjects next to a social partner, who was always another individual from the subject's social group. The partner received either the same reward (equitable condition) or a better reward (inequitable condition; a grape is the better reward and a similarly sized piece of cucumber is the less-good reward) for performing the same task, a simple exchange. In both species, subjects responded negatively to the situation in which a partner got a better reward as compared to the situation in which both individuals received the same rewards. These reactions included refusing to participate in the exchange, refusing to accept the lesser-value reward, and throwing away the rewards or tokens. These results indicate that both capuchin monkeys and chimpanzees meet the second stage in the evolution of inequity responses, or responding negatively to inequity.

Of course, to demonstrate a negative response to inequity, it is not enough that the subject responds in the above situation. The subject must also respond more strongly to a situation in which their partner gets a better reward than to a situation in which a better reward is available, but not given to the other primate. This is the separation of 'envy' (the former) from 'greed' (the latter). To control for this, another condition was included in which subjects both saw a better reward, a grape, before they had to complete the exchange, for which they received a cucumber. Critically, no primate ever received the grape, so subjects saw no other individual receive a grape; they only saw that it was present. In this condition, subjects were much less likely to respond negatively to receiving their cucumber than in the previous condition in which their partner received the grape (Brosnan & de Waal, 2003a; Brosnan et al., 2005; van Wolkenten, Brosnan, & de Waal, 2007).

Another possibility is that subjects were simply frustrated not to receive the grape, which is essentially a contrast between the current reward and that received in a previous session or test (Brosnan & de Waal, 2006; Reynolds, 1961; Roma, Silberberg, Ruggiero, & Suomi, 2006; Tinklepaugh, 1928). In the 1920s, Tinklepaugh demonstrated that such contrast effects exist in monkeys, when he surreptitiously switched the monkeys' rewards to less preferred ones (Tinklepaugh, 1928). To examine this, we compared capuchin monkeys' reactions in sessions which were immediately preceded by those in which they received a grape to sessions which were preceded by only cucumber rewards. If subjects are experiencing frustration, they are expected to respond much more strongly in the first case, in which the session was preceded by a grape-earning session. However, subjects showed no change in response, indicating that previous rewards do not affect results in this test (van Wolkenten et al., 2007).

In humans, effort also plays a role in how inequity is perceived. For instance, in the Ultimatum Game,[3] human proposers make much smaller offers and responders accept them if the proposer has earned the right to be the first mover (Hoffman et al., 1994). In our early work on distributional inequity, we included a condition in which responders had to work harder but received less, essentially doubling the inequity. Chimpanzees responded to this as they had for the distributional inequity task; however in monkeys, unequal effort appeared to enhance the response to unequal distributions, making subjects who received less reward for more effort respond even more negatively than when they received less reward for the same amount of effort. A follow-up study done with capuchin monkeys emphasizes this role of effort (van Wolkenten et al., 2007). When rewards are very good, an effort differential makes little difference; monkeys will do more work for the better reward. Furthermore, when the effort difference is large, it makes little difference whether the partner gets the same small reward as the partner or a much larger one; monkeys are much more likely to refuse to participate. However, when the effort difference is small, whether the rewards are equal or not make a big difference in response, with subjects responding much more negatively to unequal rewards than to equal (small) ones. Thus, effort seems to moderate the response to distributional inequity, but subjects' responses are apparently based on their own experience of effort, rather than on their effort as compared to their partners (see also Fontenot, Watson, Roberts, & Miller, 2007). Thus, unlike humans, monkeys may not titrate their response to take into account relative levels of deservedness.

These studies are very similar to the Impunity Game (IG), an economic game that is closely related to the Ultimatum Game (see Fig. 1). In the IG, after the proposer makes the split, the responder must either accept the division or refuse. However, in the IG, refusal means that the proposer still receives their money, while the responder receives nothing. It is often assumed that no rational responder would ever refuse; nonetheless, as many as 40% of responders choose to do so (Horita & Yamagishi, 2007; Yamagishi, Horita, & Takagishi, 2008; Yamagishi, 2007, but see also Bolton & Zwick, 1995). The situation which we presented to the monkeys is very similar to the situation faced by the responder in the IG – they must decide whether to accept a reward, but their action does not affect their partner's outcome. The critical difference between the human and nonhuman primate versions of the game is that, for the primates, the distribution is determined by the experimenter rather than the partner. This was done intentionally, as it is extremely difficult to verify that a primate understands the contingency between their partner's actions and their current constellation of choices in such experimental tasks. The responses of humans and nonhumans to this game vary widely among conditions and populations, but this variability within species is greater than that between species. The fact that all are within the same range indicates a shared evolutionary background (Table 1).

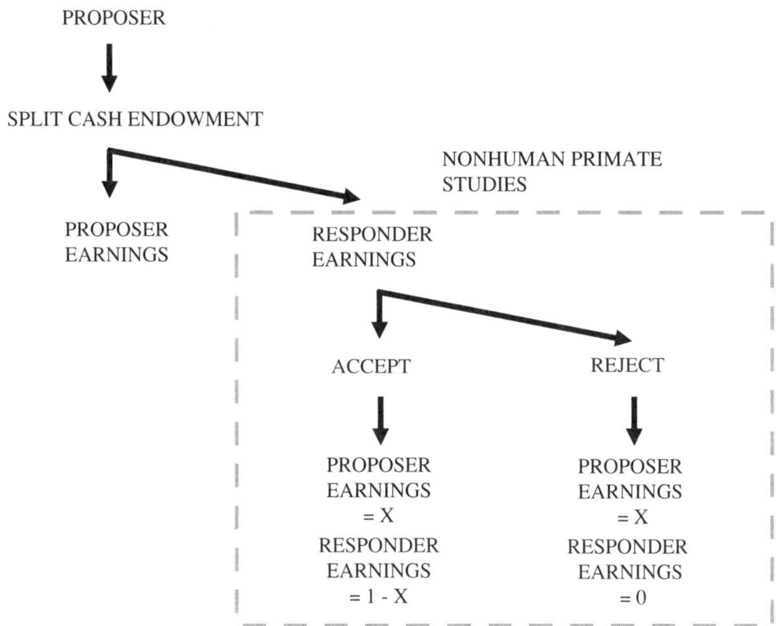

Fig. 1. A Schematic Diagram of the Impunity Game, an Economic Game which is Similar in Structure to the Ultimatum Game. The Part of the Game Completed by the Nonhuman Primates is Boxed with the Dashed Line. Because of the Difficulty in Verifying that the Nonhuman Primates Understand the Contingency of their Choices Now Being Constrained by Their Partners' Previous Choices, We Chose to Have the Experimenter Set the Inequity Rather than the Social Partner.

Table 1. Level of Refusals to the Impunity Game (see Fig. 1) by Humans and Nonhuman Primates.

Species Studied	Percent Refusals	Study
Humans	Almost 0	Bolton & Zwick (1995)
Humans	31	Fukuno and Ohbuchi (2001, in Japanese)
Humans	38	Horita and Yamagishi (2007)
Capuchin monkeys (second half of game)	42	Brosnan and de Waal (2003a)
Capuchin monkeys (second half of game)	20	van Wolkenten, Brosnan, and de Waal (2007)
Chimpanzees (second half of game)	25 (~0–65)	Brosnan, Schiff, and de Waal (2005)

Of course, an obvious question is why there is such a large range of responses within a species. This variability indicates that other factors are modulating the effects of basic inequity. In humans, social and contextual factors play a large role in responses to inequity. For instance, individuals from different cultures respond very differently when asked to play the Ultimatum Game (Henrich et al., 2001). Thus, we further investigate the various social and contextual factors which may affect the level of response in chimpanzees and capuchin monkeys.

SOCIAL AND CONTEXTUAL EFFECTS ON THE INEQUITY RESPONSE

Perhaps the most obvious sources of variation between individuals are gender and rank; yet, we found no effect of either of these variables on reactions to inequity in either species. We had predicted that more dominant individuals would be more upset by being treated inequitably (as compared to a subordinate) than their more subordinate counterparts. The reason is that even in these relatively tolerant species, the dominants are accustomed to receiving a greater share. One possible explanation for our findings is that the subjects perceived that the inequity was brought on not by their partner, but by the human experimenter. In support of this, any negative behavioral reactions (e.g., threats) were directed at the experimenter and not at the partner. Thus, there was no retaliation against the primate who received the better reward following the experiment.

For chimpanzees, but not capuchin monkeys, there was a strong effect of social group membership on response (Brosnan et al., 2005). In both species, individuals from multiple groups were tested. The capuchins came from two different social groups, and the level of response did not differ between the two groups. The chimpanzees also came from two social groups, and responses did vary between them. One group had been housed together for more than 30 years (i.e., long-term social group), and all subjects but one were born and reared within the group; the exceptional subject was present at the group formation and was the alpha female at the time of testing. The other social group had been put together a mere eight years before the study (i.e., short-term social group; Seres, Aureli, & de Waal, 2001). Thus, no subject had been born in the group and most individuals had been introduced as adults. We also used two pair-housed pairs of chimpanzees who had the same diet, enrichment, care, and availability of outdoor access as the subjects housed in larger groups.

The pair-housed chimpanzees and those from the short-term social group showed a strong response to inequity, similar to that of the capuchins. However, chimpanzees from the long-term group showed virtually no response to inequity. Given that the other groups all reacted to inequity, it seems unlikely that this group does not notice when the situation is to their disadvantage. Instead, it seems that they do not react to this negative situation. Intriguingly, those individuals who always completed the interaction also took about half the amount of time to do so, as compared to those chimpanzees which frequently refused to exchange. This is true in all cases, including the equity test, indicating that the speed of interaction is not related to the distribution of food rewards. From this test we cannot determine causation, yet it is intriguing that those individuals who take more time, and thus may have more opportunity to evaluate the situation, are more likely to react to inequity.

This response to inequity fits well with other data from these groups. Aside from their response to inequity, the long-term social group in our study shows high levels of reciprocity in food sharing and grooming (a behavior that is presumably associated with equity; de Waal, 1997), extensive reconciliation after fights (Preuschoft, Wang, Aureli, & de Waal, 2002), and a tendency to avoid confrontation (Hare et al., 2000). Those in the short-term group were still working out social issues four years after their formation (Seres et al., 2001). Although one test is insufficient to understand all of the contingencies of how relationships affect responses to inequity, it is interesting that individuals who had grown up together and had social interactions implying harmony showed communal orientation to the inequity test while those from the less stable situations showed more contingent rules. Furthermore, it is known that chimpanzees will alter their behavior depending upon the current social situation (Brosnan & de Waal, 2003b), housing situation (Aureli & de Waal, 1997; Baker, Seres, Aureli, & de Waal, 2000), or social group (Whiten et al., 1999). However, due to the scarcity of chimpanzees, most behavioral testing utilizes individuals from only a single social group (or chimpanzees from pair- or single-housed situations).

These data also fit well with current understanding of social relationships on behavior in humans. Current theory proposes that individuals in close or positive relationships follow communal rules that do not pay overt attention to fairness, whereas those in less stable relationships utilize contingent rule-based behavior such as equity or inequality (Clark & Grote, 2003; Loewenstein, Thompson, & Bazerman, 1989). Such committed relationships are also highly correlated with willingness to sacrifice (van Lange et al., 1997).

If our long-term group of chimpanzees has similarly close relationships, the inequity presented to them may be largely irrelevant within the context of their relationships. Further study of multiple social groups is certainly warranted, both in primates and in other species, so that we get a full picture of responses.

We also see variation in responses based upon the context in which inequity occurs. Inequity likely arose as subjects compared their payoffs to their efforts in cooperative and other joint tasks. Outside of this context, behavior may be quite different. In our earlier studies, effort was added with the use of a simple exchange task. This task was chosen because it is easily visible by the partner and is a correlate to the social exchange seen in many nonhuman primate species. However, following the initial investigation, several studies on both chimpanzees and capuchin monkeys found different responses when no task was performed (Bräuer, Call, & Tomasello, 2006; Dindo & de Waal, 2006; Dubreuil, Gentile, & Visalberghi, 2006). Such differences can be due to factors like social situation and subject housing; however, in one case the same capuchin monkey subjects' responses to their partner receiving a better food depended on the task. These subjects responded negatively when the interaction involved a task (exchange) and failed to respond when the food was simply handed to the subjects (Brosnan & de Waal, 2003a; Dindo & de Waal, 2006; van Wolkenten et al., 2007).

Thus, the presence of a task seems to be crucial to activate inequity. Further work needs to be done to determine the situations in which inequity is important and the situations in which subjects are willing to tolerate inequitable outcomes. We hypothesize that inequity responses evolved in the context of cooperation (Brosnan, Freeman, & de Waal, 2006; van Wolkenten et al., 2007), because it is critical for individuals to compare their efforts and rewards to those of their cooperative partners to verify that they should continue the interaction. If this is correct, we are more likely to find responses in situations such as the exchange, which evoke cooperation, than in those which do not. We further investigate this with a study of cooperation in which subjects work for unequal payoffs in a mutualism task.

DOES THE PARTNER'S BEHAVIOR MATTER?

If responses to inequity evolved in the context of cooperation, we might expect stronger responses when monkeys do need to work together to obtain food rewards (Brosnan et al., 2006). In the previous experiments (described earlier), monkeys worked next to each other, but did not actually work together. For the current study, monkeys had to cooperate in a mutualism task to obtain rewards. However, we varied whether or not the rewards were the same for each player. Critically, we did not determine beforehand which monkey received which reward. Instead, we let the monkeys work it out themselves when deciding whether or not to cooperate. Thus, we were able to examine how monkeys resolve a situation in which they can (1) cooperate, with one individual receiving more than the other (unequal outcome); (2) cooperate and share access to better rewards (equal outcome over the long term, both benefit); or (3) fail to cooperate, blocking both individuals from rewards (equal outcome, neither benefit).

This was done using a mutualistic barpull task, which has been used extensively to test cooperation and altruism in these capuchin monkeys (Brosnan & de Waal, 2002; de Waal & Berger, 2000; de Waal & Davis, 2002; Mendres & de Waal, 2000). In this study, a tray was weighted such that no capuchin could pull it in by themselves. Working together, two individuals could bring it in. On the tray were rewards for the pullers, one on each side of the apparatus. The barpull tray was baited with either two low-value (apple) rewards, two high-value (grape) rewards, or an inequitable distribution of one low and one high-value reward. We knew from previous studies that each monkey would obtain the food that is in front of the bar they were pulling, and neither individual would be able to monopolize it and take both rewards (de Waal & Davis, 2002). Monkeys were unrestrained during the study and could choose which of the bars they were willing to pull. Thus, the experimenter could manipulate rewards so that one individual received more, but the experimenter could not determine which individual would receive which reward. The monkeys' interactions determined the outcome.

We predicted that individuals would be best at pulling for two rewards of the same value, independent of reward quality (apple or grape), since these equal reward divisions are the easiest to negotiate. We further hypothesized that individuals would pull least often for the unequal rewards, since this would require one individual to receive a less valuable reward than the other. Nonetheless, we found that individuals did not vary their pulling based on the distribution of the rewards; they were equally likely (or unlikely) to pull in all three conditions. However, not all pairs pulled with the same frequency. Some pairs succeeded in obtaining the rewards almost all of the time, while others succeeded only occasionally. Again, within these groups all options (equal low, equal high, unequal) were pulled with the same frequency. The critical factor we uncovered was how often each member of the partnership obtained the better reward in the unequal trials. When one monkey dominated the better reward (taking it almost 80% of the time on average), the pair's success rate was quite low – about 30%. However, partnerships in which neither monkey claimed the better reward more than about half of the time were more than twice as successful, cooperating about 70% of the time. This indicates that the monkeys were not choosing whether or not to pull based on the distribution of the rewards, but were instead choosing whether or not to pull based on whether their partner dominated the better reward, or allowed them to receive it about as often. Thus willingness to pull was determined by one's partner's behavior, not the initial reward distribution.

These results indicate that capuchin monkeys are willing to sacrifice an absolute gain to prevent a partner from getting a larger one. This is the third proposed stage in the evolution of the inequity response. Additionally, there are three major implications of these results that should be noted. First, it appears that when the individuals have some control over the outcome, their cooperative interactions are not limited by the possibility of unequal outcomes, but instead by whether their partner's behavior ameliorates this inequality. Note that this means that on any given 'unequal' trial (baited with one apple and one grape), one individual will receive less. However, over the long run, individuals' rewards were approximately the same. Thus, they appear to be judging the interaction over a longer time frame than trial by trial, and are evaluating whether or not to continue participating based on the history of the relationship rather than the outcome of any single trial. This has profound implications for cooperative group activities, such as cooperative hunts, in which many individuals participate but the reward is not readily divisible for any given interaction.

Second, note that for those pairs in which the rate of cooperation was low, it was low for *all* trials, not just the trials in which the initial distribution was unequal (apple/grape). Thus, subjects were turning down good rewards even in situations in which inequitable outcomes were impossible (apple/apple and grape/grape trials). If the monkeys are really responding based solely on the equality (or not) of the outcome, they should be more than willing to pull when both partners will receive the same reward. This may indicate that the mechanism these monkeys are using to make decisions about whether or not to cooperate is based on an emotional response to the partner, rather than a calculated determination of one's potential rewards. In the latter case, we would expect individuals to participate regardless of their partner's behavior in the two conditions in which the rewards are identical, because both relative and absolute outcomes will be the same between partners, and only refrain from cooperating when the partner has the opportunity claim relatively more. Perhaps in neither monkeys nor humans can we expect responses to be maximizing at all times. Preferences for the partner can affect even interactions that seem to have no possibility for an unfair outcome.

Finally, in order to obtain the most rewards, a dominant individual needs to keep track of whether their partner is receiving sufficient incentive to stay involved (remember, the dominant can obtain nothing without the subordinate's help). This may not require exact calculations on the part of the dominant, but it does require that dominants are sensitive to cues about their partners' needs and occasionally respond by allowing their partner to receive more. This requires the ability to – when it is in one's long-term interest – make a decision that benefits another more than oneself. Even though the long-term gain is still self-interested, it may be difficult to overcome the desire to obtain the better reward. This is an element of the fourth level of response to inequity, or the response to overcompensation. However, while these monkeys have the ability to respond to overcompensation, it is unknown whether they will do so in situations in which longer-term gains are less directly tied to their short-term responses.

The same study has not yet been done with chimpanzees, although several studies indicate that they may respond similarly. For instance, we know that chimpanzees are much more likely to cooperate with a tolerant partner (e.g., one who shares rewards more equitably; Melis, Hare, & Tomasello, 2006b) and, when given the chance, will recruit a partner who is tolerant over one who is not (Melis, Hare, & Tomasello, 2006a). Counter to these results, a recent study purporting to replicate the Ultimatum Game in chimpanzees finds that chimpanzees are 'rational maximizers,' 'accepting' almost any offer in the responder position (Jensen, Call, & Tomasello, 2007). However, there are several problems with this study (Brosnan, 2008; Visalberghi & Anderson, 2008). Subjects played repeatedly, indicating the possibility that reciprocity was involved. Moreover, no controls were run to verify that the chimpanzees understood how the apparatus worked; 56% of them 'accepted' the offer by pulling in a tray even when they received no reward whatsoever. Related to this, there were no controls to verify that the responder understood that their partner had determined their choices. Given that humans respond quite differently when unequal outcomes are due to chance (or computer) versus another individual's conscious choice (Blount, 1995; Knoch, Pascual-Leone, Meyer, Treyer, & Fehr, 2006), this is a critical omission. This study needs to be replicated with more rigor before such conclusions can be drawn.

RESPONSES TO OVERCOMPENSATION IN NONHUMAN PRIMATES

Finally, we have completed a series of studies to investigate whether chimpanzees make 'prosocial' choices, or those which benefit a partner when there is no benefit to the self. Although none of the studies discussed earlier were explicitly designed to investigate how subjects respond when they are the advantaged partner, they do shed some light on the question. In the first inequity studies discussed, the advantaged partner, who received the grape, could have equalized the situation by sharing the grape. In fact, neither species showed this behavior. Some capuchin monkeys did share their (inferior) cucumber, but none shared their grape. In five instances (of 2000), chimpanzees shared their grape; however this represents a great deal less sharing than is typical of these groups. On the other hand, the results of the cooperative barpull study, discussed immediately earlier, indicate that in at least some situations, monkeys are willing to let their partner have a better reward. As discussed, this requires an ability to recognize when one is compensated more than a partner and rectify the situation. However, this study only addresses behavior which assists another in a purely self-interested situation (in which doing so directly affects one's long-term payoffs). Humans have been argued to exhibit such tendencies even when there is no direct benefit to them for doing so (Gintis, Bowles, Boyd, & Fehr, 2003).

My colleagues and I recently completed a series of studies examining whether chimpanzees would bring food to unrelated members of their group in the absence of opportunities for reciprocity (Silk et al., 2005; Vonk et al., 2008). This study was done with two groups of chimpanzees with very different rearing histories. This allowed us to compare responses across different environments and social situations.[4] For the first study, subjects were paired with another member of their social group and given the opportunity to choose between an option that brought a piece of food only to them and an option which brought a piece of the same quantity and type of food to each of the chimpanzees. In order to verify that the subjects were not simply confused and choosing the option with two pieces of food because it was more numerous (even though subjects could access only one piece), we compared their responses in sessions in which a partner was present to sessions in which they were adjacent to an empty cage. All 18 subjects from both facilities showed the same responses, regardless of whether another chimpanzee was present (Silk et al., 2005). Not only did they fail to discriminate between the presence and absence of a partner, but they chose between the two options at chance levels in all cases. Shortly after this study was published, a very similar study showed the same results for a third group of captive chimpanzees (Jensen, Hare, Call, & Tomasello, 2006). Taken together, this is very good evidence that chimpanzees are not inclined to bring their partner rewards in this sort of experimental task.

However, it is possible that the subjects were simply so excited by the prospect of receiving food that they made a choice for themselves without attending to the possibility of rewarding a partner. To address this possibility, we ran a second study with the same subjects. Again the chimpanzee had two options, but this time could choose either one or both of them. One option brought a food reward to only the subject and the other brought an identical food reward to only the partner. Thus, subjects could obtain their reward and, after they were no longer focused on their outcome, could choose to obtain a reward for their partners. Again, subjects were tested adjacent to both a partner and an empty cage.

The majority of the subjects showed no tendency to obtain a reward for their partner at any higher rate than they obtained a reward for the empty cage. This implies again that they do not choose to reward others. However, there were a few clues that chimpanzees may respond differentially in at least some situations; one female from the Bastrop colony was significantly prosocial, obtaining rewards for her partner at a much higher rate when a partner was actually present than when next to an empty cage. Also, on their initial session, the subjects from Bastrop chose the prosocial option more often when a partner was present. These data certainly do not indicate robust prosocial preferences. Nonetheless, they do indicate that in certain situations, some chimpanzees have the capacity to make prosocial choices. Recent evidence also demonstrates that chimpanzees may make more prosocial decisions in helping tasks, where subjects can perform an action to assist another chimpanzee or the human experimenter, outside of the context of food (Warneken, Hare, Melis, Hanus, & Tomasello, 2007; Warneken & Tomasello, 2006). Perhaps food is such a salient good that it affects individuals' responses. More investigation is clearly required, to determine in which situations and with which individuals these prosocial choices occur.

HUMAN HEALTH, DECISION-MAKING, AND INEQUITABLE BEHAVIOR

Humans have a strong sense of fairness, which takes into account not only situations in which they are treated inferiorly, but also those in which they are overcompensated relative to their partners. Nonhuman primates, too, recognize and exhibit strong negative reactions to inequity, indicating that they have achieved at least the first two stages in my proposed model for the evolution of inequity responses. Capuchin monkeys are also willing to sacrifice a desirable reward in order to keep their partner from getting more than they do. This demonstrates the third level of the model, sacrificing gains to rectify inequity. Thus, it appears that humans' responses to being treated inequitably are an evolutionarily robust strategy which is, at minimum, rooted deeply in the primate lineage.

More research is needed to determine whether these subjects respond to overcompensation, the fourth level. Capuchins sometimes allow their partners to obtain better rewards in a cooperative task, when it benefits them (in the longer term) to do so. Chimpanzees do not give food rewards to their partners in an experimental task, although they do help each other in non-food related tasks. Thus, more evidence needs to be gathered to clarify our understanding of how nonhuman primates respond to overcompensation. This may represent the greatest difference between human and nonhuman primates, perhaps indicating that a response to overcompensation is a response which developed most fully in the human lineage.

Studying the reaction of nonhuman primates to inequity illuminates the situations in which negative reactions may occur in humans. It also helps us understand the origin of these behaviors. By understanding the evolution of the behaviors, we are in a better position to address them effectively in humans. Research on capuchin monkeys and chimpanzees tells us that there are at least two aspects of the reaction to inequity that we must take into account when thinking about humans: distress over inequitable distributions of rewards and distress over inequitable behavior by the partner. Each of these will be important in different situations.

First, in situations in which individuals lack any power to alter outcomes, the most important factor in their decisions about whether to respond negatively is the equitability of the distribution. In these situations, individuals are likely to bow out and refuse to participate (that is, find a new situation) rather than suffer a relatively inferior outcome to that of a partner in the current situation – even if that outcome would have represented an absolute gain over what they receive by no longer participating. Note that this response is often considered 'irrational,' as the individual may end up both absolutely and relatively less well off than they would have been had they accepted the outcome. Nonetheless, valuing relative equity – here achieved by leaving an inequitable situation – over absolute gains is likely a robust evolutionary strategy. Given that in most situations what matters from an evolutionary perspective is one's fitness *relative* to others of one's species or group, this emphasis on relative over absolute gains makes sense. (To paraphrase the aphorism, it is not necessary to outrun the tiger, just the person next to you!) However, when discussing humans, it is often assumed that individuals will always try to maximize their outcomes in an absolute way. Making such an assumption may be inaccurate, and detrimental to policies and procedures. Relative outcomes should always be considered when calculating how individuals will respond in a situation.

Second, in situations in which the individuals involved do have some control, the original distribution of the rewards may be less important than the behavior of the other players. In this case, it is okay if one set of payoffs is unequal, as long as each individual feels as if they benefit at some point. Note, too, the flip side of this; if an individual feels that another is not treating them equitably, they may cease interacting with them, regardless of the payoffs. This may occur even in situations in which the relative outcomes of a given interaction are guaranteed to be equal. In fact, in situations in which individuals feel cheated or taken advantage of, it may be extremely difficult to get them to voluntarily re-join participation. This, too, must be taken into account when designing policies and procedures that involve human behavior.

Finally, the social environment may be as important as the structure of the institution or interaction. Remember that the results in the abovementioned distributional inequity test varied dramatically between social groups of chimpanzees, even though nothing about the experimental situation was changed. Individuals may be less likely to respond negatively to individuals to whom they are close. Of course, this also means that individuals are likely to be very focused on differences in efforts and outcomes with individuals who they know only superficially or not at all. A challenge in a large group is to set up the social environment appropriately to elicit the more communal approach that is shown by individuals who know each other well.

Earlier I posed the question whether looking at monkeys and apes was a good way to learn about human decision-making and health. I see two ways in which the lessons from nonhuman primates are of utmost importance for health. The first is in setting up our institutions, such as a healthcare system. In order to function successfully, both the distributions *and* the behavior of those involved must be perceived as fair by those participating in the system, and the social structure surrounding the system needs to be carefully designed. Another lesson from monkeys is that it may be quite difficult to regain people's trust in the system after they have evaluated it as 'unfair.' This is vital to keep in mind as the US faces its current situation of determining how to set up a healthcare system that guarantees equal access and treatment for all people. Any initiative will ultimately fail if it is not equitable to all (both those who currently lack good access and those who currently are satisfied). Likewise, it will be difficult to regain people's trust after an initial failure. This makes institutional design more difficult, as there may not be the ability to adjust after an initial failure.

A second lesson is simply the toll that inequitable treatment takes on health. This has significant negative consequences both emotionally and physically, and humans who are suffering from inequity suffer far worse health and longevity than those who are better off (Wilkinson, 2006). However, by studying the situations that cause inequity, and making an effort to determine how such inequity can be relieved, we may find ways to improve lives and long-term health. Remember, again, the lessons from the primates. Things do not always need to be fair in the short term, and procedures and intentions may be just as important as absolute outcomes. Capuchin monkeys will accept the inequitable outcome on occasion (that fifty-cent cup of coffee), as long as they sometimes get the better deal (the cappuccino). Thus, our aim is not the impossible task of giving everyone the better deal all the time, but to set up situations where, over the long-term, equity reigns.

NOTES

1. Note that humans' complex cultural capability is an evolved characteristic, which is shared at least to some extent with nonhuman primate species.
2. This indicates the phylogenetic Order, used in the taxonomy of each species. Primates share labels at the levels of Kingdom, Phylum, Class, and Order (Animalia, Chordata, Mammalia, Primates, respectively), and vary at the levels of Family, Genus, and Species.
3. In the Ultimatum Game, one individual of a pair, the proposer, makes a decision about how to divide a pot of money. The second individual in the pair, the responder, then gets to determine whether to accept the proposed split, in which case both individuals receive their money, or refuse it, in which case neither individual receives anything. For more information, see Camerer (2003).
4. One group collected data at the Michale E. Keeling Center for Comparative Medicine and Research of the University of Texas M.D. Anderson Cancer Center from six corral-housed social groups of chimpanzees. These groups were all multi-male, multi-female, and many contained infants and juveniles. The majority of individuals were mother reared. Moreover, these groups had had very little previous experience with behavioral or cognitive testing. Finally, the sample size was sufficiently large that we were able to test 11 pairs without re-using subjects and without testing pairs in both directions. Thus, there was no opportunity for reciprocity within the experimental situation. The second group collected data on a

group of chimpanzees at the Cognitive Evolution Group of New Iberia Primate Center. This group, which has a single adult male, has had extensive cognitive and behavioral testing since the chimpanzees were very young. Given that there were only seven potential subjects, all chimpanzees were tested with each available partner; thus, the potential for long-term reciprocity did exist.

ACKNOWLEDGMENT

This work was supported by a Human Social Dynamics grant from the National Science Foundation (SES 0729244) to S.F.B. and an NIH IRACDA grant to Emory University.

REFERENCES

Andreoni, J., Brown, P. M., & Vesterlund, L. (2002). What makes an allocation fair? Some experimental evidence. *Games and Economic Behavior*, *40*, 1–24.

Aureli, F., & de Waal, F. B. M. (1997). Inhibition of social behavior in chimpanzees under high-density conditions. *American Journal of Primatology*, *41*, 213–228.

Baker, K., Seres, M., Aureli, F., & de Waal, F. B. M. (2000). Injury risks among chimpanzees in three housing conditions. *American Journal of Primatology*, *51*, 161–175.

Beran, M. J. (2002). Maintenance of self-imposed delay of gratification by four chimpanzees (*Pan troglodytes*) and an orangutan (*Pongo pygmaeus*). *Journal of General Psychology*, *129*(1), 49–66.

Blount, S. (1995). When social outcomes aren't fair: The effect of causal attributions on preferences. *Organizational Behavior and Human Decision Processes*, *63*(2), 131–144.

Boehm, C. (1999). *Hierarchy in the forest: The evolution of egalitarian behavior*. Cambridge, MA: Harvard University Press.

Boesch, C. (1994). Cooperative hunting in wild chimpanzees. *Animal Behavior*, *48*, 653–667.

Bolton, G. E., & Zwick, R. (1995). Anonymity versus punishment in ultimatum game bargaining. *Games and Economic Behavior*, *10*, 95–121.

Bräuer, J., Call, J., & Tomasello, M. (2006). Are apes really inequity averse? *Proceedings of the Royal Society of London. Series B*, *273*, 3123–3128.

Brosnan, S. F. (2006a). At a crossroads of disciplines. *Social Justice Research*, *19*, 218–227.

Brosnan, S. F. (2006b). Nonhuman species' reactions to inequity and their implications for fairness. *Social Justice Research*, *19*, 153–185.

Brosnan, S. F. (2008). The ultimatum game and nonhuman primates. Scientific American Mind "Mind Matters" blog. Available at http://science-community.sciam.com/blog-entry/Mind-Matters/Chimps-Rational-Humans/300009942

Brosnan, S. F., & de Waal, F. B. M. (2002). A proximate perspective on reciprocal altruism. *Human Nature*, *13*(1), 129–152.

Brosnan, S. F., & de Waal, F. B. M. (2003a). Monkeys reject unequal pay. *Nature*, *425*, 297–299.

Brosnan, S. F., & de Waal, F. B. M. (2003b). Regulation of vocal output by chimpanzees finding food in the presence or absence of an audience. *Evolution of Communication*, *4*(2), 211–224.

Brosnan, S. F., & de Waal, F. B. M. (2004a). Reply to Henrich and Wynne. *Nature*, *428*, 140.

Brosnan, S. F., & de Waal, F. B. M. (2004b). Socially learned preferences for differentially rewarded tokens in the brown capuchin monkey, *Cebus apella. Journal of Comparative Psychology*, *118*(2), 133–139.

Brosnan, S. F., & de Waal, F. B. M. (2006). Partial support from a non-replication: Comment on Roma, Silberberg, Ruggiero, and Suomi (2006). *Journal of Comparative Psychology*, *120*(1), 74–75.

Brosnan, S. F., Freeman, C., & de Waal, F. B. M. (2006). Partner's behavior, not reward distribution, determines success in an unequal cooperative task in capuchin monkeys. *American Journal of Primatology*, *68*, 713–724.

Brosnan, S. F., Schiff, H. C., & de Waal, F. B. M. (2005). Tolerance for inequity may increase with social closeness in chimpanzees. *Proceedings of the Royal Society of London. Series B*, *1560*, 253–258.

Camerer, C. (2003). *Behavioral game theory: Experiments in strategic interaction*. Princeton: Princeton University Press.

Clark, M. S., & Grote, N. K. (2003). Close relationships. In: T. Millon & M. J. Lerner (Eds), *Handbook of psychology: Personality and social psychology* (Vol. 5, pp. 447–461). New York: Wiley.

Custance, D., Whiten, A., & Fredman, T. (1999). Social learning of an artificial fruit task in capuchin monkeys (*Cebus apella*). *Journal of Comparative Psychology*, *113*(1), 13–23.

Dana, J. D., Weber, R. A., & Kuang, J. (2003). *Exploiting moral wriggle room: Behavior inconsistent with a preference for fair outcomes*. Carnegie Mellon Behavioral Decision Research Working Paper no. 349. Available at http://ssrn.com/abstract = 400900

Dawes, C. T., Fowler, J. H., Johnson, T., McElreath, R., & Smirnov, O. (2007). Egalitarian motives in humans. *Nature*, *446*, 794–796.

de Waal, F. B. M. (1997). The chimpanzee's service economy: Food for grooming. *Evolution and Human Behavior*, *18*, 375–386.

de Waal, F. B. M., & Berger, M. L. (2000). Payment for labour in monkeys. *Nature*, *404*, 563.

de Waal, F. B. M., & Brosnan, S. F. (2006). Simple and complex reciprocity in primates. In: P. Kapeller & C. P. van Schaik (Eds), *Cooperation in primates and humans: Evolution and mechanisms*. Berlin: Springer.

de Waal, F. B. M., & Davis, J. M. (2002). Capuchin cognitive ecology: Cooperation based on projected returns. *Neuropsychologia*, *1492*, 1–8.

Diekmann, K. A., Samuels, S. M., Ross, L., & Bazerman, M. H. (1997). Self-interest and fairness in problems of resource allocation: Allocators versus recipients. *Journal of Personality and Social Psychology*, *72*(5), 1061–1074.

Dindo, M., & De Waal, F. B. M. (2006). Partner effects on food consumption in brown capuchin monkeys. *American Journal of Primatology*, *69*, 1–6.

Dubreuil, D., Gentile, M. S., & Visalberghi, E. (2006). Are capuchin monkeys (*Cebus apella*) inequity averse? *Proceedings of the Royal Society of London. Series B*, *273*, 1223–1228.

Evans, T. A., & Westergaard, G. C. (2006). Self-control and tool use in tufted capuchin monkeys (*Cebus apella*). *Journal of Comparative Psychology*, *120*(2), 163–166.

Fehr, E., & Gachter, S. (2002). Altruistic punishment in humans. *Nature*, *415*, 137–140.

Fehr, E., & Rockenbach, B. (2003). Detrimental effects of sanctions on human altruism. *Nature*, *422*, 137–140.

Fehr, E., & Schmidt, K. M. (1999). A theory of fairness, competition, and cooperation. *The Quarterly Journal of Economics*, *114*, 817–868.

Fontenot, M. B., Watson, S. L., Roberts, K. A., & Miller, R. W. (2007). Effects of food preferences on token exchange and behavioural responses to inequality in tufted capuchin monkeys, *Cebus apella*. *Animal Behavior*, *74*, 487–496.

Frank, R. H. (1988). *Passions within reason: The strategic role of the emotions*. New York: W. W. Norton & Company.

Frank, R. H. (2001). Cooperation through emotional commitment. In: R. M. Nesse (Ed.), *Evolution and the capacity for commitment* (pp. 57–76). New York: Russell Sage Foundation.

Fukuno, M., & Ohbuchi, K. (2001). Respondent's rejection of unequal offer as protection of one's identity in ultimatum bargaining. *Japanese Journal of Social Psychology*, *26*, 131–144.

Gintis, H., Bowles, S., Boyd, R., & Fehr, E. (2003). Explaining altruistic behavior in humans. *Evolution and Human Behavior*, *24*, 153–172.

Hare, B., Call, J., Agnetta, B., & Tomasello, M. (2000). Chimpanzees know what conspecifics do and do not see. *Animal Behaviour*, *59*(4), 771–785.

Hatfield, E., Walster, G. W., & Berscheid, E. (1978). *Equity: Theory and research*. Boston: Allyn and Bacon.

Henrich, J., Boyd, R., Bowles, S., Camerer, C., Fehr, E., Gintis, H., & McElreath, R. (2001). In search of homo economicus: Behavioral experiments in 15 small-scale societies. *American Economic Review*, *91*, 73–78.

Hoffman, E., McCabe, K., Shachat, K., & Smith, V. (1994). Preferences, property rights and anonymity in bargaining games. *Games and Economic Behavior*, *7*, 346–380.

Horita, Y., & Yamagishi, T. (2007). *Rejection of unfair offers in the ultimatum game for maintaining self-image*. Presentation at the 12th International Conference of Social Dilemmas, July 8–12, Seattle, WA, USA.

Jensen, K., Call, J., & Tomasello, M. (2007). Chimpanzees are rational maximizers in an ultimatum game. *Science*, 107–109.

Jensen, K., Hare, B., Call, J., & Tomasello, M. (2006). What's in it for me? Self-regard precludes altruism and spite in chimpanzees. *Proceedings of the Royal Society of London*. (Series B, 271, pp. 1013–1021). Published online (10.1098/rspb.2005.3417).

Kahneman, D., Knetsch, J. L., & Thaler, R. (1986). Fairness as a constraint on profit seeking: Entitlements in the market. *The American Economic Review*, *76*, 728–741.

Knoch, D., Pascual-Leone, A., Meyer, K., Treyer, V., & Fehr, E. (2006). Diminishing reciprocal fairness by disrupting the right prefrontal cortex. *Science*, *314*, 829–832.

Lowenstein, G. F., Thompson, L., & Bazerman, M. H. (1989). Social utility and decision-making in interpersonal contexts. *Journal of Personality and Social Psychology*, *57*(3), 426–441.

McGrew, W. C. (2004). *The cultured chimpanzee: Reflections on cultural primatology*. Cambridge, UK: Cambridge University Press.

Melis, A. P., Hare, B., & Tomasello, M. (2006a). Chimpanzees recruit the best collaborators. *Science*, *311*, 1297–1300.

Melis, A. P., Hare, B., & Tomasello, M. (2006b). Engineering cooperation in chimpanzees: Tolerance constraints on cooperation. *Animal Behavior*, *72*, 275–286.

Mendres, K. A., & de Waal, F. B. M. (2000). Capuchins do cooperate: The advantage of an intuitive task. *Animal Behaviour*, *60*(4), 523–529.

Preuschoft, S., & van Hooff, J. A. R. A. M. (1995). Homologizing primate facial displays: A critical review of methods. *Folia Primatologica*, *65*(3), 121–137.

Preuschoft, S., Wang, X., Aureli, F., & de Waal, F. B. M. (2002). Reconciliation in captive chimpanzees: A reevaluation with controlled methods. *International Journal of Primatology*, *23*, 29–50.

Reynolds, G. S. (1961). Behavioral contrast. *Journal of the Experimental Analysis of Behavior*, *4*, 441–466.

Roma, P. G., Silberberg, A., Ruggiero, A. M., & Suomi, S. J. (2006). Capuchin monkeys, inequity aversion, and the frustration effect. *Journal of Comparative Psychology*, *120*(1), 67–73.

Rose, L. M. (1997). Vertebrate predation and food-sharing in *Cebus* and *Pan*. *International Journal of Primatology*, *18*(5), 727–765.

Sanfey, A. G., Rilling, J. K., Aronson, J. A., Nystrom, L. E., & Cohen, J. D. (2003). The neural basis of economic decision-making in the ultimatum game. *Science*, *300*, 1755–1758.

Seres, M., Aureli, F., & de Waal, F. B. M. (2001). Successful formation of a large chimpanzee group out of two preexisting subgroups. *Zoo Biology*, *20*, 501–515.

Silk, J. B., Brosnan, S. F., Vonk, J., Henrich, J., Povinelli, D. J., Richardson, A. S., Lambeth, S., Mascaro, J., & Schapiro, S. J. (2005). Chimpanzees are indifferent to the welfare of unrelated group members. *Nature*, *437*, 1357–1359.

Tinklepaugh, O. L. (1928). An experimental study of representative factors in monkeys. *Journal of Comparative Psychology*, *8*, 197–236.

Van Lange, P. A. M., Drigotas, S. M., Rusbult, C. E., Arriaga, X. B., Witcher, B. S., & Cox, C. L. (1997). Willingness to sacrifice in close relationships. *Journal of Personality and Social Psychology*, *72*(6), 1373–1395.

van Wolkenten, M., Brosnan, S. F., & de Waal, F. B. M. (2007). Inequity responses in monkeys are modified by effort, but not other individual factors. *Proceedings of the National Academy of Sciences*, *104*(47), 18854–18859.

Visalberghi, E., & Anderson, J. R. (2008). Fair game for chimpanzees. *Science*, *319*, 282–283.

Vonk, J., Brosnan, S. F., Silk, J. B., Henrich, J., Richardson, A. S., Lambeth, S. L., Schapiro, S., & Povinelli, D. J. (2008). Chimpanzees do not take advantage of very low cost opportunities to deliver food to unrelated group members. *Animal Behaviour*, *75*(5), 1757–1770.

Warneken, F., Hare, B., Melis, A. P., Hanus, D., & Tomasello, M. (2007). Spontaneous altruism by chimpanzees and young children. *PLoS Biology*, *5*(7), e184.

Warneken, F., & Tomasello, M. (2006). Altruistic helping in human infants and young chimpanzees. *Science*, *311*, 1301–1303.

Whiten, A. (1998). Imitation of the sequential structure of actions by chimpanzees (*Pan troglodytes*). *Journal of Comparative Psychology*, *112*(3), 270–281.

Whiten, A., Goodall, J., McGrew, W. C., Nishida, T., Reynolds, V., Sugiyama, Y., Tutin, C. E. G., Wrangham, R. W., & Boesch, C. (1999). Cultures in chimpanzees. *Nature*, *399*, 682–685.

Wilkinson, R. G. (2006). The impact of inequality. *Social Research*, *73*(2), 711–732.

Wrangham, R., & Peterson, D. (1996). *Demonic males*. Boston: Hougton Mifflin Company.

Xiao, E., & Houser, D. (2005). Emotional expression in human punishment behavior. *Proceedings of the National Academy of Sciences*, *102*(20), 7398–7401.

Yamagishi, T. (2007). Reciprocity, strong reciprocity, and fairness. Paper presented at the Society for Experimental Social Psychology, Chicago, IL.

Yamagishi, T., Horita, Y., & Takagishi, H. (2008). *Strong reciprocity and reputation management*. Center for Experimental Research in Social Science Working Paper no. 83.

Zizzo, D. J., & Oswald, A. (2001). Are people willing to pay to reduce other's incomes? *Annales d'Economie et de Statistique*, *63–64*, 39–62.

ON THE NATURE, MODELING, AND NEURAL BASES OF SOCIAL TIES

Frans van Winden, Mirre Stallen and K. Richard Ridderinkhof

ABSTRACT

Purpose – *This chapter addresses the nature, formalization, and neural bases of (affective) social ties and discusses the relevance of ties for health economics. A social tie is defined as an affective weight attached by an individual to the well-being of another individual ('utility interdependence'). Ties can be positive or negative, and symmetric or asymmetric between individuals. Characteristic of a social tie, as conceived of here, is that it develops over time under the influence of interaction, in contrast with a trait like altruism. Moreover, a tie is not related to strategic behavior such as reputation formation but seen as generated by affective responses.*

Methodology/approach – *A formalization is presented together with some supportive evidence from behavioral experiments. This is followed by a discussion of related psychological constructs and the presentation of suggestive existing neural findings. To help prepare the grounds for a model-based neural analysis some speculations on the neural networks involved are provided, together with suggestions for future research.*

Neuroeconomics
Advances in Health Economics and Health Services Research, Volume 20, 125–159

ISSN: 0731-2199/doi:10.1016/S0731-2199(08)20006-3

Findings – *Social ties are not only found to be important from an economic viewpoint, it is also shown that they can be modeled and related to neural substrates.*

Originality/value of the *chapter – By providing an overview of the economic research on social ties and connecting it with the broader behavioral and neuroeconomics literature, the chapter may contribute to the development of a neuroeconomics of social ties.*

1. INTRODUCTION

Interpersonal attachments appear to play a key role in human life. As extensively documented by Baumeister and Leary (1995), people form social attachments readily and resist the dissolution of existing bonds. A broad assortment of psychological evidence pleads in favor of the hypothesis put forward by these authors that the desire for affective interpersonal relationships is a fundamental human motivation. From an evolutionary viewpoint this readiness to form groups makes sense, for example, as a behavioral mechanism to protect against external threats. Furthermore, in line with the hypothesis, there are many studies indicating that mental and physical health problems are more common among people who lack close personal relationships, that is, if they involve positive interaction (*op. cit.*, pp. 508–511; see also Berscheid & Reiss, 1998). For instance, without bonds marked by positive concern and caring, people are more likely to be unhappy, depressed, and anxious. Apart from being important for health and subjective well-being, interpersonal attachments – or, social ties, as we will call them below – show significant cognitive and emotional effects related to their tendency to blur the boundaries between the relationship partner and the self ('to include the other in the self').

Notwithstanding this wealth of evidence, processes of interpersonal attachment have been neglected in formal models of social interaction. This also holds for recent models in behavioral economics and game theory that allow for other-regarding preferences (like inequity aversion or reciprocity), as we will discuss in greater detail below. What is missing is the incorporation of affective processes providing the 'social glue' for attachment. Note that doing so would give relations an individualized, historical, and context-dependent content. This would further help to bridge the gap between an 'undersocialized' and an 'oversocialized' account of human behavior that characterizes many models (Granovetter, 1985). The former is characteristic for neoclassical economic models assuming narrowly selfish behavior, while the latter characterizes models in economics and sociology assuming agents with fully internalized social norms (like fairness or equity). In both cases, behavior is atomized in the sense that it is not embedded in culture as an ongoing process that is continuously constructed and reconstructed during interaction.

The significance of affect in interpersonal relationships is increasingly acknowledged also in economics (see e.g., Elster, 1998; Loewenstein, 2000). This tendency is reinforced by recent neuroscientific findings and the concomitant rise of social neuroeconomics (Fehr & Camerer, 2007; Sanfey, 2007). Already, a few models have been developed formalizing interpersonal behavior as the outcome of interacting affective and deliberative systems (Loewenstein & O'Donoghue, 2007; van Dijk & van Winden, 1997; van Winden, 2001). In this chapter, we will focus on the dual-system model of van Dijk and van Winden (1997), which explicitly deals with the affective processes involved in interpersonal attachment.

The organization of this chapter is as follows. After a brief summary of the state of the art in the (economic) modeling of social interaction, Section 2 presents an outline of the social ties model of van Dijk and van Winden (1997) and shortly reports on the behavioral experimental evidence regarding this model. Section 3 is concerned with an exploration of what we know at this stage about the neural substrates of ties, based on the existing literature, paying special attention to the constructs of empathy and sympathy. It also provides some speculations on the neural correlates of social ties. Section 4 concludes.

2. SOCIAL TIES

2.1. Social Ties: Introduction

Economists are well aware that for a variety of strategic and non-strategic reasons individuals may show behavior that seems to conflict with the assumed behavior of *homo economicus* – the fully rational and narrowly selfish agent populating most economic models (see e.g., Fehr & Schmidt, 2005; Sobel, 2005). One strategic reason is that such behavior may help to build up a *reputation* (e.g., of being cooperative) which is expected to further one's selfish interests in the future, even though it hurts these interests in the short-run. While this is still compatible with narrowly selfish behavior, this is not the case with another (non-strategic) reason that regularly pops up in the literature, which is *altruism*, that is, behavior that is costly to the actor and beneficial to the recipient. *Envy* or *spitefulness*, defined as costly behaviors that are also costly for the recipient, have received some attention too, albeit to a much lesser extent. Both types of (unconditional) behavior are assumed to stem from other-regarding preferences, formalized through interdependent utility functions, where, in the case of altruism (envy), a positive (negative) weight is attached to the utility or welfare of other individuals.

More recently, another type of other-regarding preference, related to *inequity aversion*, has attracted much attention. In that case, an individual's utility function is embellished with an argument representing differences in payoffs with other individuals. A different strand of recent models focuses on intention-based *reciprocity*, defined as costly (un)kind behavior in response to the (un)kind behavior of another person. This is modeled by incorporating beliefs about the intentions or about the (kindness of the) type of the other person into the individual's utility function. We will return to these models in the next section. Here, we would like to emphasize that in these revisions of the *homo economicus* model, only stable other-regarding preferences have been accounted for, which show no time dependency. Furthermore, there is hardly any serious attempt to explicitly deal with the affective processes involved.[1] This brings us to our discussion of affective social ties, where both these aspects of existing models will be challenged.

To explain how social interactions can influence economic interactions through the development of affective ties, we need to become more specific about the notion of a social tie (a formal representation is given in the next section). Basically, a social tie refers to a caring about the interests of a specific other person, based on feelings experienced while interacting with that other person. Sentiments are the affective component of interpersonal attachments and are considered to be a key element of a social tie (Baumeister & Leary, 1995; see also Granovetter, 1973). Feelings that individuals have with respect to specific others are related to the extent they care about the welfare of those others. The more they care in a positive way, the stronger the affective bond and 'we' feeling is supposed to be. However, it is important to note that a social tie is not simply determined by the weight that an individual attaches to the welfare of another person.

In general, if positive or negative sentiments are maintained towards others, a social tie can only be said to exist if the weight attached to this specific other's well-being differs from the weight given to the well-being of a 'generalized other (van Dijk & van Winden, 1997).' Furthermore, the strength and the valence of a tie are supposed to depend on the interaction between the individuals concerned, which can be experienced as more or less beneficial or harmful. It is the accumulated affective experience that is taken to matter for the sign and size of the weight attached to the specific other's interests. In this respect, a social tie is like a capital good (a stock variable), built up through investments over time. This makes the development of a social tie inherently dynamic and its strength subject to change. In this process, differences in personality are likely to play a role. Individual differences in tolerance, rationality, altruism, or emotionality may be crucial for the speed with which positive or negative ties develop, and their mutuality (symmetry).

2.2. Social Ties: A Formal Model

In this section we present a formalization of social ties based on van Dijk and van Winden (1997), in the sequel referred to as the vDvW-model. An important advantage of formalization is that it enables the development of rigorous theory and a coherent framework for testable hypotheses. Its relevance will be illustrated in the context of the voluntary provision of a public good.

A public good is characterized by the fact that no one can be excluded from its consumption while, in addition, its consumption by someone does not rival with the consumption by someone else. A classic example concerns the defence of a country against external aggressors. However, here, we are more interested in local public goods, like for small communities, neighborhoods, social networks, or groups. Relevant examples are the provision of security, a healthy, clean or pleasant environment, common information, or the establishment and maintenance of social norms (through sanctions).

The following simple public good game captures the essence of the voluntary provision of a public good. Suppose there are two players, A and B, both endowed with an amount of money of y euros. The money can be spent on private goods and a public good. Let js contribution to the public good be denoted by g_j (with $j = A, B$). Normalizing the price of both the private and the public good to one, the consumption of private goods by j, denoted as x_j, equals: $x_j = y - g_j$, while the consumption of the public good, indicated by g, equals $g = g_A + g_B$ for both players. The welfare, or utility, derived from the consumption of x_j and g is denoted by $U_j(x_j, g)$. For illustration, suppose that both players have the same linear utility function: $U_j(x_j, g) = x_j + mg\ [= y - g_j + m(g_A + g_B)]$, where m stands for the marginal per capita return on public good contributions. Typically, it is assumed for these games that $0<m<1$ and $nm > 1$, with n the number of players. Thus, in our case, let $2m > 1$ and assume that both players have to decide only once (one-shot game). Then, it is easily seen that a rational and selfish (own utility maximizing) player will not contribute to the public good ($g_j = 0$, leading to a utility of y), even though both players would be better off if they would contribute all their money ($g_j = y$, rendering a utility of $2my$, which is larger than y). Whatever the other player is expected to do, it is always in one's (selfish) interest not to contribute. More generally, the private provision of public goods seems to be haunted by a 'free-riding' problem, in the sense that all want to benefit from the contributions by others without putting an own effort into it which is adequate from a social point of view (i.e., taking the benefits for others into account).

According to the general standard model of public goods (see Bergstrom, Blume, & Varian, 1986), the welfare losses to a social group from free-riding tend to become larger the bigger the group.[2] Moreover, generally, the equilibrium public good level turns out to be invariant to the distribution of the endowments (income) and also to an income tax financed public provision of some of the good. In the latter case, public provision simply replaces (crowds out) private provision, one for one. Theoretically, socially better outcomes can be obtained if the game is not one-shot, but repeatedly played over an infinite or uncertain time span, basically because players (may) perceive sufficient opportunity to punish uncooperative behavior (see e.g., Fudenberg & Tirole, 1991). In case of a finitely repeated game, with a known fixed ending, larger contributions can be sustained if the likelihood exists that some players (for whatever reason) are cooperative but will negatively react to free-riding (like tit-for-tat players, see Kreps, Milgrom, Roberts, & Wilson, 1982). In that event, even a selfish player might want to build up a reputation for being cooperative, for some time. However, evidence from laboratory experiments shows that substantial contributions occur even in a one-shot linear public good game, like the one discussed above, or in the last round of such a game, where zero contributions are predicted (for a survey, see Ledyard, 1995; see also Cox & Sadiraj, 2007). To explain these 'anomalous' experimental findings, over the last decade or so several models have been proposed that incorporate some kind of other-regarding preferences (see the previous section). These preferences may relate to an interest in the distribution of *outcomes* (like altruism or inequity aversion) or to reciprocity based either on the (un)kindness of other players' behavioral *intentions* (e.g., fairness) or the *type* of the other players (e.g., selfish, altruistic, or spiteful).[3] For example, it is easy to see that even in a one-shot linear public good game, sufficiently inequity-averse individuals may contribute to the public good if others contribute as well.

Three important characteristics of these new models are that they (1) assume stable other-regarding preferences; (2) do not specify any emotional mechanisms that are, at least implicitly, referred to (as in intention-based models); and, (3) focus on static equilibria. The vDvW-model differs in these respects because of its focus on affect as a driving factor of other-regarding preferences and its explicitly dynamic nature. The model concerns a finitely repeated two-person (non-linear) public good game. For notational convenience, using the notation introduced in the example above, we will focus on player A in the game and leave out the time index. As argued in the previous section, the affective component is taken to be a key element of a social tie. The feelings a person (consciously or unconsciously) experiences with respect to the specific other in a tie are related to the extent s/he cares about the well-being of that specific other person. Staying close to traditional economic modeling this is formalized through an interdependent utility function,

$$V_A = \ln U_A + \alpha_A \ln U_B \tag{1}$$

and similarly for B, where $U_j(x_j, g)$, $y_j = x_j + g_j$ $(j = A, B)$, and $g = g_A + g_B$.[4] Furthermore, the weight α_A attached to the utility of B represents As tie with B; that is, the valence and the intensity of the sentiment that A experiences with respect to B. *Mutatis mutandis*, the same holds for α_B. Based on empirical evidence (Goeree, Holt, & Laury, 2002; Liebrand, 1984; Sawyer, 1966), it is assumed that $-1<\alpha_j<1$ $(j = A, B)$. Note that B need not necessarily maintain a similar tie with A; that is, α_A need not be equal to α_B.[5]

Let us focus first on some stark cases when α_j is *fixed*. If $\alpha_j = 0$, we are back to the standard economic model with selfish preferences. If $\alpha_j \to 1$, approximately, an equal weight becomes attached to both own and other's well-being, inducing fully cooperative behavior (efficiency). In sharp contrast, if $\alpha_j \to -1$, behavior becomes maximally uncooperative, inducing a minimal contribution level. Consequently, the existence of social ties can dramatically influence the private provision of a public good. Furthermore, with fixed social ties, government provision financed through an income tax would lead to a one-for-one crowding out of private provision, as in the standard model without social ties. Interestingly, some experimental support has been provided for the predictive power of the (log-linearized) Cobb–Douglas specification of V_A represented by (1) in explaining contributions in (one-shot) linear public good games (Goeree et al., 2002).[6] In addition, this study finds substantial heterogeneity of α_j across individuals, with estimates ranging between –0.5 and +0.5. Cox and Sadiraj (2007) show that this type of model can explain several stylized facts regarding last-round contributions in linear public good games (where reputation and future reciprocity cannot play a role), in contrast with inequity aversion models.

As mentioned above, existing models of other-regarding preferences are typically static, not allowing for any intertemporal effects.[7] Although such preferences may be genetically and/or culturally determined (via the instillment of norms), the vDvW-model focuses on a mechanism that is intrinsically dynamic and non-strategic, involving autonomic affective responses in the limbic system of the brain. Based on (social) psychological findings,[8] this model assumes that ties develop as an unconscious by-product of prolonged interaction which generates positive (negative) sentiments if valued positively (negatively), and that they may decay over time. In the context of a public good game, the valuation of the interaction is likely to depend on the contributions to the public good. In the model this is captured for A by the 'impulse':

$$G_A = g_B - \varepsilon_A g_A \tag{2}$$

and similarly for B, where ε_A reflects As tolerance or reference level regarding Bs contribution. For example, if $\varepsilon_j = 0$ ($j = A$, B), then any contribution by the other player is positively valued, whereas it should at least match js own contribution if $\varepsilon_j = 1$. Taking into account the possibility of attrition, the development of a tie over time is formalized for A by the following differential equation:

$$\mathrm{d}\alpha_A/\mathrm{d}t = f_A(G_A, \alpha_A) \tag{3}$$

and similarly for B. Fig. 1 presents a phase diagram of Eq. (3), assuming a diminishing marginal impact of the impulse.[9]

If ties do not decay over time, then stationarity ($\mathrm{d}\alpha_A/\mathrm{d}t = f_A = 0$) is compatible with any α_A if the impulse G_A is zero (horizontal part of dashed line b), whereas for positive (negative) values of the impulse the tie grows to its upper (lower) bound of 1 (–1). With attrition, the upward sloping solid line a shows the level of the impulse G_A required to compensate for the decay such that a particular value of α_A can be sustained. Specifically, note that a sustained impulse $G_A \neq 0$ is required for $\alpha_A \neq 0$. To analyze the dynamics of tie formation, the vDvW-model makes the simplifying assumption that individuals are myopic. This implies that they do not take into account the potential impact of their contributions on their own future feelings and the feelings of others towards them. Although perhaps not

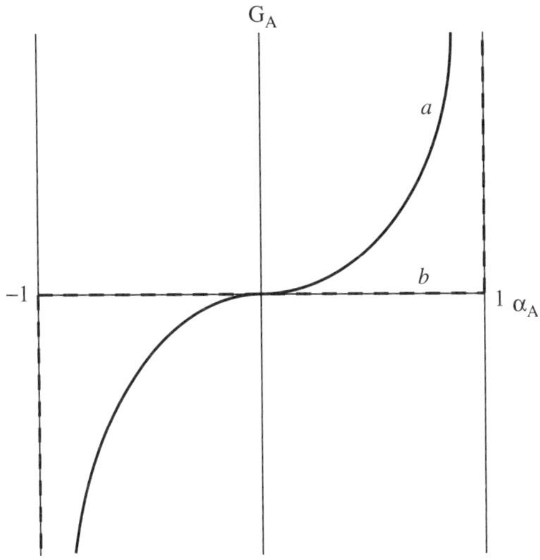

Fig. 1. Phase Diagram of Eq. (3): (a) with Decay, (b) without Decay.

completely realistic, this assumption finds some empirical support in the evidence that people show a tendency to underweight their own and others' future emotions (Loewenstein, 1996; Loewenstein & Schkade, 1999). As a consequence, the dynamics can be modeled as a sequence of contribution decisions connected by the development of the tie over time. To illustrate, we assume that players are identical (and $0<\varepsilon_j<1$).[10] Fig. 2 shows the phase diagram.[11]

For explanation, suppose we have a negative value of α_A. Decay over time would make α_A less negative. For stationarity, that is, to keep α_A from becoming less negative, this decay effect needs to be offset by a sufficiently negative value of G_A, requiring that *A*s contribution is larger than *B*s (since $\varepsilon_A<1$; see Eq. (2)). But, this implies that α_B would have to be more negative than α_A, which explains why the *A*-curve (where $f_A=0$) is located below the dashed line in the 3rd quadrant of the diagram. Similarly, for $\alpha_A=0$ stationarity demands that $G_A=0$, which again implies that α_B would have to be smaller than α_A, and negative. When α_A becomes positive, G_A must also be positive to compensate for the attrition (which would now decrease the value of α_A). Consequently, for stationarity (see again the *A*-curve) α_B increases and switches sign. As α_A becomes more and more positive, α_B must become larger than α_A at some point, due to the assumed declining marginal impact of larger values of G_A. Because individuals are assumed to be

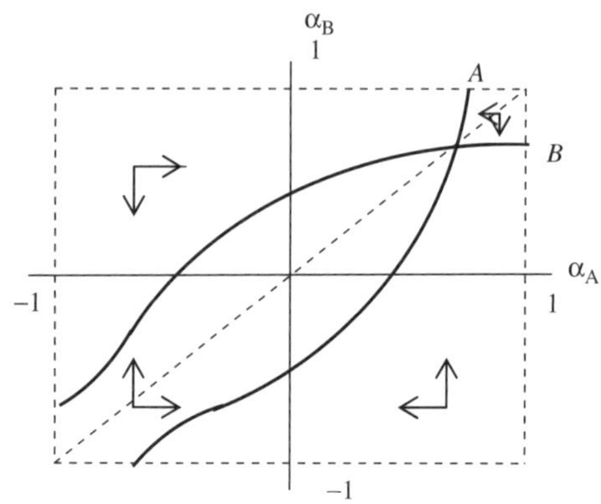

Fig. 2. Phase Diagram of Eq. (3) with Identical Individuals (Using $G_A(\alpha_A, \alpha_B)$ and $G_B(\alpha_B, \alpha_A)$), with A: $f_A = 0$, B: $f_B = 0$.

identical, the A-curve and the B-curve (where $f_A = 0$ and $f_B = 0$, respectively) are symmetric and cross where $\alpha_A = \alpha_B$. The arrows in the diagram show the direction of movement of the ties (α_A and α_B) in that particular region of the diagram. Eventually, one will end up in this case at the intersection of the two solid curves.

Some of the main results of the vDvW-model, focusing on the impact of differences in income and preferences for public and private goods, are the following. First of all, a unique social ties equilibrium exists.[12] With equal preferences and incomes, the ties are symmetric and positive ($\alpha_A = \alpha_B > 0$), boosting the voluntary provision of the public good. In case of different preferences or income levels, the ties are asymmetric ($\alpha_A \neq \alpha_B$) and the one with the lower value may be negative, in which event contributions are lowered, against one's own direct interests, to hurt the person concerned. Furthermore, with different incomes, the provision level of public goods may be lower than the level derived from the standard model due to the potential development of negative ties.

In contrast with the invariance result of the standard model of public goods, in case of social ties, government intervention need no longer be neutral with respect to the provision level of the public good. If some of the public good is provided by the government (and financed by an income tax), the total provision level may go down, because of a crowding out of intrinsic motivation through a negative effect on social ties. However, for similar reasons, government intervention can have a positive impact on the provision of public goods if a community is characterized by negative ties or facing substantial mobility or migration which breaks up existing networks. Also, note that a reduction in public provision will not immediately be taken over by private provision (if at all), because the formation of ties takes time.

2.3. Social Ties: Evidence from the Lab

In this section we present some behavioral experimental support for the social ties mechanism formalized by the vDvW-model. The tool used in these behavioral experiments to measure social ties is based on the psychological 'Ring-test of social value orientation (Liebrand, 1984).' In this test each participant is randomly coupled with an anonymous other participant, and has to choose repeatedly between two 'self-other' payoff combinations. Each such combination allocates a positive or negative number of points (to be exchanged for real money at the end of the experiment) between the decision-maker and the participant s/he is matched with. All payoff combinations lie on a circle with the origin as center (which explains the name of this test), with on the horizontal axis points allocated to the decision-maker him- or herself (Self) and on the vertical axis points allocated to the other person (Other). Each allocation pair can be seen as a vector. Fig. 3 presents an example.[13] Adding all the choices of a participant renders an aggregate vector. The angle of this vector with the horizontal axis provides a measure of the extent to which this participant cares about a 'generalized other,' that is, his or her 'social value orientation.' The predictive validity of people's social value orientation has been shown by many studies (see e.g., Rusbult & van Lange, 1996).

However, a tie refers to a specific other, not a generalized other. Therefore, to measure a social tie van Dijk, Sonnemans, and van Winden (2002) applied

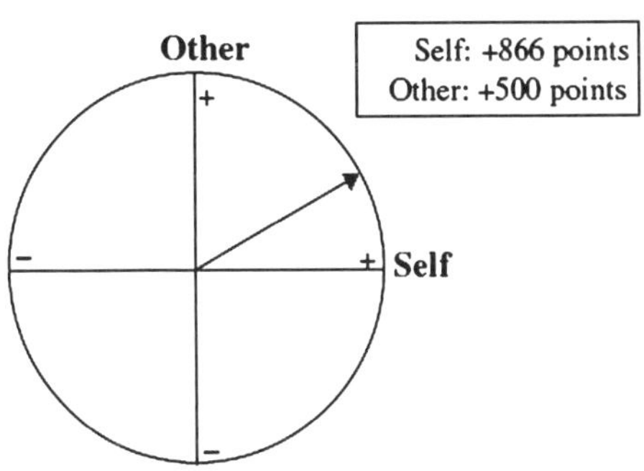

Fig. 3. Example of Self-Other Payoff Combination in the Ring-Test.

the test twice: once before social interaction, and a second time after the interaction. In the second case, the participant is no longer linked with a randomly selected other but with the participant s/he interacted with. The sign and the size of the difference in the aggregate vectors (angles) thus determined, respectively, represent the valence and the strength of the social tie established through the interaction. Without correcting for social value orientation – measured by the angle of the vector obtained from the first test – the angle from the second test would reflect the more general sentiment of an individual with respect to the specific other interacted with.[14] Applying this procedure in a repeated two-person non-linear public good game experiment[15], they obtained the following results. First of all, they found a mean angle of the first Ring-test equal to 3°, with a large majority (95%) of the individual angles being located between –45° and +45°. This implies that the absolute weight attached to the Other's payoff was almost never larger than 1 (providing some additional empirical support for the plausibility of the assumption that $-1<\alpha_j<1$). Second, the social value orientations thus measured appeared to be correlated with individual contributions to the public good, particularly in the beginning of the interaction, confirming the validity of this measure. Third, individuals typically responded to an increase (decrease) in the contribution by the partner with an increase (decrease) in their own contribution. This reciprocity can be interpreted as providing evidence of a continuous development of social ties (with sentiments being correlated with observed contributions), but it may also (partly) reflect some kind of strategic behavior (like conditional cooperation, see Keser & van Winden, 2000). Fourth, using earnings in the public good game as an indicator of successful interaction (as they are positively related to the contributions by the partner), a clear impact on the angle of the second Ring-test was found, given the individual's initial angle (social value orientation); Table 1.

In this case, the second Ring-test was applied unexpectedly after 25 periods of play (out of a total of 32 periods). Similar results were obtained in an experiment with the second test being applied at the end, after the same number of periods. This suggests that ties are developed continuously. Also, different measures of success did not qualitatively affect the findings.[16]

Sonnemans, van Dijk, and van Winden (2006) extended the experimental study of van Dijk et al. (2002) to a similar public good game with four instead of two players. To avoid an excessive time consumption by the second Ring-test (unexpectedly applied after 25 periods), where now each participant would have to make multiple (in fact 32) self-other payoff allocation decisions concerning, successively, each of the three partners in

Table 1. Linear Regressions with Angle from Second Ring-Test as Dependent Variable and, as Independent Variables, Social Value Orientation (Angle from First Ring-Test) and Earnings in the Last Five Periods of the Public Good Game.

	B	SE *B*	Beta	*t*	Sign. *t*
Social value orientation	0.715	0.141	0.564	5.056	0.000
Earnings period 21–25	0.048	0.019	0.283	2.536	0.015
Constant	−33.074	14.661		−2.256	0.029
Multiple *R*: 0.712					
Adjusted R^2: 0.484					

Source: Reprinted from Frans van Dijk et al. (2002), with permission from Elsevier.

Table 2. Attitudes of Participants Towards Others.

	Positive	Neutral[a]	Negative	Total
Social value orientation (first Circle-test)	26 (47%)	28 (51%)	1 (2%)	55
Sentiments towards specific other (second Circle-test)	80 (48%)	73 (44%)	12 (8%)	165
Social ties (difference in Circle-tests)	41 (25%)	76 (46%)	48 (29%)	165

[a]Neutral attitudes correspond to Circle-test angles between −5° and +5°.
Source: Reprinted from Joep Sonnemans et al. (2006), with permission from Elsevier.

the game, they applied a simpler technique: the Circle-test. In the Circle-test, participants have to make a self-other payoff allocation only *once* by clicking on a circle, like in Fig. 3. With groups, this technique is much more convenient, although it is obviously noisier due to the single decision that is to be made. Their main findings are the following: On average, it turns out that contributions are quite similar to what is observed in the two-player game. However, a large variance is observed between groups, with some groups being highly successful, and others failing strongly in the provision of the public good. Table 2 shows the outcomes of the different attitude (Circle-test) measures. Almost all participants showed a non-negative social value orientation, with almost half of them maintaining a positive attitude towards a generalized (randomly selected and anonymous) other. As observed for the two-player game, almost always the first Circle-test angle is between −45° and +45° (98% of the cases). Sentiments towards the specific others interacted with – measured by the second Circle-tests, after the game – turn out to be more negative. Finally, in terms of social ties – measured by the difference in the angles derived from the second and the first Circle-tests – an almost equal percentage is observed for positive and negative ones. About half of the participants with a neutral (zero) first angle developed at least some tie with the others interacted with.

In support of the vDvW-model it is further found that differences in the second Circle-test angles with respect to specific others are correlated with the differences in their contributions, which suggests that during the game participants have built bonds with specific group members, rather than a general 'group cohesion.' Also, responses in the debriefing questionnaire to the question of whether one would want to continue the game with a specific partner (asked separately for each of the three partners) are strongly correlated with sentiments and ties. This speaks for the validity of the social ties measure. Interestingly, mutually positive or negative ties are observed in only 15% of the cases (mutual neutrality in 19% of the cases). Apparently, even an environment in which participants have equal endowments and payoff structures, individual differences in social value orientation and behavioral response patterns result in complex dynamics, mostly generating asymmetric ties. These results would seem to qualify the suggestion borne out by the 'minimal group paradigm' and social identity theory (Tajfel & Turner, 1986; Taylor & Moghaddam, 1994) that social cohesion is easily established.[17]

Up to now, the support for the vDvW-model of social ties has been only indirect in the sense that no direct evidence has been provided for the affective mechanism assumedly underlying social ties.[18] A recent experimental study by Brandts, Riedl, and van Winden (2007) fills this gap. One of their experiments concerns a repeated social dilemma game, where each of the two players can either choose to cooperate or not to cooperate. As in a linear public good game it is a dominant strategy in the stage (one-shot) game not to cooperate, even though they would obtain a higher payoff if both would cooperate. The authors used the Circle-test before and after the interaction, to measure social value orientation and the ex post sentiment towards the other player. In addition, after the interaction but before the second Circle-test, they measured the positive and/or negative emotions participants experienced (like anger, joy, guilt, etc.) and with what intensity, using self-reports.[19]

Their main findings are, first, that interaction success (in terms of earnings) is clearly positively (negatively) correlated with the positive (negative) emotions participants experienced after the interaction. However, it turns out that interaction success does not help much to explain sentiment towards the partner as measured by the second Circle-test. In a regression model with social value orientation and interaction success as other explanatory variables, only emotions show a clear impact (as does the individual's social value orientation) and significantly improve the fit of the model. More specifically, guilt and surprise show a positive impact, whereas a strongly negative effect is observed from contempt. Thus, it appears that interaction success triggered (some) emotions, which in turn produced a positive or negative social tie with the individual interacted with. These experimental results indeed suggest that the development of ties is mediated by emotions, as hypothesized in the vDvW-model.

3. TOWARDS THE NEUROECONOMICS OF SOCIAL TIES

The experimental support found for the vDvW-model depends for the affective part on the validity of the self-report measures that were used. Although there is evidence showing that self-reports in economic game experiments correlate with physiological measures of emotionality (see e.g., Ben-Shakhar, Bornstein, Hopfensitz, & van Winden, 2007), there are clear limitations to this often-used technique of measuring emotions. One example is the fact that it relies on consciously experienced feelings and honest reporting. Therefore, it would be interesting to see what evidence can be mustered from modern neuroscientific methods like brain imaging. This would fit into the gradually emerging interdisciplinary field of neuroeconomics (Camerer, Loewenstein, & Prelec, 2005; Rustichini, 2005; Sanfey, Loewenstein, Mcclure, & Cohen, 2006). Within this approach, researchers combine traditions from human and animal experimental psychology and cognitive neuroscience with mathematical decision models, often using simple experimental games, like the prisoner's dilemma game[20] (see Fehr & Camerer, 2007; Sanfey, 2007).

To prepare the grounds for a model-based neural analysis, in this section, after a short reminder of the nature of social ties and a discussion of related constructs, we will review the existing evidence of neural correlates. Several cognitive and affective processes may underlie or be involved in social tie formation, each perhaps playing a role at different moments of the social interaction. Below, the processes that may be relevant for the development of a social tie in a public good game will be evaluated, and we will discuss and speculate on the possible neural bases of these processes and their dynamics.

3.1. Constructs Related to Social Ties

An important feature of a social tie is its dynamic stock-variable nature. While social ties are presumed to be nonexistent when individuals meet for the first time, they are taken to develop rapidly during a relatively short period of interaction (minutes to hours). Affective feelings towards the other may start to develop already during the initial moments of social interaction. Whether these affective feelings result in a positive or negative tie will depend on one's appraisal of the other's behavior. If the other's behavior is in line with one's interests, this can be considered as an impulse for the development of a positive social tie. A positive social tie in the two-person public good game exists to the extent that one positively cares about the payoff of the other player in excess of one's care for a 'generalized other.' Formally, this is captured by a weight attached to the other's welfare, which is net of the weight representing one's social value orientation. A negative social tie develops when the behavior of the other is not in line with one's own interests. A social tie is not necessarily symmetric: one may be concerned about the payoff of the other in the public good game, while the other is not concerned (as much) about your welfare.

Of the numerous concepts that are used to describe social behavior in psychology, the notions of empathy and sympathy seem of particular relevance here. *Empathy*, which roughly refers to the ability to 'put oneself into another's shoes,' is commonly considered to have three characteristics (Lamm, Batson, & Decety, 2007): (1) affective sharing, that is, an affective response to another person which may entail sharing that person's (imagined) emotional state; (2) perspective taking, involving a cognitive capacity to take the other person's perspective; and (3) cognitive appraisal, involving monitoring mechanisms that keep track of the origins (self vs. other) of the experienced feelings. The third property refers to the generally accepted view that empathy requires a link, but no confusion, between the self and other (Decety & Hodges, 2006). This property seems to dissociate empathy from the concept of a (positive) social tie, which involves a kind of merger between the self and the other into some shared identity, accompanied by a ('we') feeling of bonding.

Empathy further appears to be subject to contextual appraisal and modulation, and supposedly exists because it facilitates social communication and helps forecast other people's needs and actions (de Vignemont & Singer, 2006). These properties are clearly important for the development of social ties. However, negative experimental findings concerning the presumed link between empathy and altruism (the capacity to act selflessly) point again at an important difference with (positive) social ties. According to (Maner et al., 2002; Cialdini, Brown, Lewis, Luce, & Neuberg, 1997), the relation with helping put forward in the literature appears to be due to two concomitant non-altruistic factors: perceived oneness and experienced negative affect (which in turn mediates helping). Oneness (merged identity with the person in need) stimulates emphatic concern as well as helping, which may further function as an emotional signal of oneness.

Consequently, while empathy can be regarded as an important factor in the development of social ties, it particularly differs from the latter construct in the motivational role that the other plays. During social tie development, the cognitive capacity to understand the mental state of the other plays an important role as the capacity of perspective taking is accompanied by feelings of attachments (e.g., friendship, familiarity, and similarity, see also Cialdini et al., 1997) or aversion. Taking the perspective of the other while at the same time attending to the other's behavior can lead to an empathic affective response (which does not require any direct emotional stimulation). However, empathy is not identical to a social tie as perceived here, because the merger of self and other in some shared identity is absent in empathy, where the self and the other remain separate entities.

The concept of *sympathy* seems more closely related to a (positive) social tie. Most scholars seem to agree that sympathy is an affective response that frequently stems from empathy and consists of feelings of concern for another person. According to Decety and Chaminade (2003), sympathetic concern indicates that there is affinity, agreement, and association with someone. Anything that affects oneself is supposed to similarly affect the other. This is in line with our description of a (positive) social tie. To the extent that interactions between individuals are experienced as positive (assumedly fostering a positive social tie), feelings of affinity, agreement, and association are likely to grow as well. However, it is important to note that the opposite may also occur; namely, negatively experienced social interactions (inducing feelings of antipathy, dislike, and dissociation with the other) may foster the development of a negative tie.

Interestingly, the founding father of economics as a science, Adam Smith, referred to (habitual) sympathy as an underlying factor driving affective (kin and non-kin) relationships representative of social ties (Smith, 1759). Furthermore, in his view, social ties abound even in competitive business environments, as illustrated by the following quote (*op. cit.*, p. 224): 'Colleagues in office, partners in trade, call one another brothers; and frequently feel towards one another as if they really were so. Their good agreement is an advantage to all (. . .).'[21]

3.2. Neural Correlates of Constructs Related to Social Ties

With respect to the dynamic formation of social ties, the key features of empathy and sympathy appear to be perspective taking, cognitive appraisal, and concern about the other's well-being. The first two components encompass factors such as 'mentalizing' and 'theory of mind' and entail the processing of norms like fairness. The latter component may encompass processes related to altruism, generosity, reciprocity, oneness, and so on. Below, we will selectively review the literature on the neural bases of each of these three components.

3.2.1. Perspective Taking – What would the Other Think?

Especially during the first rounds of the public good game, the capacity to take the perspective of the other is essential for both players. This capacity (often referred to as 'mentalizing') enables one to explain and predict the emotions and actions of the other. This cognitive capacity of perspective taking is also known as 'theory of mind.' Having a theory of mind (ToM) means that one recognizes that the other has a different perspective of the world than oneself, and that his or her behavior may be determined by different goals than one's own. Understanding the actions of someone facilitates the effective development of a social tie.

Functional neuroimaging has been invoked to help identify neural mechanisms underlying ToM. Evidence from such studies highlights the role of a number of areas in the brain (e.g., Gallagher & Frith, 2003; Saxe, 2006). However, most of these studies did not involve actual social interactions. Instead, in these experiments participants were asked to reason about the mental states of characters that were presented in stories, cartoons, or photographs (Baron-Cohen et al., 1999; Brunet, Sarfati, Hardy-Bayle, & Decety, 2000; Gallagher et al., 2000). Only few studies examined the neural correlates of mentalizing in participants who were immersed in actual social interactions, or in which participants believed they were interacting with a real human being while in actuality responses of the partner were generated and administered by a computer algorithm (Gallagher, Jack, Roepstorff, & Frith, 2002; McCabe, Houser, Ryan, Smith, & Trouard, 2001; Rilling, Sanfey, Aronson, Nystrom, & Cohen, 2004a). These studies show that two brain areas are particularly important for mentalizing in fictive situations and are associated with ToM in actual social interactions. These brain areas are the anterior paracingulate cortex (APCC) and the posterior superior temporal sulcus (pSTS).

Anterior Paracingulate Cortex. McCabe et al. (2001) reported dorsomedial prefrontal regions to be activated when subjects were playing a 'trust game' with a human partner. In this two-person sequential game, the first mover could decide to either end the game (which leads to a fixed equal payoff to both players) or to let the other player (the trustee) choose between an option where both players would be better off and an option where only the second player would benefit but the first player would lose, compared to their payoffs when the game is ended by the first mover (the trustor). Of most interest, McCabe et al. (2001) observed that the APCC is activated when trustees make cooperative decisions, that is, when they choose not to be selfish but go for the option where both players benefit. The authors suggest the APCC to be an 'active convergence zone that binds joint attention to mutual gains with sufficient inhibition of immediate reward gratification to allow cooperative decisions.'

Krueger et al. (2007) replicated and extended this finding using a similar, albeit non-anonymous, sequential reciprocal trust game in which partnership building and maintenance became essential. The APCC was shown to be critically involved in building a trust relationship by inferring another person's intentions to predict subsequent behavior.

In a study by Rilling et al. (2004a), the APCC is also reported as an important neural correlate of ToM. In their experiment the APCC was activated when participants were playing a series of a one-shot ultimatum game[22] and a series of a one-shot sequential prisoner's dilemma game. In both games, participants observed their partner's decision before they had to respond (with either acceptance or rejection of the offer in the ultimatum game, and with cooperation or defection in the prisoner's dilemma game). The decision a participant makes depends on how s/he interprets the action of the partner.

Posterior Superior Temporal Sulcus. In addition to the APCC, Rilling et al. (2004a) also found the pSTS to be more active when participants believed they were playing these games against a human being instead of a computer. Studies that examined the ToM ability by asking participants to mentalize about characters (instead of real human beings) consistently activated the STS area (Brunet et al., 2000; Castelli, Happe, Frith, & Frith, 2000; Gallagher et al., 2000). It has been suggested that the role of the STS is related to an initial analysis of social cues to provide a signal of the intention of another individual (Allison, Puce, & McCarthy, 2000).

3.2.2. Appraisal – Is the Behavior of the other in Line with One's Own Interests? Some people may readily develop a social tie, while others need more time to develop affective feelings towards the other player in the public good game. Whether one cares about the other's concerns will depend on the perceived importance of the other person's behavior for one's own concerns, including internalized social norms (Montague & Lohrenz, 2007). If the other behaves according to one's social norms, then this may function as an impulse for the development of a positive social tie. Fairness norms, in particular, play a role in the modulation of social relations (Dawes, Fowler, Johnson, McElreath, & Smirnov, 2007). The implementation of fairness norms in the public good game leads one to expect the other to reciprocate investments in the public good. In the case that a player plays unfairly (i.e., does not contribute to the public good), this may indulge negative feelings in the other towards this player. Brain areas that play a role in the implementation of fairness-related behavior are discussed below.

The Striatum. The striatum appears to be involved in monitoring the other's decision to reciprocate cooperation or not, presumably in order to facilitate learning who can and who cannot be trusted as a social partner. In a prisoner's dilemma game, each participant probably makes an estimate of the likelihood that his or her cooperation will be reciprocated, even though this estimate is unlikely to be correct. The discrepancy between the actual choice of cooperation (0 or 1) and the probability with which cooperation by the other player is predicted is the reward prediction error. Positive reward prediction errors (as elicited by reciprocated cooperation) have been found to correlate with increased activity in the striatum, while negative reward prediction errors (elicited by unreciprocated cooperation) were associated with a decreased activation (Rilling et al., 2002; Rilling, Sanfey, Aronson, Nystrom, & Cohen, 2004b). Thus, the striatum appears to register social prediction errors (and perhaps encodes the positive feeling garnered by mutual cooperation) to guide decisions about reciprocity (Sanfey, 2007).

King-Casas et al. (2005) found that activity in the caudate nucleus (part of the striatum) was modulated by reciprocity in a multi-round trust game. Benevolent reciprocity (when the trustor is generous in response to a defection by the trustee in the previous round) was associated with greater activity of the caudate nucleus in the trustee's brain than malevolent reciprocity (when the trustor repays the generosity of the trustee with selfishness). These results confirm the suggestion that the striatum registers the benevolence of the other's decision and guides decisions about reciprocity. Furthermore, in the beginning of the trust game, the caudate was most active after the decision of the trustor was revealed, but as the game progressed, activity in the caudate shifted its time of occurrence to a time before that decision. Thus, the dynamics of activation patterns in the caudate reveal that as the social interactions progress, the trustee learns to develop intentions to trust or distrust the other player.

Anterior Insula. Experiments with the ultimatum game suggest that activation seen in the insula reflects one's negative emotional response to 'unfair' offers, that is, offers where one gets less than an even-split (Sanfey, Rilling, Aronson, Nystrom, & Cohen, 2003). The insula is a brain region that is often associated with negative emotional states (Calder, Lawrence, & Young, 2001; Damasio et al., 2000). In the study by Sanfey et al. (2003), activity in the anterior insula is greater when participants in the ultimatum game are offered unfair instead of fair splits of money. Furthermore, activity in this brain area was predictive of the decision to reject unfair offers, with rejections associated with significantly higher activation than acceptances. The anterior insula has been suggested to encode the social interaction as aversive, serving to discourage trust and positive responses (Sanfey, 2007), or, alternatively, to encode the degree of unfairness of the other's offer, that is, how much the offer differs from some norm (Montague & Lohrenz, 2007).

Anterior Cingulate Cortex. Activity in the anterior cingulate cortex (ACC), a brain area involved in processing signals that register as a risk (Ridderinkhof, Ullsperger, Crone, & Nieuwenhuis, 2004), is also involved in the decision to accept or reject unfair offers in the ultimatum game (Sanfey et al., 2003). The ACC is known for its role in cognitive conflict and its activation may reflect the tension between cognitive and emotional motivations when persons consider rejecting an unfair offer. Using an iterated trust game, Tomlin et al. (2006) found two distinct agent-specific response types in the ACC, one consistent with decisions that signal 'me' and another consistent with decisions that signal 'not me.'

Dorsolateral Prefrontal Cortex. Besides the influence of emotional states on the decision to accept or reject unfair behavior (as reflected by insular activity), cognitive processes are also of importance in this decision. Sanfey et al. (2003) observed that the dorsolateral prefrontal cortex (DLPFC), a region usually linked to cognitive control processes such as goal maintenance (Miller & Cohen, 2001), plays a role during the ultimatum game. Possibly, competition between the anterior insula and the DLPFC is important in the decision to accept or reject an unfair offer. Activity in the DLPFC was higher than activity in the anterior insula when participants decided to accept unfair offers, while unfair offers that were rejected showed instead greater activity in the insula than in the DLPFC.

Studies using transcranial magnetic stimulation (TMS) have elaborated on the role of the DLPFC in the decision to accept or reject unfair behavior (Knoch, Pascual-Leone, Meyer, Treyer, & Fehr, 2006; van 't Wout, Kahn, Sanfey, & Aleman, 2005). These studies suggest that the DLPFC is involved in overriding selfish impulses in order to reject offers that are perceived as unfair. Disrupting brain activity in the DLPFC by the administration of a brief TMS pulse caused a greater number of unfair offers to be accepted in this group of participants compared to the control group.[23]

3.2.3. Beneficial Behavior – Care about the Other's Welfare

Both processes discussed so far, the ability to reason about one's partner's intentions and the impulse that determines if a social tie may start to develop, are important for the development of a social tie between participants in the public good game. Neural correlates of these processes have been suggested. However, what happens in the brain when one indeed has started to care about the other player?

ACC and Insula. Results of an experimental study with an iterated one-shot trust game by Singer et al. (2006) showed that neuronal activity in the ACC and in the anterior insula are modulated as a function of whether the subjects liked or disliked their partner in the game. In the second part of this experiment, participants observed partners who had played fair and unfair strategies (i.e., reciprocated with large and small amounts, respectively) receiving painful stimulation. Unfair players were rated as less likeable than fair players. Activity in pain-related brain areas (the anterior insula and the ACC) was attenuated by the knowledge that an unfair player was in pain. The finding that responses to fair and unfair behavior are related to the affective feelings one has towards another lends support to the notion that brain activity in the public good game may be modulated as a function of a social tie.[24] In this respect, the activation of the anterior insula might be a case in point. Its putative role in risk prediction (Knutson & Bossaerts, 2007; Kuhnen & Knutson, 2005) and in signaling norm violations (Montague & Lohrenz, 2007) suggests that under the formation of a positive social tie its role in social decision-making will diminish,[25] whereas under the formation of a negative social tie it will be more active. The latter is suggested also by the role of anterior insula activation in frustration (Abler, Walter, & Erk, 2005).

Orbitofrontal Cortex. Arranging and experiencing mutual cooperation in economic interactions has been related to the reception of reward. Cooperative behavior in an iterated one-shot prisoner's dilemma game has been found to elicit increased activity in reward-related areas such as the striatum (caudate nucleus, nucleus accumbens, and putamen), the ventromedial prefrontal cortex (VMPFC), and the orbitofrontal cortex (OFC) (Rilling et al., 2002; Rilling et al., 2004b). These areas receive mesencephalic dopamine projections and play an essential role in the processing of rewards, such as food, drugs, sex, and money (Moll, Zahn, De Oliveira-Souza, Krueger, & Grafman, 2005; Schultz, Dayan, & Montague, 1997; Tanaka et al., 2004). Regarding the OFC, there is general agreement on a medial to lateral functional specialization within the OFC on behavior that is related to reward and punishment. The lateral OFC has been linked to punishment and associated with social aversion (Kringelbach, 2005; Moll et al., 2005). The medial part of the OFC is suggested to be more important for reward-related behavior (Kringelbach, 2005). Although the OFC was activated during cooperation in the prisoner's dilemma game, its response was not dependent on the context, that is, whether the partner was a computer or a human being. In contrast, increased activation in the striatum and VMPFC after a cooperative outcome was only elicited when a human partner reciprocated cooperation, but not in the case of a computer partner (or when an equivalent amount of money was simply provided). These results indicate that successful interaction with human partners is particularly rewarding.[26]

Striatum and Septal Area. Activation of the striatum is modulated by several factors that might be related to the strength of social ties. For instance, Fließbach et al. (2007) showed that responses in the ventral striatum are modulated by social comparison. Rewards that were equal in absolute magnitude elicited smaller responses in the striatum when the reward was less than that received by a second person. Harbaugh, Mayr, and Burghart (2007) observed that donations to charity goals elicit activity in the ventral striatum, but more so when these donations were voluntary than when they were mandatory. Moreover, the striatal response to the charity's financial gains predicted voluntary giving.

Delgado, Frank, and Phelps (2005) examined how prior social and moral information about someone modulated striatal activity. They replicated earlier findings in that activity in the caudate nucleus differentiated between reciprocated and unreciprocated cooperation in the trust game (cf. Rilling et al., 2004b). However, when information was provided about the character of the partner, either good or bad, this differential response in the striatum between positive and negative feedback was absent. This suggests that perceptions of moral character can diminish reliance on feedback mechanisms in an area that is involved in social reward learning.

More generally, the striatum is seen as part of a modality-independent network of reward structures that is specialized to mediate attachment (Bartels & Zeki, 2004, see also above). This network is generally rich in receptors of oxytocin, a neuropeptide that is well-known for its relationship with attachment and caring behavior (Insel & Young, 2001).[27] Zak, Stanton, and Ahmadi (2007) found that participants infused (via nasal administration) with oxytocin exhibited greater generosity in dictator as well as ultimatum games.[28] Kosfeld, Heinrichs, Zak, Fischbacher, and Fehr (2005), using a similar technique, found a substantial increase in trusting behavior in a trust game, but no difference in the acceptance of financial risks, suggesting an essential role for oxytocin as biological basis for a pro-social approach.

In their reciprocal trust game study, Krueger et al. (2007) observed for non-defectors (who never defected on the partner's decision to trust), after a 'building' stage where the paracingulate cortex was relatively active, that their unconditional trust selectively activated the septal area (relative to defectors) during the subsequent 'maintenance' stage. This brain region, linked to social memory and learning, contains oxytocin receptors and is putatively involved in controlling the release of oxytocin.[29] Furthermore, behavioral ratings revealed that only non-defector pairs felt closer to each other and ranked themselves as being more of a partner to the other person after the experiment. According to the authors, this brain area may be involved in encoding goodwill. Also, some evidence exists showing that oxytocin can be enhanced by receiving signals of trust in a trust game, which in turn may lead to greater trustworthiness (Zak, Kurzban, & Matzner, 2005).

3.3. Neural Bases of Social Ties: Some Speculations

Based on the findings summarized in the previous subsection, it seems that a social tie can show up in various ways. In general, it may manifest itself in an increased activation in some brain region (like the striatum), in a changing timing and/or location of the activation within some region (like the striatum with learning[30]), in the involvement of new regions (like the septal area, linked to attachment), or a diminished involvement of some regions (like the paracingulate cortex). Regarding the last point, Bartels and Zeki (2004) speak of human attachment as a 'push-pull mechanism' that overcomes social distance by deactivating neural networks used for critical social judgment and negative emotions while bonding individuals through the reward circuitry. Therefore, it seems likely that the weight that is attached to the well-being of another person is represented by a compound neural network rather than some specific brain area. Nevertheless, some brain regions may be critical, like the amygdala and the VMPFC that appear to be essential for the activation and successful integration of emotion-related memories (e.g., of sanctions) in the anticipation of future consequences of actions (see e.g., Bechara & Damasio, 2005; Güroğlu et al., 2008).

Although we do not know at this stage what this network precisely looks like, we can speculate regarding its nature, under the usual caveat implied by such speculations. We assume, for simplicity, two players in a public good game who are initially complete strangers to each other (no existing ties), and we neglect any social value orientation (we will return to that later). Furthermore, for expositional reasons, we focus on the development of a positive tie.

Our discussion in the previous subsection suggests three key facets of the development of an affective social tie: perspective taking, appraisal, and care.[31] Particularly in the beginning of the game, players are likely to be engaged with fathoming the situation the other is in and what the other will think. Two brain areas have been particularly associated with this 'mentalizing,' the APCC and the pSTS. Behavioral expectations on the basis of norms or other reference levels may be generated. In terms of the simple ties model presented in section 2, this might shape the tolerance or reference level ε_A (see Eq. (2)). Appraisals of the other's behavior during the game in light of one's concerns (including internalized norms) and adjusting beliefs are important for the further cognitive and affective encoding of the signals extracted from the social interaction. Brain areas expected to be particularly involved in these appraisal processes are related to reward prediction and learning (striatum), norm violations (anterior insula), cognition-emotion conflict (ACC), and cognitive control (DLPFC). In the formal model this facet of tie formation is, as a first approach, represented in a simplistic way by the 'impulse' G_A. Personality traits (e.g., related to emotionality) may cause a substantial heterogeneity among individuals in the way these appraisals are made and elaborated. Both processes of perspective taking and appraisal, finally, may set in motion a growing appreciation (care) for the concerns of the partner in the game, which is represented in the model by the (stock) variable α_A attached to the utility of the other individual. Brain areas presumably implicated once an individual has started to (positively) care about the other individual[32] are the striatum, the VMPFC,[33] and the septal area. In the next, concluding section several issues for future research will be indicated.

4. CONCLUDING REMARKS

In this article we have addressed the economic importance, formalization, and the psychological and neural correlates of affective social ties. We hope to have shown the promising nature of this topic and conclude with some important issues for future research.

First of all, it is now important to link up the parameters of formal models of social ties with neural activity, for example, through model-based fMRI studies. In this way, a systematic and empirical data-based approach is obtained that lends itself for the generation of a coherent set of hypotheses and the development of a well-founded neuroeconomics of social ties.

Secondly, a dynamic model of social ties is needed because emotion is all about transition and more related to homeodynamics (behavioral adjustment) than homeostasis (Damasio, 2003). In this respect, the dual-system vDvW-model discussed above seems a good starting point for the study of voluntary public good provision. However, a more flexible model, for example, allowing for some foresight or the influence of moods or personality traits, may be desirable.

Thirdly, because the state of the art in neuroeconomics is such that no definitive answers are to be expected from whichever method or technique one uses, it is important to exploit as many research tools as possible. This includes not only various neuroscientific techniques like TMS, physiological measures (e.g., skin conductance or heart rate), the administration of substances (like oxytocin), or the use of individuals with brain lesions, but also questionnaires (e.g., for the measurement of traits, particular emotional states, or expectations). Furthermore, the simultaneous investigation of interacting brains through hyperscanning may deliver important additional information, for example, in relation to the issue of oneness in case of social ties (Krueger et al., 2007). In the context of social ties, oneness (or 'me-other' merger) would seem to imply that one's own payoff should show up as being similarly rewarding as the other's payoff. However, the fact that one cares about the other also implies that, when appropriate, one tries to figure out what is best for the other, involving perspective taking and mentalizing, which means a differentiation between self and even a close other (cf. Heatherton et al., 2006).

Fourthly, among the important (additional) issues to be studied are the impact of the mode and the frequency of interaction. For example, to what extent is interaction with others through political participation to provide a public good different from decentralized provision via voluntary contributions? Apart from the frequency of interaction, factors determining emotional intensity, such as proximity and anonymity, would seem to be important here.

Another interesting issue concerns the equilibration of a social tie. The vDvW-model allows for an equilibrium state with a social tie, where the decay of the tie is just compensated by the impulse. However, if emotion is indeed all about transition and homeodynamics, it is not immediately clear whether an affective tie is compatible with an equilibrium state where nothing unexpected happens. This is not the place to go more deeply into this issue. Note, however, that the incorporation of randomness in the model – which may be appropriate because of the stochasticity in neural firing rates, for example (Glimcher, Dorris, & Bayer, 2005) – would imply some unpredictability of behavior.

Fifthly, what is the relationship, if any, between social value orientation and social ties? To what extent is it simply an aggregate (weighted) representation of one's (past and present) social ties?[34]

Finally, in view of the observed similarities between romantic love and addiction regarding the use of reward structures in the brain, it seems of interest to investigate the (dis)similarities between addiction and different forms of attachment, including social ties. In all these cases, affective impulses (like an investment) are feeding an intertemporal stock variable. On a different and more speculative note, a similar production process seems to take place in case of the internalization of a social norm, where through the application of sanctions (punishments and rewards) a concern or interest is instilled in the individual. Therefore, it might be interesting to include the internalization of norms into this investigation as well.

NOTES

1. An exception is Loewenstein and O'Donoghue's (2007) dual-system model of altruism.

2. In the standard model the individually optimal contribution level need not be zero (but falls short of the socially optimal level).

3. Regarding outcome-based models, see Fehr and Schmidt (1999), Bolton and Ockenfels (2000). For intention-based models, see Rabin (1993), Dufwenberg and Kirchsteiger (2004). For mixed models, see Charness and Rabin (2002), Falk and Fischbacher (2006). Levine (1998) presents a 'types' model.

4. Without loss of generality, we use here a logarithmic transformation of the multiplicative Cobb–Douglas specification in the vDvW-model. Note furthermore that if V_B would be substituted for U_B in Eq. (1) the model's results mentioned below would not be affected in a qualitative sense.

5. For simplicity, we neglect for the moment the possibility of a general attitude towards other people, which is to be distinguished from a social tie concerning a specific other person. See the next subsection.

6. Cox, Friedman, and Gjerstad (2007) apply a (CES) generalization of this specification to the data sets of several experimental studies concerning a variety of games (other than public good games). Their estimates show that in most cases (5 out of 7) a Cobb–Douglas specification cannot be rejected. For a similarly specified model incorporating emotions, see van Winden (2001).

7. This also holds for the model of Cox et al. (2007) where α (the 'emotional state') is supposed to depend on a reciprocity variable (related to payoffs) and relative status.

8. See e.g., Homans (1950), Frijda (1986), Coleman (1990), and the wealth of studies surveyed in Baumeister and Leary (1995).

9. Reprinted from Frans van Dijk and Frans van Winden (1997), with permission from Elsevier.

10. Furthermore, an interior equilibrium, with $g_j > 0$, is assumed if $\alpha_j = 0$.

11. Same as footnote 9.

12. Because van Dijk and van Winden (1997) prove that the equilibrium of their model is locally stable (based on the Jacobean of the system at its equilibrium), in general, convergence is (only) assured for 'small' departures from the equilibrium.

13. Reprinted from Joep Sonnemans et al. (2006), with permission from Elsevier.

14. By applying this procedure to a control group, which faced an individual decision task without social interaction between the two tests, van Dijk et al. (2002) found the Ring-test to be a reliable test also in this context.

15. In this experiment each participant, randomly matched with another participant, received an endowment of 10 markers to be allocated to a private account (with a monetary payoff of $28*i - i^2$ cents for i markers) and a public account (with a fixed payoff of 14 cents per marker); in addition there was a fixed cost of 110 cents. This game was repeated for a fixed number of rounds, with the same partner. Assuming rational and selfish players, the game has an interior Nash-equilibrium where 7 markers are put in the private account, and the remainder of the endowment is put in the public account (for any endowment larger than 7), whereas contributing all markers to the public account is group optimal (efficient).

16. Another interesting observation is that in an experiment with unequal endowments (with one player having 8 markers and the other player 12 markers) they found that the contributions by participants with the higher endowment (in excess of the Nash-equilibrium prediction) were significantly less, in line with the predictions of the vDvW-model.

17. The results also plead against inequity aversion. In only 4% of the cases positive–negative combinations of sentiments are observed, while such combinations should occur if indeed a participant with large earnings in the game (a free rider) would typically give (+) to a little earning participant (who contributed a lot) and the latter would typically take (–) from the former.

18. Another important issue that is awaiting investigation is to what extent behavior indeed converges as suggested by the model.

19. Subjects only learned the nature of a specific part of the experiment once that part started.

20. A prisoner's dilemma game can be seen as a simple two-player public good game with only two choices available to the players, either to 'cooperate' (equivalent to contributing one's endowment to the public good)) or to 'defect' (not contributing to the public good).

21. Later, Edgeworth (1881) called a parameter similar to our α a 'coefficient of effective sympathy,' in a footnote (p. 53) in his classic book *Mathematical Psychics*.

22. An ultimatum game is a two-player game where one player gets the opportunity to make an offer regarding the division of an amount of money given by the experimenter and the other player can either accept or reject. In the latter case both players get nothing (Güth, Schmittberger, & Schwarze, 1982).

23. As noted by Knoch et al. (2006), these findings run counter to the interpretation of Sanfey et al. (2003) that the DLPFC is crucial in overriding fairness impulses (to reject unfair offers).

24. In fact, in male participants the effect was accompanied by increased activity in reward-related areas (striatum), which was correlated with an expressed desire for revenge. These findings are suggestive of a negative tie, as these participants appear to experience the loss in well-being of the person in pain as rewarding.

25. Instead, evidence from studies on maternal and romantic love relationships points at a potentially increasing role of the medial insula in that case (Aron et al., 2005; Bartels & Zeki, 2004). The medial insula is considered to be a pathway for 'limbic touch,' evoking pleasant feelings of touch and regulating affiliative responses.

26. This finding may be related to a positive social tie, because an extra reward is obtained from the presence of a human partner with whom one interacted successfully. Using fMRI with a social interaction simulation task, Güroğlu et al. (2008) find that interacting with friends specifically involves the VMPFC and the nucleus accumbens. In addition, they find friend-specific involvement of the amygdala and the hippocampus, which may indicate the spontaneously greater retrieval of emotionally salient memories in case of the interaction with friends.

27. Oxytocin is also implicated in addiction. There seem to be similar pathways for social attachment and psychostimulants (Insel & Young, 2001).

28. A dictator game differs from an ultimatum game in that the second mover can only accept what the first player 'proposes.'

29. From a learning perspective, it is interesting to note that whereas the septal area as well as the pallidum have been found to play a role in early-stage romantic love relationships, the pallidum appeared to gain in importance in relationships of longer duration (Aron et al., 2005; Bartels & Zeki, 2004).

30. Regarding the former, see King-Casas et al. (2005), and, with respect to the latter, Haruno and Kawato (2006).

31. The neural circuits involved in perspective taking and appraisal will likely involve common areas irrespective of whether the social tie will develop positively or negatively. Below we will speculate on the potentially differential involvement of brain areas in the third phase of positive and negative tie formation.

32. We can speculate that the development of negative ties involves several areas. First, as in positive tie formation, the striatum is expected to be involved as it detects unreciprocated cooperation in the trust game (Delgado et al., 2005; Rilling et al., 2004b). Also, increased activity of the striatum was correlated with observed physical pain in a disliked individual (Singer et al., 2006), suggesting a rewarding experience (like 'sweet' revenge), as one would expect in case of a negative tie. Second, as the anterior insula is implicated in signaling norm violations (Montague & Lohrenz, 2007) and in encoding aversive interaction (Sanfey, 2007), it is likely to be more active under the formation of negative social ties, as suggested also by the role of anterior insula activation in frustration (Abler et al., 2005).

33. A recent study (Jenkins, Macrae, & Mitchell, 2008) suggests that the VMPFC is similarly engaged by mentalizing about oneself as by mentalizing about similar others. To the extent that a positive tie makes people feel more similar this finding would add to the role of the VMPFC.

34. For some empirical support, see van Lange, Agnew, Harinck, and Steemers (1997).

ACKNOWLEDGMENTS

Support by the Netherlands Organisation for Scientific Research (NWO) and the European Union through the research network ENABLE is gratefully acknowledged. We are further thankful to an anonymous referee and participants of the Arne Ryde Workshop on Neuroeconomics (Lund), in particular our discussants Georgio Coricelli and Erik Mohlin, for their useful comments.

REFERENCES

Abler, B., Walter, H., & Erk, S. (2005). Neural correlates of frustration. *Neuroreport*, *16*(7), 669–672.

Allison, T., Puce, A., & McCarthy, G. (2000). Social perception from visual cues: Role of the STS region. *Trends in Cognitive Sciences*, *4*(7), 267–278.

Aron, A., Fisher, H., Mashek, D. J., Strong, G., Li, H., & Brown, L. L. (2005). Reward, motivation, and emotion systems associated with early-stage intense romantic love. *Journal of Neurophysiology*, *94*(1), 327–337.

Baron-Cohen, S., Ring, H. A., Wheelwright, S., Bullmore, E. T., Brammer, M. J., Simmons, A., & Williams, S. C. (1999). Social intelligence in the normal and autistic brain: An fMRI study. *European Journal of Neuroscience*, *11*(6), 1891–1898.

Bartels, A., & Zeki, S. (2004). The neural correlates of maternal and romantic love. *Neuroimage*, *21*(3), 1155–1166.

Baumeister, R. F., & Leary, M. R. (1995). The need to belong: Desire for interpersonal attachments as a fundamental human motivation. *Psychological Bulletin*, *117*(3), 497–529.

Bechara, A., & Damasio, A. R. (2005). The somatic marker hypothesis: A neural theory of economic decision. *Games and Economic Behavior*, *52*(2), 336–372.

Ben-Shakhar, G., Bornstein, G., Hopfensitz, A., & van Winden, F. (2007). Reciprocity and emotions in bargaining using physiological and self-report measures. *Journal of Economic Psychology*, *28*(3), 314–323.

Bergstrom, T., Blume, L., & Varian, H. (1986). On the private provision of public goods. *Journal of Public Economics*, *29*(1), 25–49.

Berscheid, E., & Reiss, H. T. (1998). Attraction and close relationships. In: T. Gilbert, S. T. Fiske & G. Lindzey (Eds), *The handbook of social psychology* (4th ed., pp. 193–281). New York: Mc Graw-Hill.

Bolton, G. E., & Ockenfels, A. (2000). ERC: A theory of equity, reciprocity, and competition. *The American Economic Review*, *90*(1), 166–193.

Brandts, J., Riedl, A., & van Winden, F. (2007). *On competition and well-being: An experimental investigation into rivalry, social disposition and subjective well-being*. Working paper, University of Amsterdam.

Brunet, E., Sarfati, Y., Hardy-Bayle, M. C., & Decety, J. (2000). A PET investigation of the attribution of intentions with a nonverbal task. *Neuroimage*, *11*(2), 157–166.

Calder, A. J., Lawrence, A. D., & Young, A. W. (2001). Neuropsychology of fear and loathing. *Nature Reviews Neuroscience*, *2*(5), 352–363.

Camerer, C., Loewenstein, G., & Prelec, D. (2005). Neuroeconomics: How neuroscience can inform economics. *Journal of Economic Literature*, *43*(1), 9–64.

Castelli, F., Happe, F., Frith, U., & Frith, C. (2000). Movement and mind: A functional imaging study of perception and interpretation of complex intentional movement patterns. *NeuroImage*, *12*(3), 314–325.

Charness, G., & Rabin, M. (2002). Understanding social preferences with simple tests. *The Quarterly Journal of Economics*, *117*(3), 817–889.

Cialdini, R. B., Brown, S. L., Lewis, B. P., Luce, C., & Neuberg, S. L. (1997). Reinterpreting the empathy-altruism relationship: When one into one equals oneness. *Journal of Personality and Social Psychology*, *73*(3), 481–494.

Coleman, J. S. (1990). *Foundations of Social Theory*. Cambridge: Harvard University Press.

Cox, J. C., Friedman, D., & Gjerstad, S. (2007). A tractable model of reciprocity and fairness. *Games and Economic Behavior*, *59*(1), 17–45.

Cox, J. C., & Sadiraj, V. (2007). On modeling voluntary contributions to public goods. *Public Finance Review*, *35*(2), 311–332.

Damasio, A. R. (2003). *Looking for Spinoza: Joy, sorrow and the feeling brain*. Orlando, FL: Harcourt.

Damasio, A. R., Grabowski, T. J., Bechara, A., Damasio, H., Ponto, L. L., Parvizi, J., & Hichwa, R. D. (2000). Subcortical and cortical brain activity during the feeling of self-generated emotions. *Nature Neuroscience*, *3*(10), 1049–1056.

Dawes, C. T., Fowler, J. H., Johnson, T., McElreath, R., & Smirnov, O. (2007). Egalitarian motives in humans. *Nature*, *446*(7137), 794–796.

De Vignemont, F., & Singer, T. (2006). The empathic brain: How, when and why? *Trends in Cognitive Sciences*, *10*(10), 435–441.

Decety, J., & Chaminade, T. (2003). Neural correlates of feeling sympathy. *Neuropsychologia*, *41*(2), 127–138.

Decety, J., & Hodges, S. D. (2006). The social neuroscience of empathy. In: P. A. M. van Lange (Ed.), *Bridging social psychology: Benefits of transdisciplinary approaches* (pp. 103–109). Mahwah: Erlbaum.

Delgado, M. R., Frank, R. H., & Phelps, E. A. (2005). Perceptions of moral character modulate the neural systems of reward during the trust game. *Nature Neuroscience*, *8*(11), 1611–1618.

Dufwenberg, M., & Kirchsteiger, G. (2004). A theory of sequential reciprocity. *Games and Economic Behavior*, *47*(2), 268–298.

Edgeworth, F. Y. (1881). *Mathematical psychics*. London: Kegan Paul.

Elster, J. (1998). Emotions and economic theory. *Journal of Economic Literature*, *36*(1), 47–74.

Falk, A., & Fischbacher, U. (2006). A theory of reciprocity. *Games and Economic Behavior*, *54*(2), 293–315.

Fehr, E., & Camerer, C. F. (2007). Social neuroeconomics: The neural circuitry of social preferences. *Trends in Cognitive Sciences*, *11*(10), 419–427.

Fehr, E., & Schmidt, K. M. (1999). A theory of fairness, competition, and cooperation. *The Quarterly Journal of Economics*, *114*(3), 817–868.

Fehr, E., & Schmidt, K. M. (2005). *The economics of fairness, reciprocity and altruism-Experimental evidence and new theories*. Working paper, University of Zurich.

Fließbach, K., Weber, B., Trautner, P., Dohmen, T., Sunde, U., Elger, C. E., & Falk, A. (2007). Social comparison affects reward-related brain activity in the human ventral striatum. *Science*, *318*(5854), 1305–1308.

Frijda, N. H. (1986). *The emotions*. Cambridge: Cambridge University Press.

Fudenberg, D., & Tirole, J. (1991). *Game theory*. Cambridge: MIT Press.

Gallagher, H. L., & Frith, C. D. (2003). Functional imaging of 'theory of mind'. *Trends in Cognitive Sciences*, *7*(2), 77–83.

Gallagher, H. L., Happe, F., Brunswick, N., Fletcher, P. C., Frith, U., & Frith, C. D. (2000). Reading the mind in cartoons and stories: an fMRI study of 'theory of mind' in verbal and nonverbal tasks. *Neuropsychologia*, *38*(1), 11–21.

Gallagher, H. L., Jack, A. I., Roepstorff, A., & Frith, C. D. (2002). Imaging the intentional stance in a competitive game. *Neuroimage*, *16*(3 Pt 1), 814–821.

Glimcher, P. W., Dorris, M. C., & Bayer, H. M. (2005). Physiological utility theory and the neuroeconomics of choice. *Games and Economic Behavior*, *52*(2), 213–256.

Goeree, J. K., Holt, C. A., & Laury, S. K. (2002). Private costs and public benefits: Unraveling the effects of altruism and noisy behavior. *Journal of Public Economics*, *83*(2), 255–276.

Granovetter, M. S. (1973). The strength of weak ties. *The American Journal of Sociology*, *78*(6), 1360–1380.

Granovetter, M. S. (1985). Economic action and social structure: The problem of embeddedness. *The American Journal of Sociology*, *91*(3), 481–510.

Güroğlu, B., Haselager, G. J., van Lieshout, C. F., Takashima, A., Rijpkema, M., & Fernandez, G. (2008). Why are friends special? Implementing a social interaction simulation task to probe the neural correlates of friendship. *Neuroimage*, *39*(2), 903–910.

Güth, W., Schmittberger, R., & Schwarze, B. (1982). An experimental analysis of ultimatum bargaining. *Journal of Economic Behavior & Organization*, *3*(4), 367–388.

Harbaugh, W. T., Mayr, U., & Burghart, D. R. (2007). Neural responses to taxation and voluntary giving reveal motives for charitable donations. *Science*, *316*(5831), 1622–1625.

Haruno, M., & Kawato, M. (2006). Different neural correlates of reward expectation and reward expectation error in the putamen and caudate nucleus during stimulus-action-reward association learning. *Journal of Neurophysiology*, *95*(2), 948–959.

Heatherton, T. F., Wyland, C. L., Macrae, C. N., Demos, K. E., Denny, B. T., & Kelley, W. M. (2006). Medial prefrontal activity differentiates self from close others. *Social Cognitive and Affective Neuroscience*, *1*(1), 18–25.

Homans, G. C. (1950). *The human group*. New York: Harcourt, Brace and World.

Insel, T. R., & Young, L. J. (2001). The neurobiology of attachment. *Nature Reviews Neuroscience*, *2*(2), 129–136.

Jenkins, A. C., Macrae, C. N., & Mitchell, J. P. (2008). Repetition suppression of ventromedial prefrontal activity during judgments of self and others. *Proceedings of the National Academy of Sciences USA*, *105*(11), 4507–4512.

Keser, C., & van Winden, F. (2000). Conditional cooperation and voluntary contributions to public goods. *Scandinavion Journal of Economics*, *102*(1), 23–39.

King-Casas, B., Tomlin, D., Anen, C., Camerer, C. F., Quartz, S. R., & Montague, P. R. (2005). Getting to know you: reputation and trust in a two-person economic exchange. *Science*, *308*(5718), 78–83.

Knoch, D., Pascual-Leone, A., Meyer, K., Treyer, V., & Fehr, E. (2006). Diminishing reciprocal fairness by disrupting the right prefrontal cortex. *Science*, *314*(5800), 829–832.

Knutson, B., & Bossaerts, P. (2007). Neural antecedents of financial decisions. *Journal of Neuroscience*, *27*(31), 8174–8177.

Kosfeld, M., Heinrichs, M., Zak, P. J., Fischbacher, U., & Fehr, E. (2005). Oxytocin increases trust in humans. *Nature*, *435*(7042), 673–676.

Kreps, D. M., Milgrom, P., Roberts, J., & Wilson, R. (1982). Rational cooperation in the finitely repeated prisoners' dilemma. *Journal of Economic Theory*, *27*(2), 245–252.

Kringelbach, M. L. (2005). The human orbitofrontal cortex: Linking reward to hedonic experience. *Nature Reviews Neuroscience*, *6*(9), 691–702.

Krueger, F., McCabe, K., Moll, J., Kriegeskorte, N., Zahn, R., Strenziok, M., Heinecke, A., & Grafman, J. (2007). Neural correlates of trust. *Proceedings of the National Academy of Sciences USA*, *104*(50), 20084–20089.

Kuhnen, C. M., & Knutson, B. (2005). The neural basis of financial risk taking. *Neuron*, *47*(5), 763–770.

Lamm, C., Batson, C. D., & Decety, J. (2007). The neural substrate of human empathy: Effects of perspective-taking and cognitive appraisal. *Journal of Cognitive Neuroscience*, *19*(1), 42–58.

Ledyard, J. (1995). *Public goods: A survey of experimental research*. Princeton: Princeton University Press.

Levine, D. K. (1998). Modeling altruism and spitefulness in experiments. *Review of Economic Dynamics*, *1*(3), 593–622.

Liebrand, W. B. G. (1984). The effect of social motives, communication and group size on behaviour in an N-person multi-stage mixed-motive game. *European Journal of Social Psychology*, *14*(3), 239–264.

Loewenstein, G. (1996). Out of control: Visceral influences on behavior. *Organizational Behavior and Human Decision Processes*, *65*(3), 272–292.

Loewenstein, G. (2000). Emotions in economic theory and economic behavior. *The American Economic Review*, *90*(2), 426–432.

Loewenstein, G., & O'Donoghue, T. (2007). *The heat of the moment: Modeling interactions between affect and deliberation*. Working paper, Carnegie Mellon University.

Loewenstein, G., & Schkade, D. (1999). Wouldn't it be nice? Predicting future feelings. In: D. Kahneman, E. Diener & N. Schwartz (Eds), *Well being: The foundations of hedonic psychology*. New York: Russell Sage Foundation.

Maner, J. K., Luce, C. L., Neuberg, S. L., Cialdini, R. B., Brown, S., & Sagarin, B. J. (2002). The effects of perspective taking on motivations for helping: Still no evidence for altruism. *Personality and Social Psychology Bulletin*, *28*(11), 1601–1610.

McCabe, K., Houser, D., Ryan, L., Smith, V., & Trouard, T. (2001). A functional imaging study of cooperation in two-person reciprocal exchange. *Proceedings of the National Academy of Sciences USA*, *98*(20), 11832–11835.

Miller, E. K., & Cohen, J. D. (2001). An integrative theory of prefrontal cortex function. *Annual Review of Neuroscience*, *24*(No.), 167–202.

Moll, J., Zahn, R., De Oliveira-Souza, R., Krueger, F., & Grafman, J. (2005). Opinion: The neural basis of human moral cognition. *Nature Reviews Neuroscience*, *6*(10), 799–809.

Montague, P. R., & Lohrenz, T. (2007). To detect and correct: Norm violations and their enforcement. *Neuron*, *56*(1), 14–18.

Rabin, M. (1993). Incorporating fairness into game theory and economics. *The American Economic Review*, *83*(5), 1281–1302.

Ridderinkhof, K. R., Ullsperger, M., Crone, E. A., & Nieuwenhuis, S. (2004). The role of the medial frontal cortex in cognitive control. *Science*, *306*(5695), 443–447.

Rilling, J., Gutman, D., Zeh, T., Pagnoni, G., Berns, G., & Kilts, C. (2002). A neural basis for social cooperation. *Neuron*, *35*(2), 395–405.

Rilling, J. K., Sanfey, A. G., Aronson, J. A., Nystrom, L. E., & Cohen, J. D. (2004a). The neural correlates of theory of mind within interpersonal interactions. *Neuroimage*, *22*(4), 1694–1703.

Rilling, J. K., Sanfey, A. G., Aronson, J. A., Nystrom, L. E., & Cohen, J. D. (2004b). Opposing BOLD responses to reciprocated and unreciprocated altruism in putative reward pathways. *Neuroreport*, *15*(16), 2539–2543.

Rusbult, C. E., & van Lange, P. A. M. (1996). Interdependence processes. In: E. T. Higgins & A. Kruglanski (Eds), *Social psychology: Handbook of basic principles* (pp. 564–596). New York: Guilford.

Rustichini, A. (2005). Neuroscience: Emotion and reason in making decisions. *Science*, *310*(5754), 1624–1625.

Sanfey, A. G. (2007). Social decision-making: Insights from game theory and neuroscience. *Science*, *318*(5850), 598–602.

Sanfey, A. G., Loewenstein, G., Mcclure, S. M., & Cohen, J. D. (2006). Neuroeconomics: Cross-currents in research on decision-making. *Trends in Cognitive Sciences*, *10*(3), 108–116.

Sanfey, A. G., Rilling, J. K., Aronson, J. A., Nystrom, L. E., & Cohen, J. D. (2003). The neural basis of economic decision-making in the Ultimatum Game. *Science*, *300*(5626), 1755–1758.

Sawyer, J. (1966). The altruism scale: A measure of co-operative, individualistic, and competitive interpersonal orientation. *The American Journal of Sociology*, *71*(4), 407–416.

Saxe, R. (2006). Uniquely human social cognition. *Current Opinion in Neurobiology*, *16*(2), 235–239.

Schultz, W., Dayan, P., & Montague, P. R. (1997). A neural substrate of prediction and reward. *Science*, *275*(5306), 1593–1599.

Singer, T., Seymour, B., O'Doherty, J. P., Stephan, K. E., Dolan, R. J., & Frith, C. D. (2006). Empathic neural responses are modulated by the perceived fairness of others. *Nature*, *439*(7075), 466–469.

Smith, A. (1759). *The theory of moral sentiments*. Indianapolis: Liberty Fund.

Sobel, J. (2005). Interdependent preferences and reciprocity. *Journal of Economic Literature*, *43*(2), 392–436.

Sonnemans, J., van Dijk, F., & van Winden, F. (2006). On the dynamics of social ties structures in groups. *Journal of Economic Psychology*, *27*(2), 187–204.

Tajfel, H., & Turner, J. C. (1986). The social identity of inter-group behavior. In: S. Worchel & L. W. Austin (Eds), *Psychology of intergroup relations*. Chicago: Nelson Hall.

Tanaka, S. C., Doya, K., Okada, G., Ueda, K., Okamoto, Y., & Yamawaki, S. (2004). Prediction of immediate and future rewards differentially recruits cortico-basal ganglia loops. *Nature Neuroscience*, *7*(8), 887–893.

Taylor, D. M., & Moghaddam, F. M. (1994). *Theories of intergroup relations: International social psychological perspectives*. New York: Praeger.

Tomlin, D., Kayali, M. A., King-Casas, B., Anen, C., Camerer, C. F., Quartz, S. R., & Montague, P. R. (2006). Agent-specific responses in the cingulate cortex during economic exchanges. *Science*, *312*(5776), 1047–1050.

van Dijk, F., Sonnemans, J., & van Winden, F. (2002). Social ties in a public good experiment. *Journal of Public Economics*, *85*(2), 275–299.

van Dijk, F., & van Winden, F. (1997). Dynamics of social ties and local public good provision. *Journal of Public Economics*, *64*(3), 323–341.

van Lange, P. A. M., Agnew, C. R., Harinck, F., & Steemers, G. E. M. (1997). From game theory to real life: How social value orientation affects willingness to sacrifice in ongoing close relationships. *Journal of Personality and Social Psychology*, *73*(6), 1330–1344.

van 't Wout, M., Kahn, R. S., Sanfey, A. G., & Aleman, A. (2005). Repetitive transcranial magnetic stimulation over the right dorsolateral prefrontal cortex affects strategic decision-making. *Neuroreport*, *16*(16), 1849–1852.

van Winden, F. (2001). Emotional hazard exemplified by taxation-induced anger. *Kyklos*, *54*(2-3), 491–506.

Zak, P. J., Kurzban, R., & Matzner, W. T. (2005). Oxytocin is associated with human trustworthiness. *Hormones and Behavior*, *48*(5), 522–527.

Zak, P. J., Stanton, A. A., & Ahmadi, S. (2007). Oxytocin increases generosity in humans. *PLoS ONE*, *2*(11), e1128.

EMOTION EXPRESSION, DECISION-MAKING AND WELL-BEING

Erte Xiao

ABSTRACT

Purpose – *This chapter discusses the role of emotion expression in decision-making. To understand connections between emotion and decision it is helpful first to differentiate between emotion experience and emotion expression. Understanding how emotion expression influences decision-making is important as a practical matter. However, in contrast to emotion experience, economic research has paid little attention to the significance of emotion expression in decision-making.*

Approach – *I review recent studies on emotion expression, paying specific attention to possible connections between emotion expression, punishment, fair economic exchange, and well-being.*

Practical implications – *In contrast to emotions, which are typically difficult to control, I suggest that opportunities for emotion expression can feasibly be manipulated through appropriately designed policies. I further suggest that this approach may have the ability to positively affect well-being and economic outcomes.*

Value of the *chapter – The chapter provides new perspectives on how policy-makers can benefit by understanding the effect of emotion expression in decision-making. The chapter also suggests future research to improve our understanding of emotion expression.*

Neuroeconomics
Advances in Health Economics and Health Services Research, Volume 20, 161–178

ISSN: 0731-2199/doi:10.1016/S0731-2199(08)20007-5

> *"I'm all tied up ... And tied up ... Yes! You said it! I'm all tied up inside!*
> *Okay! I'm all tied up inside ... and those dirty bombs mean that ...*
> *If I don't ... Untie myself inside the emotional knots ... I'm goanna explode!*
> *Yeah! Oh it's so simple! And so brilliant!*
> *Ok Doctor M.! I Get it!*
> *Baby Step. Untie your knots! Free! Free! Free!*
>
> – Bob Wiley in "What About Bob"

Humans differ from other creatures in the variety and complexity of their emotions. The existence of emotions means that individual decision-making is much more complicated than rationality theorists might hope. Consequently, a significant interdisciplinary effort has been undertaken to unravel the complexity of connections between emotion and decision (see, e.g. Frijda, 1986; Damasio 1994; Elster, 1999; Frank, 2002; Baumeister, Vohs, DeWall, & Zhang, 2007; Gigerenzer, 2007).

To understand connections between emotion and decision it is helpful to first differentiate between emotion experience and emotion expression. Emotion experience refers to the intrapersonal, internal response to an emotion-eliciting stimulus (see, Kennedy-Moore & Watson, 1999). For example, when a person is treated unfairly, the corresponding negative emotional reaction, such as anger or sadness, becomes part of her emotional experience. Economists in past decades have paid significant attention to the effect of emotion experience in decision-making (see, e.g. Loewenstein, 2000).

Emotion expression, however, refers to observable verbal and nonverbal behaviors that communicate and/or symbolize emotional experience. With or without self-awareness, individuals experiencing emotions often desire to express those emotions. This desire for emotion expression can also potentially affect decision-making. An implication, as we discuss below, is that the constraints on emotion expression can have behavioral consequences. This is especially true when one is consciously aware of the desire to express her feelings.[1]

In comparison to emotion experience, emotion expression is simpler to measure and quantify. As I discuss below, understanding how emotion expression influences decision-making is important as a practical matter. However, in contrast to emotional experience, economic research has paid much less attention to the significance of emotion expression in decision-making. In this chapter I discuss recent economic research on the behavioral consequences of the desire for emotion expression. I focus particularly on the area of social norms and stress potential implications for policy-making. Also, an inescapable aspect of emotion expression is its impact on health. For this reason I discuss implications of emotion expression for well-being.

EMOTION EXPRESSION AS A MOTIVE FOR PUNISHMENT

Economists study how incentives can be used to affect decisions and promote the efficient allocation of limited resources. In a social dilemma environment, the individual's self-interest conflicts with the interest of the broader community. For this reason, an individual often needs an exogenous incentive to encourage decisions that are consistent with the interest of society. Previous experimental research has shown that individuals often incur cost to punish self-interested behavior. In a public goods game, subjects often impose a costly punishment upon free-riders who do not cooperate (see, e.g. Fehr & Gächter, 2000). Further investigation has found that negative emotions seem to be a key motivation for such punishment (Masclet & Villeval, 2006).

Emotion is used to explain costly punishment behavior in ultimatum games. In this game, one subject (the proposer) starts with $20, for example. The other subject (the responder) begins with nothing. The proposer suggests dividing the $20 between the two subjects, and the responder decides whether to accept the proposed split. If the responder accepts the proposal, the money is split accordingly; if not, both subjects earn nothing. Consequently, an income-maximizing responder should accept any positive offer, and an income-maximizing proposer should offer the responder the smallest possible positive amount.

Nonetheless, decades of data from ultimatum games show that responders who are offered approximately 20% of the total amount choose to reject the offer about half the time. Rejection rates increase as the responder's proposed share becomes smaller (Camerer, 2003). Using an fMRI imaging study, Sanfey, Rilling, Aronson, Nystrom, and Cohen (2003) found that rejections are tightly connected to emotions.

Most of these studies, however, have focused on the experience of negative emotion as a source for punishment decisions. In those experiments, communication is usually not allowed. Subjects are also separated into different rooms from their counterpart during the experiment. These features ensure that individuals have no opportunity to express their emotions other than indirectly through the decisions they make in the experiment. This raises the question of the extent to which costly punishment behavior can be attributed to constraints on expressing negative emotion. Are people less likely to choose costly punishment when they can convey their feelings about misbehavior to wrong-doers in an alternative and less expensive way?

To investigate this question, Xiao and Houser (2005) conducted a version of the ultimatum game in which they allowed the responder to write a message to the proposer. The baseline of the experiment is the standard ultimatum game as previously described. Thus, in the standard treatment, rejecting or accepting the offer is the only way for the responder to display a reaction to her proposer about the offer. In the emotion expression treatment, everything is kept exactly the same as the baseline; however, the responder is allowed, not required, to write a message to the proposer at no pecuniary cost to themselves. Any message is delivered to the proposer concurrently with the responder's decision.

This Xiao and Houser (2005) design ensures that proposers make their decisions before they see the responders' messages. In addition, because all experiments take place anonymously, and because each pair of subjects plays the game exactly once, the messages can have no strategic implications. Rather, a message provides an opportunity for a responder to voluntarily express her feelings regarding her proposer's division decision.

Xiao and Houser's specific hypothesis is that responders in the emotion expression treatment will use written messages to express emotions, and also reject unfair offers less frequently than in the baseline treatment. They report support for this hypothesis. First, 87% of all responders wrote a message. The emotional content of these messages was evaluated in a new experiment with saliently rewarded participants who were blind to the research hypotheses. The results were that 79% (15 out of 19) of responders who received allocations of 20% or less wrote a message expressing negative emotions. When responders were offered at least half of the total amount, 81% (29 out of 36) displayed positive emotions.

Furthermore, rejection rates of unfair offers (20% of the surplus or less) were significantly lower in the emotion expression treatment than in the baseline treatment (32% vs. 60%, respectively, $p = 0.04$). Most of the data are from cases where the responder is offered 20% ($4). This occurs 14 times in the baseline, with 7 responders (50%) choosing to reject. In contrast, only 3 out of 15 responders (20%) do so in emotion expression treatment. This difference is statistically significant ($p = 0.05$, Fig. 1).

These data show that people seem more willing to accept pecuniary inequality when they can express emotions to their counterpart. When direct channels for emotion expression are either impossible or undesirable, humans might instead resort to indirect or even costly punishment methods to convey negative feelings. This highlights the importance of the desire of emotion expression in motivating behavior.

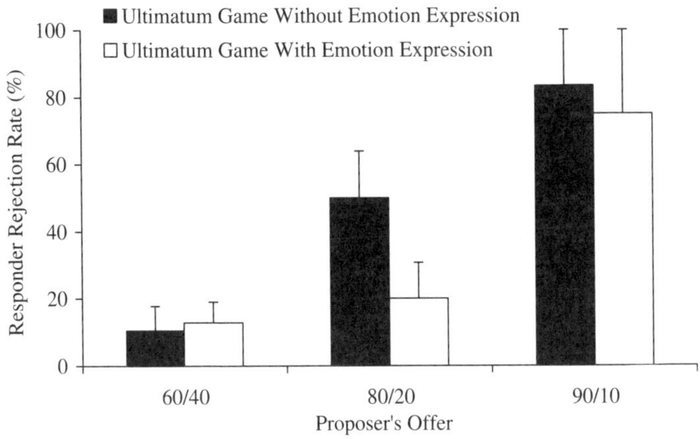

Fig. 1. Rejection Rates when Responders Offer Less than 50% (from Xiao & Houser, 2005).

As noted above, constraints on emotion expression are often a common feature of experimental environments, including highly studied trust, public goods, and bargaining games. These results raise the question of how the opportunity for emotion expression might change subjects' decisions. For example, subjects in public goods games are generally found to decrease their contribution to the public goods when others contribute little (see, e.g. Fehr & Gächter, 2000; Kurzban & Houser, 2005; Andreoni, 1990). If these decisions are partially motivated by a desire to express unhappiness to free-riders, then such reductions might be less common if subjects were provided an alternative way to express their feelings.

In addition to negative emotion expression, Xiao and Houser (2005) also found that about 80% of responders displayed positive emotions toward proposers when they received fair offers. Presumably, a demand to express positive emotions can also affect decisions. For example, in a typical "trust" game (see, e.g. Camerer & Weigelt, 1988; Berg, Dickhaut, & McCabe, 1995), where the investor transfers part of her endowment to a trustee, the only way for the trustee to say "thank you" is to reciprocate and return some amount to the investor. If this reciprocity is indeed motivated by human demand to express positive emotions (such as happiness or appreciation), then measured trustworthiness (amounts returned to investors by trustees) might decrease when trustees are given an alternative, less-costly channel to express their appreciation. It would be useful to more fully explore this area, particularly with efforts aimed at eliciting the "demand curve" for both positive and negative emotion expression.

The Xiao and Houser findings leave open the question of why emotion expression opportunities reduce the frequency of punishment. One possible answer is that expressive writing can help proposers mitigate their negative feelings (see, Pennebaker, 1997, for a review on expressive writing) and therefore make them less likely to punish. However, a survey conducted after the experiment indicated that most responders wrote the messages after they made their decisions. This suggests that a change of experienced emotion seems unlikely to be the explanation. Another possible reason is that responders believe accepting a low offer would be interpreted by the proposer as indicating acceptance of an inferior position. By expressing anger or disapproval toward the low offer, responders can deny this interpretation. However, if the interaction is anonymous and occurs only once, why does the responder care about how the proposer interprets her decision?

It is also possible that sending messages of disapproval directly to one's proposer might be a satisfying alternative form of punishment, and, due to this alternative form of punishment, the proposer will not decrease their offer to the responder even if they expect the responder is less likely to reject low offers. In fact, Xiao and Houser (2005) report the distribution of offers in the standard ultimatum game does not differ significantly from that in the emotion expression treatment. I next discuss studies which support the idea that expression of negative emotions such as anger or disapproval can work as an informal punishment to enforce norms such as fairness and cooperation.

EXPRESSION OF NEGATIVE EMOTIONS AS INFORMAL PUNISHMENT

Another interesting question is whether the expression of emotion would impose any effect on the recipient of emotion expression. Masclet, Noussair, Tucker, and Villeval (2003) conducted a lab experiment to test their hypothesis that peer-to-peer expressions of disapproval (referred to as non-monetary punishment) can promote cooperation in social dilemma environments. Subjects participated in a public goods experiment similar to those studied by Fehr and Gächter (2000). In one group, members could assign costly monetary fines to each other. The second game was identical, with the exception that punishment consisted of "disapproval points" instead of monetary fines. Participants were told that points represented the level of a sender's disapproval regarding a target's behavior. Participants also knew that disapproval points were costless to send, and receiving them had no payoff consequences. Masclet et al.'s key finding was that non-monetary sanctions had a significant positive impact on cooperation.

There are many reasons that emotion expression might promote cooperation. For example, in cases of repeated interaction, expressing emotion can be a method of communication, sending signals of members' intentions to coordinate with each other. The expressed disapproval or anger might also make the target individuals feel shame or guilt and therefore result in increased cooperation (see, e.g. Miller, Butts, & Rode, 2002; Masclet et al., 2003). The possibility I explore, however, is that emotional expressions of disapproval are an informal punishment that people prefer to avoid, and as such can perhaps be effective even in one-shot environments.

Disapproval avoidance seems plausible. The reason is that an individual who wants to selfishly maximize earnings might also be expected to feel guilt or shame from doing so. Cognitive dissonance theory (see, e.g. Festinger, 1957; Tesser & Achee, 1994; Aronson, 1995; Akerlof & Dickens, 1982; Rabin, 1994; Konow, 2000) posits that people experience an unpleasant "tension" stemming from these opposite motivations (a desire to maximize earnings vs. a belief in fairness). One strategy to reduce this tension is to self-deceive by manipulating one's own beliefs in such a way that guilt is reduced and selfishness is supported. For example, one could choose to believe that one's counterpart would make a selfish decision if the situations were reversed. However, if one knows her counterpart has an opportunity to express disapproval, and so reveal her true preferences, then it is no longer possible to avoid guilt by manipulating one's own beliefs.

Xiao and Houser (2008) conducted experiments to test the hypothesis that ex-post opportunities for emotion expression can promote fair economic outcomes, even in a one-time anonymous exchange. Their experiment is based on standard dictator games where one participant (the dictator) determines how to divide a sum of money between herself and another anonymous participant, the receiver. They conducted another treatment in which receivers were given an opportunity to write messages, in natural language, to their respective dictators. The messages were not monitored by the experimenters, and could have no effect on dictators' division decisions or ultimate earnings. Importantly though, dictators were informed before they made their decision that the receiver could write a message after they learned of the dictator's allocation.

Fig. 2 describes the distribution of dictators' offers in each treatment. In both treatments, about half of the dictators offer 40% or more (defined as fair) to the receiver and the other half offer 20% or less (defined as unfair). The distribution of fair offers is similar in the two treatments. In both treatments, about 30% of participants offer half or more, and 20% of participants offer 40%. However, the distribution of unfair offers differs between the two treatments. In the standard dictator game, significantly more dictators choose 10%, the minimum amount, than 20% (47% of participants vs. 9% of participants, $p<0.01$, two-tailed Mann-Whitney test). The reverse is true in the emotion expression treatment: more dictators choose to send 20% than 10%, though this difference is not significant (28% and 25% of participants, respectively). The reduced frequency of offers at the 10% level in the emotion expression treatment is statistically significant ($p = 0.028$, one-tail Mann-Whitney test).

Ellingsen and Johannesson (2008) conducted a closely related independent investigation to answer a similar question. In their study, different than Xiao and Houser (2008), dictators were allowed to take more than 90% and receivers were allowed to use foul language in the messages. In addition, dictators in their study were explicitly told to read the messages.

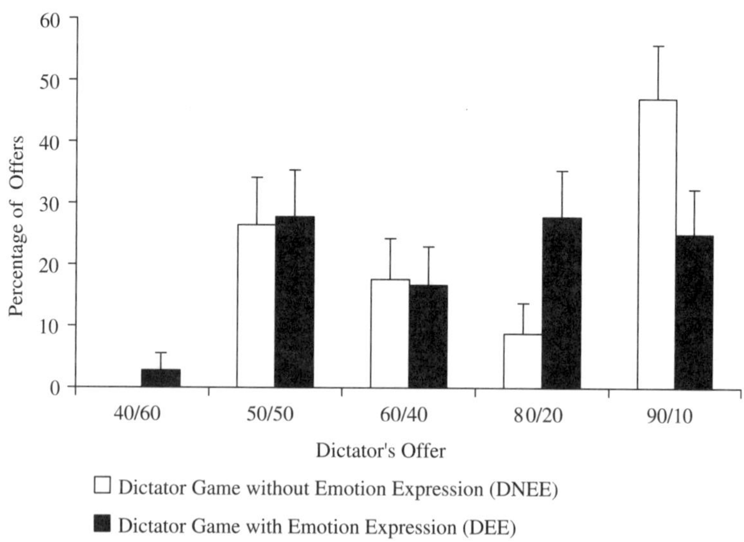

Fig. 2. Distribution of Dictators' Offers. *Note:* Offers are Denoted X/Y, where X is the Proposer's (Fig. 1) or Dictator's (Fig. 2) Percentage Share, and Y the Responder's (Fig. 1) or Receiver's (Fig. 2) Share (from Xiao & Houser, 2008).

Therefore, they studied a stronger condition of ex-post emotion expression than that studied in Xiao and Houser (2008). Interestingly, Ellingsen and Johannesson also found that anticipating this stronger form of emotion expression from receivers had a significant effect on dictators' behavior but with larger magnitude. In particular, they found a significantly higher proportion of fair splits when emotion expression was allowed.

These results are relevant to economic institution design for the reason that institutional frameworks can provide varying opportunities for expressions of disapproval. This is in contrast to emotion, which is difficult to manipulate or control. As we discuss in more detail below, if people make systematic efforts to avoid disapproval then mechanisms can be designed to discourage norm violations even within economic contexts that include partially anonymous trade with strangers (e.g. some types of internet exchange).

EMOTION EXPRESSION IN APOLOGIES

We have discussed the effect of a victim's emotion expression on herself and on those who offended her. One can also consider the impact of emotion expression on the offenders themselves. In particular, an individual who commits a bad or improper behavior might also incur negative emotions, such as regret or guilt, if she realizes that she violated a norm and caused harm to others. Under this situation, the wrongdoer might desire to express these negative emotions and apologize to the victim. The victim will also often desire to receive this apology. Indeed, much research regarding emotion expression by offenders has focused on the role of apologies in social relationships.

The rule violator's desire to apologize can be both spontaneous and strategic. The spontaneous desire for emotion expression can be caused by the experience of emotions such as guilt. Previous studies have found that guilt motivates a desire to repair, confess, apologize, or make amends. Shame is another negative emotion that often follows wrongdoing. In contrast to guilt, shame motivates individuals to hide themselves from others (see, e.g. Lewis, 1971; Wicker, Payne, & Morgan, 1983; Tangney, Wanger, Fletcher, & Gramzow, 1992).

Other studies have found that despite the shamed individual's desire to avoid social contact, she will nonetheless often share the shameful event with other people, particularly friends, acquaintances, and colleagues (see, Rimé, Mesquita, Philippot, & Boca, 1991). This sharing of shame should be treated differently from apology. While the latter is often expressed to the victim or disapproving others, the former is often conveyed to people who the shamed individual believes might sympathize. Thus, the expression of these two types of emotions can have different consequences in an individual's social relationships.

Apology can also be strategic if it can bring a subject some benefit. Plaintiffs often want apologies from their offenders, and whether or not they receive those apologies can affect their litigation decisions. If plaintiffs are more likely to forgive wrongdoing after receiving apologies, then apologies might be able to reduce the need for lawsuits (see, e.g. Cohen, 1999). An apology signals to the receiver that the apologizer recognizes the legitimacy of the norm that she violated, and moreover admits her fault and responsibility. For this reason legal counsel often discourage apologies. As a result of this paradox many psychologists and legal scholars have investigated empirical evidence regarding how an apology affects relationships between offenders and recipients of apologies.

Previous psychology studies have found that apologies generally affect recipients favorably. Apologies have been found to change recipients' perceptions of the offenders and their affective reactions (see, e.g. Gold & Weiner, 2000; Hodgins & Liebeskind, 2003; Bennett & Earwaker, 1994). However, the effect of an apology often depends on its type. For example, Gold and Weiner (2000) conducted interviews and found that whether someone shows remorse in a confession has a powerful effect on social judgments when a rule is broken. If the offender shows remorse toward the previous misconduct, people expect that she will be less likely to misbehave in the future. Robbennolt (2006) found that full apologies which clearly accept responsibility have a favorable effect on victims' attributions regarding the offender. In these cases, victims view the offenders as experiencing more regret and being more moral. Partial apologies expressing sympathy also seem to play a positive role in settlement decision-making when responsibility is less clear or injury is relatively minor. These studies suggest that the emotion expressed in apologies may be one of the keys for determining the receiver's attitude toward the offenders. Likewise, the effectiveness of the apology also depends on context factors, including the severity of the harm and whether the offenders take full responsibility.

The effect of apologies is also studied in health care disputes. The principal-agent relationship between doctor and patient is unique in that "the doctor is dealing with the patient's body and health and may literately hold the life of the patient in his/her hands (see, May & Stengel, 1990)." This means that ethics is highly important in the health care setting.

Growing attention has been drawn to how doctors handle mistakes. Since it is often difficult to pin down the responsibilities in medical accidents, and apologizing might hurt a doctor's reputation or lead to lawsuit, doctors may have high incentives to refuse to apologize. Empirical studies have thus been conducted on whether and how to communicate with patients about medical errors.

Mazor et al. (2004) conducted a survey in which participants were asked to read a set of written vignettes describing a medical error and the physician's response. In the nondisclosure conditions, the physician expressed regret but did not accept responsibility or make an apology. In full disclosure conditions, the physician accepted responsibility and made an apology. The study showed that, in relation to nondisclosure conditions, participants in full disclosure conditions are less likely to change physicians. They also display greater satisfaction, trust, and positive emotional response toward the physicians (see Robbennolt, 2005 for a good review and discussion of related studies).

Apology can also play an important role in an economic exchange environment, especially when it involves social norms such as trust and cooperation. Ho (2006) conducted a noisy trust game in which the principal could transfer some money to the agent, the amount of which would be tripled. The agent could then decide how much money to return to the principal. However, the actual amount that the principal received would be subject to some uncertainty. In other words, the principal would not know the amount the agent actually returned. At each period, the agent was told the outcome and given an opportunity to send a message "I am sorry" at a cost. The author found that principals trusted the agent more after receiving an apology.

In sum, previous studies suggest that providing an opportunity for offenders to express emotion can benefit both parties. By expressing regret or guilt through apologies, trust can be rebuilt and the cost of punishment or a lawsuit can perhaps be avoided.

EMOTION EXPRESSION AND WELL-BEING

To this point I have considered the impact of emotion expression on decision-making in economic exchange environments and in social interactions. However, a substantial amount of research has studied the consequences of emotion expression on health. Since emotions are closely related to human mental and physical health, a critical feature of emotion expression is its effect on well-being. For this reason, I next turn briefly to effects of emotion expression on health outcomes.

Previous research has linked emotion suppression to a variety of diseases (e.g. emotion suppression has been connected to cancer (Denollet, 1998; Temoshok, 1987), asthma (Florin, Freudenberg, & Hollaender, 1985), and cardiovascular diseases (Jorgensen, Johnson, Kolodziej, & Schreer, 1996)). Mauss and Gross (2004) reviewed a series of laboratory studies suggesting that suppressing negative emotions such as sadness, or positive emotions such as amusement, leads to acute increase in sympathetic activation of the cardiovascular system. This effect might translate into longer-term threats to cardiovascular health through psychophysiological and psychosocial pathways. Pennebaker (1990) suggests that failing to express emotion may exacerbate minor ailments.

In addition to physical health, emotion suppression has also been found to impact mental health. Lepore (1997) found that participants who were instructed to write their deepest thoughts and feelings about an exam exhibited a significant decline in depressive symptoms from 1 month to 3 days before the exam. Participants in the control group, who wrote about a trivial topic, maintained a relatively high level of depressive symptoms over this same period.

This empirical evidence seems to support the venting hypothesis (Kennedy-Moore & Watson, 1999), which posits that expression diffuses negative emotional experience and distress-related physiological arousal. However, things are not necessarily this simple. Gross (2002) argues that it is important to differentiate reappraisal from suppression. Reappraisal involves strategies of emotion regulation that occur early in the emotion-generative process, while suppression involves strategies that occur later in the process. Reappraisal involves changing the way a situation is construed so as to decrease its emotional impact. Suppression, however, involves inhibiting the outward signs of inner feelings. Gross and his colleagues conducted experiments and found that reappraisal is often more effective than suppression. Reappraisal decreases emotion experience and behavioral expression, and has no impact on memory. In contrast, suppression decreases behavioral expression but fails to decrease emotion experience and seems to impair memory. Suppression likewise increases physiological responding for suppressors and their social partners.

Tavris (1989) pointed out that a number of conditions are required for anger expression to reduce arousal and mitigate feelings of anger. For example, anger expression is most likely to be beneficial when it is directed at the appropriate target. Anger should not be expressed if it leads to further retaliation by the target (e.g. expressing anger to the boss is different than blaming your subordinate). Anger is also likely to be diffused when the expression appropriately punishes the responsible party (see Kennedy-Moore & Watson, 1999 Chapter 2 for a detailed discussion surrounding when expression of distress can be beneficial and when it can lead to negative effects).

These findings have important implications for institution design. For example, allowing direct communication between customers and responsible parties in the company to a certain degree might help to improve the satisfaction of customers.

EMOTION EXPRESSION ASPECT IN POLICY DESIGN

Allowing channels for emotion expression can influence personal relationships, individual decision-making, and well-being. As previously mentioned, opportunities for emotion expression are different from experiences of emotion in that they can often be incorporated into policy. Emotion expression can therefore have important implications in policy design.

In January of 2006, BBC news reported an interesting story demonstrating how organizations can incorporate emotion expression into their policy in order to influence people's behavior. In particular, after one employee refused to smile all day, Nutzwerk, a German IT company, attempted to promote a more congenial atmosphere by instituting a policy that banned "grumpiness" at work. The new policy required employees to enter into a formal agreement to remain in a good mood all day at the office and leave complaints and gripes about co-workers and work conditions at home. The ban on complaints was taken seriously. After just a few weeks, two employees were given repeated warnings, three were dismissed, and one chose to leave voluntarily.

The Nutzwerk manager's intention was clearly to increase productivity by creating a friendly work atmosphere. A field study of this policy is difficult, since the policy might encourage certain types of people to choose this company (we have already seen that some employees chose to leave). However, the results from the studies discussed above might indicate some potential problems with this policy. For example, when employees are prohibited from expressing their emotion by complaining or communicating with their colleagues, they might look for some other channel to express their negative feelings. Also, employees might shirk responsibilities. If employees stop complaining at work by suppressing their emotions, instead of changing the way they construe the situation, the continual emotion suppression may result in harm to their well-being. This effect might not be immediately apparent, and thus might be ignored in the short term.

However, we have offered empirical evidence that when a person is given an opportunity to express her emotion she is more willing to accept an outcome that is unfavorable to her. Meanwhile, her counterpart is also more likely to cooperate, since she tends to want to avoid her partner's disapproval. Thus, policy-makers could exploit connections between ex-post complaint processes and ex-ante economic outcomes. For example, when pricing is unfair, consumers often boycott the unfairly priced products (see, e.g. Friedman, 1991; or Tyran & Engelmann, 2005). If boycotts are one method consumers use to express their negative feelings toward unfair prices, then a system facilitating expression of consumer dissatisfaction might help to reduce their occurrence. Also, if producers are aware of the possibility of receiving negative emotion expression from consumers, they might be more likely to set fair prices.

Since people usually try to avoid disapproval, the opportunity for emotion expression can play a particularly important role in one-time and anonymous interaction environments such as online markets. In the Internet market trade depends largely on the honesty of sellers or buyers. One important feature of many online markets, such as eBay and yahoo!, is that they provide a platform for the traders to leave feedback. This feedback system is useful not only for helping traders build their reputations but for helping to discourage fraud, even in a one-shot anonymous exchange. The reason is that buyers or sellers who may be tempted to treat the second party unfairly will face more inner pressure if they know the second party can leave them negative messages. The possibility of receiving a negative message could increase the expected cost of unfair transactions and discourage would-be on artists from exploiting the short-run profit.[2]

In comparison to using monetary punishment to promote norm obedience, emotion expression can be much less costly to implement and therefore more credible. Moreover, in many situations, it can be difficult to stipulate complete contracts that enforce punishment. Even when this is feasible, sanction threats can be counter-productive (see, e.g. Frey & Oberholzer-Gee, 1997; Gneezy & Rustichini, 2000; Fehr & Falk, 2002; Houser, Xiao, McCabe, & Smith, 2008). Therefore, allowing ex-post emotional reactions can be an efficient alternative means for enforcing fair economic exchange. Furthermore, emotion expression can have health benefits which might not be possible to achieve using monetary punishment.

Emotion expression can also have important implications for the design of legal systems. The theory of restorative justice emphasizes the importance of victim–offender mediation programs (VOMPs). VOMP is a process which allows crime victims to meet face-to face with their offenders to talk about the impact of the crime and to develop a restitution plan. VOMP has been a vital part of the solution to the crime problem. It provides an excellent opportunity for emotion expression: it makes the offenders directly accountable to the people they violate, and can help to restore emotional and material losses. Evidence shows that people feel as though they have been treated more fairly when they have had an opportunity to express their view about their situation (see, Lind & Tyler, 1988; Umbreit, 1995). Moreover, VOMP might be able to efficiently prevent wrong-doings by forcing wrong-doers to face the emotion expression of their victims.[3]

CONCLUSION

Substantial previous research has drawn attention to the importance of emotion expression in our daily lives. However, we continue to have only a limited understanding of its relevance to and impact in economic environments. While empirical studies have demonstrated benefits to allowing emotion expression, we also realize that different types of emotion inhibition can have different effects. Recklessly allowing complete freedom of emotion expression might have unexpected negative consequences.

This chapter focused on negative emotion expression. This is not to say that positive emotion expression is unimportant. In China, some donors decided not to continue support for needy students after they became disappointed that they never received any "thank you" notes from those who received financial aid. How can simple expressions of gratitude affect giving? Are people more cooperative when they know their cooperation will be acknowledged? Future studies of various aspects of emotion expression could help to improve our understanding of human decision-making.

NOTES

1. An interesting question is whether the desire of expressing emotion has different effects on behavior when subjects are aware of this desire than when they are not.

One hypothesis is that subjects might actively search channels even if they are costly to show their feelings when they are aware of this emotion desire. However, emotion expression, even when it is unintentional, can also effect social interaction as long as it is perceived by the counterparts.

2. eBay had recently announced that starting in May 2008, sellers would not be able to leave negative or neutral messages about buyers. Since it was always easier to deal with the fraud on the buyer's side, eBay argued that this policy was to ensure buyers that they would not be retaliated against for leaving negative feedback for sellers. However, given what we discussed here, if we assume both buyers and sellers have the same degree of desire to expression emotions, this policy might have a negative effect on the willingness of sellers to engage in trading. This can be true even though, according to ebay, only a minority of sellers leave negative feedback for buyers. The desire of emotion expression might also explain the ensuing seller boycott (see http://money.cnn.com/2008/02/15/smbusiness/ebay_strike_update.fsb/).

3. For a broader discussion of law and emotions, see O'Hara and Yarn (2002) and Marony (2006).

REFERENCES

Akerlof, G. A., & Dickens, W. T. (1982). The economic consequence of cognitive dissonance. *American Economic Review*, *72*(3), 307–319.

Andreoni, J. (1990). Impure altruism and donations to public goods: A theory of warm glow giving? *Economic Journal*, *100*, 464–477.

Aronson, E. (1995). *The social animal* (7th ed.). New York: W.H. Freeman.

Baumeister, R. F., Vohs, K. D., DeWall, C. N., & Zhang, L. (2007). How emotion shapes behavior: Feedback, anticipation, and reflection, rather than direct causation. *Personality and Social Psychology Review*, *11*(2), 167–203.

Bennett, M., & Earwaker, D. (1994). Victim's response to apologies: The effects of offender responsibility and offense severity. *Journal of Social Psychology*, *134*, 457–464.

Berg, J., Dickhaut, J., & McCabe, K. (1995). Trust, reciprocity, and social history. *Games and Economic Behavior*, *10*, 122–142.

Camerer, C. (2003). *Behavioral game theory: Experiments in strategic interaction*. Princeton, NJ: Princeton University Press.

Camerer, C., & Weigelt, K. (1988). Experimental tests of a sequential equilibrium reputation model. *Econometrica*, *56*, 1–36.

Cohen, J. R. (1999). Advising clients to apologize. *Southern California Law Review*, *72*, 1009–1069.

Damasio, A. (1994). *Descartes' error-emotion, reason and the human brain*. New-York: Grosset-Putnam.

Denollet, J. (1998). Personality and risk of cancer in men with coronary heart disease. *Psychological Medicine*, *28*, 991–995.

Ellingsen, T., & Johannesson, M. (2008). Anticipated verbal feedback induces altruistic behavior. *Evolution and Human Behavior*, *29*(2), 100–105.

Elster, J. (1999). *Alchemies of the mind: Rationality and the emotions*. Cambridge: Cambridge University Press.

Fehr, E., & Falk, A. (2002). Psychological foundations of incentives. *European Economic Review*, *46*, 687–724.

Fehr, E., & Gächter, S. (2000). Cooperation and punishment in public goods experiments. *American Economic Review*, *90*, 980–994.

Festinger, L. (1957). *A theory of cognitive dissonance*. Stanford, CA: Stanford University Press.

Florin, I., Freudenberg, G., & Hollaender, J. (1985). Facial expression of emotion and physiologic reactions in children with bronchial asthma. *Psychosomatic Medicine*, *47*, 382–393.

Frank, R. H. (2002). Cooperation through emotional commitment. In: R. M. Nesse (Ed.), *Evolution and the capacity for commitment* (pp. 57–76). New York: Russell Sage Foundation.

Frey, B. S., & Oberholzer-Gee, F. (1997). The cost of price incentives: An empirical analysis of motivation crowding-out. *American Economic Review*, *87*(4), 746–755.

Friedman, M. (1991). Consumer boycotts: A conceptual framework and research agenda. *Journal of Social Issues*, *47*, 149–168.

Frijda, N. H. (1986). *The emotions*. Cambridge, UK: Cambridge University Press.

Gigerenzer, G. (2007). *Gut feelings: The intelligence of the unconscious*. New York: Viking.

Gneezy, U., & Rustichini, A. (2000). A fine is a price. *Journal of Legal Studies*, *29*(1), 1–17.

Gold, G. J., & Weiner, B. (2000). Remorse, confession, group identity, and expectancies about repeating a transgression. *Basic and Applied Social Psychology*, *22*(4), 91–300.

Gross, J. J. (2002). Emotion regulation: Affective, cognitive, and social consequences. *Psychophysiology*, *39*, 281–291.

Ho, B. (2006). *The economics of apologies*. Working paper.

Hodgins, H., & Liebeskind, E. (2003). Apology versus defense: Antecedents and consequences. *Journal of Experimental Social Psychology*, *29*, 297–316.

Houser, D., Xiao, E., McCabe, K., & Smith, V. (2008). When punishment fails: Research on sanctions, intentions and non-cooperation. *Games and Economic Behavior*, *62*(2), 509–532.

Jorgensen, R. S., Johnson, B. T., Kolodziej, M. E., & Schreer, G. E. (1996). Elevated blood pressure and personality: A meta-analytic review. *Psychological Bulletin*, *120*, 293–320.

Kennedy-Moore, E., & Watson, J. C. (1999). *Expressing emotion: Myths, realities, and therapeutic strategies*. New York: Guilford Press.

Konow, J. (2000). Fair share: Accountability and cognitive dissonance in allocation decisions. *American Economic Review*, *90*(4), 1072–1091.

Kurzban, R., & Houser, D. (2005). An experimental investigation of cooperative types in human groups: A complement to evolutionary theory and simulations. *Proceedings of the National Academy of Sciences*, *102*, 1803–1807.

Lepore, S. (1997). Expressive writing moderates the relation between intrusive thoughts and depressive symptoms. *Journal of Personality and Social Psychology*, *73*, 1030–1037.

Lewis, H. B. (1971). *Shame and guilt in neurosis*. New York: International Universities Press.

Lind, E. A., & Tyler, T. R. (1988). *The social psychology of procedural justice (critical issues in social justice)*. New York and London: Plenum Press.

Loewenstein, G. (2000). Emotions in economic theory and economic behavior. *American Economic Review*, *90*(2), 426–432.

Marony, T. (2006). Law and emotion: A proposed taxonomy of an emerging field. *Law and Human Behavior*, *30*(2), 119–142.

Masclet, D., Noussair, C., Tucker, S., & Villeval, M-C. (2003). Monetary and non-monetary punishment in the voluntary contributions mechanism. *American Economic Review*, *93*, 366–380.

Masclet, D., & Villeval, M. (2006). *Punishment, inequality and emotions*. Working paper.

Mauss, I. B., & Gross, J. J. (2004). Emotion suppression and cardiovascular disease. In: I. Nyklíček, L. Temoshok & A. Vingerhoets (Eds), *Emotion expression and health* (pp. 61–81). Hove: Brunner-Routledge.

May, M. L., & Stengel, D. B. (1990). Who sues their doctors? How patients handle medical grievances. *Law and Society Review*, *24*, 105–120.

Mazor, K. M., Simon, S. R., Yood, R. A., Martinson, B. C., Gunter, M. J., Reed, G. W., & Gurwitz, J. H. (2004). Health plan members' views about disclosure of medical errors. *Annals of Internal Medicine*, *140*(6), 409–418.

Miller, J. H., Butts, C., & Rode, D. (2002). Communication and cooperation. *Journal of Economic Behavior and Organization*, *47*, 179–195.

O'Hara, E. A., & Yarn, D. (2002). On apology and consilience. *Washington Law Review*, *77*, 1121–1192.

Pennebaker, J. (1990). *Opening up: The healing powers of confiding in others*. New York: Morrow.

Pennebaker, J. W. (1997). Health effects of the expression (and non-expression) of emotions through writing. In: A. J. J. M. Vingerhoets, F. J. Van Bussel & A. J. W. Boelhouwer (Eds), *The (non)expression of emotions in health and disease* (pp. 267–278). Tilburg, The Netherlands: Tilburg University Press.

Rabin, M. (1994). Cognitive dissonance and social change. *Journal of Economic Behavior and Organization*, *23*(2), 177–194.

Rimé, B., Mesquita, B., Philippot, P., & Boca, S. (1991). Beyond the emotional event: Six studies of the social sharing of emotion. *Cognition and Emotion*, *5*, 435–465.

Robbennolt, J. (2006). Apologies and settlement levers. *Journal of Empirical Legal Studies*, *3*(2), 333–373.

Robbennolt, J. K. (2005). What we know and don't know about the role of apologies in resolving health care disputes. *Georgia State University Law Review*, *21*, 1009–1027.

Sanfey, A. G., Rilling, J. K., Aronson, J. A., Nystrom, L. E., & Cohen, J. D. (2003). The neural basis of economic decision-making in the ultimatum game. *Science*, *300*, 1673–1675.

Tangney, J. P., Wanger, P., Fletcher, C., & Gramzow, R. (1992). Shame into anger? Development of the self-conscious affect and attribution inventory. *Journal of Personality and Social Psychology*, *59*, 102–111.

Tavris, C. (1989). *Anger: The misunderstood emotion*. New York: Simon and Schuter.

Temoshok, L. (1987). Personality, copying style, emotion, and cancer: Toward an integrative model. *Cancer Survey*, *6*, 837–839.

Tesser, A., & Aschee, J. (1994). Aggression, love, conformity, and other social psychological catastrophes. In: R. R. Vallacher & A. Nowak (Eds), *Dynamical systems in social psychology* (pp. 96–109). New York: Academic Press.

Tyran, J., & Engelmann, D. (2005). To buy or not to buy? An experimental study of consumer boycotts in retail markets. *Economica*, *72*, 1–16.

Umbreit, M. S. (1995). *Mediating interpersonal conflicts: A pathway to peace*. Erickson Mediation Institute.

Wicker, F. W., Payne, G. C., & Morgan, R. D. (1983). Participant descriptions of guilt and shame. *Motivation and Emotion*, *7*, 25–39.

Xiao, E., & Houser, D. (2005). Emotion expression in human punishment behavior. *Proceedings of the National Academy of Sciences*, *102*(20), 7398–7401.

Xiao, E., & Houser, D. (2008). *Emotion expression and fairness in economic exchange*. Working paper.

SOURCE PREFERENCE AND AMBIGUITY AVERSION: MODELS AND EVIDENCE FROM BEHAVIORAL AND NEUROIMAGING EXPERIMENTS

Soo Hong Chew, King King Li, Robin Chark and Songfa Zhong

ABSTRACT

Purpose – *This experimental economics study using brain imaging techniques investigates the risk-ambiguity distinction in relation to the source preference hypothesis (Fox & Tversky, 1995) in which identically distributed risks arising from different sources of uncertainty may engender distinct preferences for the same decision maker, contrary to classical economic thinking. The use of brain imaging enables sharper testing of the implications of different models of decision-making including Chew and Sagi's (2008) axiomatization of source preference.*

Methodology/approach – *Using fMRI, brain activations were observed when subjects make 48 sequential binary choices among even-chance lotteries based on whether the trailing digits of a number of stock prices at*

Neuroeconomics
Advances in Health Economics and Health Services Research, Volume 20, 179–201

ISSN: 0731-2199/doi:10.1016/S0731-2199(08)20008-7

market closing would be odd or even. Subsequently, subjects rate familiarity of the stock symbols.

Findings – *When contrasting brain activation from more familiar sources with those from less familiar ones, regions appearing to be more active include the putamen, medial frontal cortex, and superior temporal gyrus. ROI analysis showed that the activation patterns in the familiar–unfamiliar and unfamiliar–familiar contrasts are similar to those in the risk–ambiguity and ambiguity–risk contrasts reported by Hsu et al. (2005). This supports the conjecture that the risk-ambiguity distinction can be subsumed by the source preference hypothesis.*

Research limitations/implications – *Our odd–even design has the advantage of inducing the same "unambiguous" probability of half for each subject in each binary comparison. Our finding supports the implications of the Chew–Sagi model and rejects models based on global probabilistic sophistication, including rank-dependent models derived from non-additive probabilities, e.g., Choquet expected utility and cumulative prospect theory, as well as those based on multiple priors, e.g., α-maxmin. The finding in Hsu et al. (2005) that orbitofrontal cortex lesion patients display neither ambiguity aversion nor risk aversion offers further support to the Chew–Sagi model. Our finding also supports the Levy et al. (2007) contention of a single valuation system encompassing risk and ambiguity aversion.*

Originality/value of chapter – *This is the first neuroimaging study of the source preference hypothesis using a design which can discriminate among decision models ranging from risk-based ones to those relying on multiple priors.*

1. INTRODUCTION

Risks figure prominently in decision-making today as well as in the distant past, when exposure to danger was commonplace. From then to now, a willingness to take risk remains essential to the human condition. Ipso facto, risk has been the focus of much research in economics. Inspired by Ramsey (1931) and De Finetti (1937), Savage (1954) developed the subjective expected utility (SEU) model, which hypothesized that individuals make decisions among options by choosing the one that provides the highest expected utility. Savage showed that both probabilities and utilities can be inferred from choices made among gambles. This model has provided the workhorse for much of the modeling of decision-making under risk in economics and related areas.

Earlier on, Knight (1921) made the distinction between measurable uncertainty or risk, which can be represented by precise probabilities, and unmeasurable uncertainty which cannot. In the same year, Keynes (1921) discussed the following: "In the first case we know that the urn contains black and white in equal proportions; in the second case the proportion of each colour is unknown, and each ball is as likely to be black as white. It is evident that in either case the probability of drawing a white ball is half, but that the weight of the argument in favor of this conclusion is greater in the first case." He argued that "If two probabilities are equal in degree, ought we, in choosing our course of action, to prefer that one which is based on a greater body of knowledge?"

Keynes' observation found its way into the celebrated paper by Ellsberg (1961) who observed that people prefer to bet on a ball drawn from the known urn rather than betting on the unknown urn. In other words, decision makers have different risk attitudes towards events with known probabilities (risk) and unknown probabilities (uncertainty). Such choice behavior (see, e.g., Camerer & Weber, 1992) is commonly referred to as ambiguity aversion and is incompatible with the SEU model of Savage (1954) or the more general definition of global probabilistic sophistication (Machina & Schmeidler, 1992; Chew & Sagi, 2006). A number of theoretical models have also been proposed to account for ambiguity aversion, including Choquet expected utility (Schmeidler, 1989), maxmin expected utility (MEU) with multiple priors (Gilboa & Schmeidler, 1989), α-maxmin (Ghirardato, Maccheroni, & Marinacci, 2004), and cumulative prospect theory (CPT) (Tversky & Kahneman, 1992).

More recently, Fox and Tversky (1995) coined the term source preference, which refers to the observation that choices between prospects depend not only on the degree of uncertainty but also on the source of uncertainty. The authors interpreted ambiguity aversion as a special case of source preference. This identification of source preference, encompassing the risk-ambiguity distinction, motivated Chew and Sagi (2008) to develop an axiomatic model of source preference, by foregoing global probabilistic sophistication while seeking smaller systems of compatible events, called *small worlds*, within which the decision maker could behave probabilistically. Their axiomatization delivers the theoretical possibility of the decision maker having different attitudes towards risks arising from distinct sources of uncertainty.

The neuroimaging experiment reported in this chapter seeks to test the implications of a number of decision models in the literature relating to source preference and ambiguity aversion. The remainder of the chapter is organized as follows. Section 2 reviews the theoretical models on ambiguity aversion and source preference alongside behavioral evidence. Section 3 discusses neuroimaging evidence on ambiguity aversion while Section 4 presents new neuroimaging results testing the source preference hypothesis. We conclude in Section 5.

2. UTILITY MODELS AND BEHAVIORAL EVIDENCE

Since the advent of probability in the 17th century, the use of mean value to assess the worth of a lottery has been commonplace. In the so-called St. Petersburg paradox, Bernoulli (1738/1954) showed that valuing lotteries strictly according to their mean values can lead one to assign an infinite value to a lottery that pays a finite amount for sure. This observation led him to hypothesize that people have diminishing marginal utility for money. He posited specifically a logarithmic utility function for money. Rather than its expected value, the utility of a lottery would be the expectation of the utilities of its outcomes with respect to the underlying probability distribution. In this case, the decision maker will be averse to risks, i.e., valuing lotteries less than their expected values.

The mean-variance model, introduced by Markowitz (1952), is an alternative approach to model the behavior of a risk-averse investor in modern financial economics. Here, variance acts as a proxy for "risk" which is considered "bad." In other words, the decision maker's "indifference curves" on a two-dimensional mean-variance space always slope upwards. For any two lotteries to be indifferent, it is necessary that the one with a lower mean must have lower variance. Yet, as shown by Borch (1969), the high-mean-high-variance lottery can be constructed in such a way that it always pays more than the low-mean-low-variance lottery, which is preferred. This casts doubt on the normative appeal of the mean-variance preference specification and to some extent also its empirical validity.

There has been a number of works, including the pioneering contribution of von Neumann and Morgenstern (1947), on the axiomatic characterization of the Bernoulli model generally known as the expected utility hypothesis. A significant advance in this strand of thinking came from the seminal work of Savage (1954) who axiomatized the so-called SEU model of choice under uncertainty in which probabilities, being inferred from revealed preference, are purely subjective. In Savage's setting, lotteries or bets are in the form of $f = (x_1, E_1; \cdots; x_n, E_n)$ for some mutually exclusive and exhaustive partition $\{E_1, \cdots, E_n\}$ of the state space Ω and (not necessarily distinct) outcomes $\{x_1, \cdots, x_n\}$ from a consequence set X. Savage's axioms imply the existence of a cardinal *utility* function u over outcomes and a subjective probability measure p over events, such that the individual evaluates such bets according to an ordinal preference specification of the form

$$\text{SEU}(x_1, E_1; \cdots; x_n, E_n) = \sum_{i=1}^{n} u(x_i)p(E_i)$$

A key characteristic of this model, which follows from the additive structure of SEU, is known as the sure-thing principle: *For all f, g, h, h′ and event E, fEh* $\succcurlyeq$ *gEh if and only if fEh′* $\succcurlyeq$ *gEh′, where fEg refers to the act which pays f(s) if s belongs to E and pays* g(*s*) *otherwise.* We use $\succ$ to denote the strict preference relation.

Despite the appeal and wide success of the SEU model in economics, finance, and other areas of the behavioral and social sciences, questions about its empirical validity have arisen especially in the work of Ellsberg (1961). In the well-known Ellsberg Paradox, there are two urns. The first contains 50 black balls and 50 red balls. The second contains 100 balls of either black or red color, with no additional information. One ball is picked at random from each urn. There are four events, denoted by R_1, B_1, R_2, B_2, where R_1 denotes the event, for instance, the event that the color of the ball chosen from urn 1 is red. On each of the events a bet is offered: \$100 if the event occurs and zero otherwise. People would generally be indifferent between betting on R_1 or B_1 (urn 1), and similarly between betting on R_2 or B_2 (urn 2). Yet, decision makers tend to prefer betting on either B_1 or R_1 to betting on either B_2 or R_2. Under SEU, indifference between betting on R_1 and B_1 and between betting on R_2 and B_2 implies that $p(B_1) = p(R_1) = 1/2 = p(B_2) = p(R_2)$. Taken together, the decision maker would be indifferent among all four bets, which does not accord well with empirical observations (Camerer & Weber, 1992).

In a 1995 paper, Fox and Tversky argued that Ellsbergian behavior may be subsumed under the more general phenomenon of source preference, in which the appeal of a prospect depends not only on the degree of uncertainty but also on the source of uncertainty. In their experiment, they assessed subject's willingness to pay (WP) for a gamble on whether the temperature of San Francisco (T_S) (or Istanbul (T_I)) is at least or less than 60° F. Should his guess be correct, the subject would win \$100. They found that

$$\mathrm{WP}(T_S \geq 60) > \mathrm{WP}(T_S < 60) > \mathrm{WP}(T_I \geq 60) > \mathrm{WP}(T_I < 60)$$

In other words, subjects are more willing to pay more to bet on the temperature of the more familiar San Francisco than the unfamiliar Istanbul. They labeled this as source preference and concluded that people may prefer to bet on a source of uncertainty where they are more familiar or knowledgeable.

A number of models have been proposed to accommodate Ellsberg-type behavior, including the Choquet expected utility model (Schmeidler, 1989), CPT (Tversky & Kahneman, 1992), MEU model (Gilboa & Schmeidler, 1989), and α-maxmin model (Ghirardato et al., 2004). More recently, Chew and Sagi (2008) offered a *small worlds* axtiomatization of source preference which encompasses the risk-ambiguity distinction.

Choquet Expected Utility, Rank-Dependent Expected Utility, and Cumulative Prospect Theory

Choquet expected utility model and its extension to CPT both satisfy a comonotonic sure-thing principle (Chew & Wakker, 1996): *For all comonotonic f, g, h, h' and event E, $fEh \succcurlyeq gEh$ if and only if $fEh' \succcurlyeq gEh'$.* (Two acts f and g are *comonotonic* if it never happens that $f(s) \succ f(t)$ and $g(t) \succ g(s)$ for some states s and t.) For $f = (x_1, E_1; \cdots; x_n, E_n)$ with $x_1 \succ x_2 \succ \cdots \succ x_n$, its *Choquet expected utility* is given by

$$\mathrm{CEU}(f) = \sum_{i=1}^{n} \left[\pi(\cup_{j=1}^{i} E_j) - \pi(\cup_{j=1}^{i-1} E_j) \right] u(x_i)$$

where π is a unique non-additive probability (or capacity) which is monotone by set inclusion and assigns zero to the empty set, and 1 to Ω. It is straightforward to see that the empirically observed choice pattern in Ellsberg's 2-urn paradox could be consistent with CEU. Specifically, $\pi(R_1) = \pi(B_1) > \pi(B_2) = \pi(R_2)$.

Rank-dependent expected utility (RDEU), axiomatized in Quiggin (1982) and Quiggin and Wakker (1994), can be viewed as a special case of the Choquet expected utility in the presence of a known underlying probability distribution p, in conjunction with an auxiliary hypothesis that relates closely to stochastic dominance: $\pi(E) = \pi(E')$ if and only if $p(E) = p(E')$ (see Chew & Wakker, 1996). The RDEU specification is defined by a non-decreasing function g: [0,1] → [0,1] with $g(0) = 0$ and $g(1) = 1$ such that $\pi(E) = g(p(E))$, for any event E. For $f = (x_1, E_1;\cdots; x_n, E_n)$ $(x_1 \preccurlyeq x_2 \preccurlyeq \cdots \preccurlyeq x_n)$ where $q_j = p(E_j)$, its RDEU is given by:

$$\sum_{i=1}^{n}\left[g\left(\sum\nolimits_{j=1}^{i} q_j\right) - g\left(\sum\nolimits_{j=1}^{i-1} q_j\right)\right]u(x_i)$$

For the case of a 2-outcome lottery which delivers a positive outcome x with probability p and zero otherwise, its RDEU has a simple expression:

$$g(1-p)u(0) + [1 - g(1-p)]u(x)$$

which can be further simplified into $\pi(p)u(x)$ with $\pi(p) = [1-g(1-p)]$ and $u(0) = 0$. Subsequently, Chew, Karni, and Safra (1987) showed that a sufficient condition for risk aversion (risk affinity) in terms of mean-preserving increase in risk (Rothschild & Stiglitz, 1970) is for both u and g functions to be concave (π convex).

CPT incorporates a status quo or reference point e and a capacity π^+ for gain-oriented uncertainties and a possibly different capacity π^- for loss-oriented uncertainties. For $f = \{x_1, E_1;\cdots; x_n, E_n\}$ where $x_1 \succ \cdots \succ x_k \succ e \succcurlyeq x_{k+1} \succ \cdots \succ x_n$, its CPT utility is given by:

$$\sum_{i=1}^{n}\left[\pi^+(\cup_{j=1}^{i} E_j) - \pi^+(\cup_{j=1}^{i-1} E_j)\right]u(x_i) + \sum_{i=k+1}^{n}\left[\pi^-(\cup_{j=i}^{n} E_j) - \pi^-(\cup_{j=i+1}^{n} E_j)\right]u(x_i)$$

As demonstrated in Chew and Wakker (1996), CPT also reduces to a globally probabilistically sophisticated counterpart, called *rank-linear utility* (Green & Jullien, 1988), under consistency with stochastic dominance.

Maxmin Expected Utility and α-Maxmin Expected Utility

Gilboa and Schmeidler (1989) introduced Maxmin Expected Utility (MEU) as

$$\text{MEU}(f) = \min_{\pi \in C}\left[\sum_{i=1}^{n} u(f_i)\pi(s_i)\right]$$

where C is a set of possible probability measures. The decision maker under MEU is extremely pessimistic in the sense that he behaves as if the worst among the possible probability distributions will take place. This model accords with Ellsberg-type behavior in the following sense. For urn 1, the probability of R_1 and B_1 are well-defined and equal half while for urn 2, the worst possible probability of drawing R_2 (resp: B_2) is zero. Consequently, the observed choice pattern – preferring to bet on urn 1 can be rationalized. However, MEU has the implausible implication that the certainty equivalent of betting on either color in urn 2 is zero.

The MEU model was further generalized by Ghirardato et al. (2004) to the α-MEU model in which decision makers evaluate each act by forming a convex combination of the best and worst expected utilities by placing a decision weight $\alpha(\in[0, 1])$ and $1-\alpha$ for the worst and the best expected utilities respectively:

$$\alpha\text{-MEU}(f) = \alpha \min_{\pi\in C}\left[\sum_{i=1}^{n} u(f_i)\pi(s_i)\right] + (1-\alpha)\max_{\pi\in C}\left[\sum_{i=1}^{n} u(f_i)\pi(s_i)\right]$$

Like MEU, α-MEU is compatible with Ellsbergian behavior and enjoys the additional advantage that the certainty equivalent of betting on R_2 or B_2 would be bounded away from zero as long as $\alpha<1$.

Source-Dependent Expected Utility (SDEU)

Chew and Sagi (2008) offered an axiomatic approach to model source preference in terms of possibly distinct attitudes towards risks arising from within each source of uncertainty. In the 2-urn Ellsberg paradox, indifference between betting on B_1 and on R_1 reveals that the decision maker has the same subjective likelihood between these two complementary events. This is similarly the case for B_2 and R_2. Yet, a strict preference in favor of betting on either B_1 or R_1 over B_2 or R_2 tells us that the decision maker exhibits greater aversion (often called ambiguity aversion) towards urn 2 bets. In other words, an individual is ambiguity averse for one source of uncertainty over another if she is more averse to risks from that source than for risks arising from another source of uncertainty. The simplest source preference model corresponds to having possibly distinct SEU preferences, with different von Neumann-Morgenstern (vNM) utility functions, for risks arising from different sources of uncertainty, e.g., u_1 for urn 1 and u_2 for urn 2. The certainty equivalents c_1 and c_2 for the bets on the two urns are given by $u_1(c_1) = 1/2u_1(100)$ and $u_2(c_2) = 1/2u_2(100)$. It follows that c_1 is greater than

c_2 if u_2 is more concave than u_1. A similar reasoning could apply to the source preference examples in Fox and Tversky (1995).

More recently, Chew, Li, Chark, and Zhong (2008) conducted a number of experiments using a Japanese ascending price clock auction design to discriminate between the Chew–Sagi approach and models based on global probabilistic sophistication or having multiple priors. To elicit subject's valuations towards different source of uncertainties, subjects bid for even-chance lotteries whose payoffs depended on whether the trailing digit of the closing price of a specific stock the following day would be odd or even. The authors used questionnaires to assess each subject's degree of familiarity with the various stocks. They tested the hypothesis, discussed earlier, that subjects would be willing to pay more for bets based on the price of a more familiar stock. Subjects' risk premia for different sources of uncertainty are found to be negatively correlated with their self-reported degrees of familiarity, a result compatible with the source preference approach. At the same time, their finding is incompatible with the implications of the α-maxmin model or any model that coincides with global probabilistic sophistication.

In the Chew–Sagi formulation, ambiguity aversion towards one source of uncertainty relative to another source arises from the decision maker having distinct attitudes towards risks from multiple sources of uncertainty. In this sense, one may expect a decision maker who is more risk averse than another decision maker in one source to also be comparatively more averse to risks arising from another source. This implication is supported by Halevy (2007) who finds positive correlation between the risk premium and ambiguity premium in the Ellsberg urns. This implication is further corroborated by the findings in Bossaerts, Ghirardato, Guarneschelli, and Zame (2007) in the setting of an experimental asset market.

3. NEUROIMAGING EVIDENCE

Identifying the brain regions that encode reward and risk has been the theme of a number of papers. Knutson, Taylor, Kaufman, Peterson, and Glover (2005) conduct an fMRI experiment to investigate the neural mechanisms that compute expected value. They find that nucleus accumbens is activated in proportion to anticipated gain magnitude while the cortical mesial prefrontal cortex is activated according to the probability of anticipated gain. In another study, activation of anterior insular and posterior inferior frontal gyrus and intraparietal sulcus correlate positively with the degree of 'uncertainty' (Huettel, Song, & McCarthy, 2005). More recently, Preuschoff,

Bossaerts, and Quartz (2006) find that activation of putamen and ventral striatum are positively correlated with the expected reward value of the gamble. On the other hand, activation of anterior insula correlates positively with the reward variance (as a proxy for risk). Anterior insula is implicated in negative somatic states (Bechara, 2001). On the other hand, Chua, Krams, Toni, Passingham, and Dolan (1999) report that the anterior insula is activated during anticipation of physical pain, which correlates with self-reported anxiety. Kuhnen and Knutson (2005) investigate the relationship between the anterior insula and risk attitude. Subjects with greater insula activation, tend to be risk neutral or risk averse in an experiment involving financial risk taking.

Smith, Dickhaut, McCabe, and Pardo (2002)

Using PET, Smith et al. (2002) conducts the first neuroimaging study on the distinction between risk and ambiguity. Subjects make binary choices between gambles involving known probabilities (risk) and gambles with unknown probabilities (ambiguity). The authors investigate how risk and ambiguity interact with gambles in the domain of gain and loss. Their design includes four conditions: risk with gains (RG), risk with losses (RL), ambiguity with gains (AG), and ambiguity with losses (AL). They find that subjects display different risk attitudes in gain and loss conditions. Subjects avoid riskier gambles in the gain domain and less so in the loss domain. Subjects also avoid ambiguity gambles in both gain and loss conditions. There is significant interaction between the gain and loss domains and the risk and ambiguity conditions. Subjects' ambiguity aversion is significantly stronger in the gain condition than it is in the loss condition.

The authors present two difference-on-difference contrasts [(RG–RL)–(AG–AL)] and [(RL–RG)–(AL–AG)] as major results. The former shows that the ventromedial network is more activated, while the latter contrast shows the dorsomedial network is more involved.

Rustichini, Dickhaut, Ghirardato, Smith, and Pardo (2005)

A more recent study by Rustichini et al. (2005) introduces gambles involving partial ambiguity. Subjects in this study make binary choices between two gambles. These gambles are classified as certain (C), risky (R), ambiguous (A), and partially ambiguous (PA). In the PA gambles treatment, experimenter tells the subjects that there are at least 10 balls of each color without the exact number of balls for each type. These four types of gambles constitute six conditions (or pairs of gambles) of which three have a R gamble as the reference gamble (RR, PAR, and AR) and the other three have a certainty amount (a C gamble) as the reference gamble (RC, PAC, and AC). According to the "choice-theoretic point of view" discussed in Rustichini et al. (2005), the partially ambiguous gambles should be in an intermediate position between risky and ambiguous gambles in terms of reaction time (RT), subject's valuation, and brain activation. Yet, the experimental result suggests otherwise.

For the completely ambiguous case, if a subject possesses α-maxmin preference, she would consider that all balls would lead to the high payoff under the best possible scenario. At the same time, she would consider that all balls would lead to the low payoff in the worst scenario. Unlike complete ambiguity, for the partially ambiguous case, neither the best scenario nor the worst scenario would be viewed as being certain. For a α-maxmin decision maker, it appears that partial ambiguity would be more involved than the complete ambiguity. It seems most straightforward for a α-maxmin decision maker to assess gambles involving pure risks (and she would behave as if she has SEU preference) and she can skip the phase of evaluating the best and worst scenarios.

The reaction time (RT) data, however, do not support the implication of the α-maxmin model. For the C reference type, AC takes subjects the least time to decide, followed by the PAC, with RC taking the most time. By contrast, for the R reference type, AR takes subjects the most time to decide, followed by the PAR, with RR taking the least time. The R gambles seem to trigger more deliberation as evident by the fact that the R-based comparisons, on average, always yield higher RT than C-based comparisons.

In the analysis of the cutoff data – that is, the threshold above which subjects will switch to C – the cutoff value is similar for AC and PAC, but strikingly different for RC. In addition, different brain regions are activated under the PAC condition relative to the AC condition. Contrasting the PAC with AC shows significant activations in the regions of middle frontal gyrus, parietal lobe, lingual gyrus, and superior frontal gyrus. The frontal lobe, occipital lobe and precuneus are more activated in the contrast of PAC–RC. The medial frontal gyrus is more activated in the RR–PAR.

In sum, these results reveal that subjects have distinct attitudes towards ambiguity, risk, and partial ambiguity, and hence reject the implications of the α-maxmin utility model, and is compatible with the implications of the source preference model.

Hsu, Bhatt, Adolphs, Tranel, and Camerer (2005)

Hsu et al. (2005) conducts a fMRI study on ambiguity aversion incorporating additionally Fox and Tversky's suggestion of source preference which encompasses the risk-ambiguity distinction. In each of the three treatments, subjects make 48 choices between certain amounts of money and bets on card decks or events. The *card-deck* treatment is similar to the urn treatment in previous studies. Researchers present subjects with a choice to bet on the color of a card drawn from two decks of cards in which the proportion of blue and red cards is known (i.e., risky) in one deck and is not known (i.e., ambiguous) in the other. In the *knowledge* treatment (adapted from Fox & Tversky, 1995), the experimenters classify events into the familiar (whether the high temperature in New York City on a particular day was above a certain level) and the unfamiliar (the high temperature in Dushanbe, Tajikistan). "Risky" bets are those placed on familiar events; "ambiguous" bets are those placed on unfamiliar events. In the third (*informed opponent*) treatment, subjects decide whether to bet against an opponent. Should their choices of color match, both receive the certainty payoff. Otherwise, the subject wins only if his or her choice of color is realized. Here, the "ambiguous" case corresponds to being disadvantaged by betting against an opponent who can see a sample of up to nine cards (with replacement) before choosing his or her color. The "risky" case corresponds to betting against an uninformed opponent who cannot view a sample of cards before choosing a color.

Under all three treatments, for risky tasks, subjects are assumed to have SEU preference with vNM utility, $u(x,\rho) = x^{\rho}$, where $\rho >$ $(=, <)$ 1 corresponds to the case of risk affinity (neutrality, aversion). For ambiguous tasks, subjects are assumed to have RDEU preference (exposited in Section 2) with probability weighting function $\pi(p,\gamma) = p^{\gamma}$. In particular, $\rho<1$ and $\gamma>1$ ($\rho>1$ and $\gamma<1$) implies risk aversion (risk affinity) in terms of mean-preserving increase in risk. Hsu et al. (2005) interprets γ as a measure of ambiguity aversion with $\gamma<(=, >)$ 1 corresponding to ambiguity affinity (neutrality, aversion). For a lottery which yields x with probability p, we have $\text{RDEU}(x, p; 0, 1-p) = p^{\gamma}x^{\rho}$, where subjects' subjective probability of winning p is assumed to be half in the unknown deck in the card-deck treatment and for all questions in both the knowledge and the informed opponent treatments.

In this analysis, the authors employ a theoretical framework which can be cast in terms of the Chew–Sagi source preference model in which subjects have distinct risk attitudes for risky and ambiguous gambles. Specifically, for ambiguous gambles, subjects have probability weighting function p^{γ} in addition to utility function x^{ρ}. For risky gambles, they have EU preference with the same utility function. In this connection, as a special case, the Chew–Sagi approach delivers a simple and tractable SDEU model with x^{ρ} as utility function for risky gambles and x^{θ} $(\theta<\rho)$ for the modeling of attitude towards ambiguous risks.

In the estimated behavioral results, reported in Table S6 of the supporting online materials in Hsu et al. (2005), they find that, on average, subjects are risk averse in the card-deck treatment while risk seeking in the knowledge treatment. In addition, they find that subjects are, on average, ambiguity seeking in the card-deck treatment while more ambiguity averse in the knowledge treatment. These observations contravene the usual findings in the literature, and suggest the need for an empirically successful model accommodate multiple levels of ambiguity aversion.

At the perception epoch, orbitofrontal cortex (OFC), amygdala, and the dorsomedial prefrontal cortex (DMPFC) are found to be more activated under the ambiguity condition than under the risk condition. The reverse contrast shows the dorsal striatum as having greater activation in response to the risk condition than to the ambiguity condition. It is noteworthy that under all treatments, the certainty payoffs for risky tasks are, on average, higher than those for the ambiguous tasks. This factor could contribute to the observed stronger striatum activation in risky–ambiguity contrast. At the decision epoch (Table S9–S10 in Hsu et al., 2005), they observe significant bilateral insula and left ventral striatum activation in the contrast of choosing to gamble over choosing certainty payoffs. Interestingly, these regions do not exhibit significant interaction with risk and ambiguity.

Since the bilateral OFC is more activated under "ambiguity" than under "risk," the authors conduct a separate behavioral experiment involving subjects with OFC lesion versus control subjects with temporal lobe lesion. The control group displays both risk aversion and ambiguity aversion while the target group displays neutrality towards risk as well as ambiguity. The authors interpret this finding as validating the necessity of the OFC in distinguishing between risk aversion and ambiguity aversion.

Huettel, Stowe, Gordon, Warner, and Platt (2006)

Using fMRI, Huettel et al. (2006) demonstrate a correlation between activations in specific brain regions and subjects' attitudes towards risk and ambiguity. They introduce gambles with certainty outcomes which enable the calibration of subjects' degrees of both risk aversion and ambiguity aversion. In each trial, subjects face one of four pair types: ambiguous gamble versus sure amount (AC), ambiguous gamble versus risky gamble (AR), risky gamble versus sure amount (RC), and risky gamble versus another risky gamble (RR). All gambles are resolved during scanning and subjects receive feedback at the end of each trial.

Huettel et al. (2006) assumes that subjects possess α-MEU with power utility function, $u(x, \rho) = x^{\rho}$. To assess risk attitudes, they calibrate this power function for each subject by finding a value of ρ that maximizes the number of correct predictions in the RC and RR trials. To assess attitude towards ambiguity, they make use of ρ estimated before in conjunction with the α-MEU function to find a value of α that maximizes the number of correct predictions in the AC and AR trials. As observed earlier, SDEU offers an alternative model for estimating subjects' source preference from choice behavior during the risky and the ambiguous trials.

The pIFS, anterior insular cortex (aINS), and posterior parietal cortex (pPAR) are significantly more activated during choices involving ambiguous gambles than those involving risky gambles. The authors also show positive correlation between subjects' degrees of ambiguity preference and the difference in pIFS activation between the average of the AC and AR trials and average of the RC and RR trials. In other words, subjects with greater increase in pIFS activation during the ambiguous trials (average of the AC and AR trials) relative to the risky trials (average of RC and RR trials) display less ambiguity aversion in their choices. At the same time, there is positive correlation between subjects' risk preferences and increases in their pPAR activation (relative to the AC and AR trials) during the RC and RR trials. The observed activation of pIFS in the ambiguous related trials is distinct from the activation in the parietal cortex in Smith et al. (2002) and Rustichini et al. (2005). The pIFS finding also agrees with findings in the neuroeconomics literature (Huettel et al., 2005) in which pIFS has been implicated in risky decision-making.

Levy, Rustichini, and Glimcher (2007); Preuschoff and Bossaerts (2008)

In two more recent studies (Levy et al., 2007; Preuschoff & Bossaerts, 2008), the researchers investigate how decision makers would respond to different degrees of ambiguity. Levy et al. (2007) focus on the question of whether there is a common neural substrate underlying the difference in choice behaviors in the presence of differing degrees of ambiguity or, as most of the previous studies suggest, if there are multiple systems that represent value under different conditions. The authors ask subjects to choose between a reference gamble and either a risky or an ambiguous gamble with different degrees of ambiguity (RR or RA). The authors find that activations in the medial prefrontal cortex, posterior cingulate, and ventral striatum correlate with the subjective risk-adjusted valuations of the risky gambles. They find the same correlation between these activations and the subjective ambiguity-adjusted valuations of ambiguous gambles. Levy et al. (2007) further argue that these results suggest a unitary system for subjective valuation for gambles spanning the whole spectrum of varying degrees of ambiguity.

Summary

On the whole, the neuroimaging evidence surveyed supports the idea of subjects having source preference encompassing the risk-ambiguity distinction. In facing pure risk, pure ambiguity, and partial ambiguity (Rustichini et al., 2005), the reaction times and brain activations data suggest that partial ambiguity is processed differently from pure risk and pure ambiguity. In this connection, the experimental designs in Huettel et al. (2005), Hsu et al. (2005), and Levy et al. (2007) enable observations of neural correlates of decision-making in the presence of multiple levels of ambiguity.

The choice of data under the knowledge treatment in Hsu et al. (2005) reveal that uncertainty associated with familiar events is preferred to those associated with unfamiliar events. Since the event's probability is not known in both cases, subjects appear to have an intrinsic source preference driven by familiarity. Moreover, the OFC-lesion data in Hsu et al. (2005) – OFC-lesion patients are ambiguity and risk neutral – hint at aversion to both risk and ambiguity as having a common root. This is compatible with the suggestion in Levy et al. (2007) of a unitary system responding to the valuations of gambles with different degrees of ambiguity. This also corroborates the Chew–Sagi model which posits that ambiguity aversion and source preference arise from the individual's risk attitude being distinct towards risks from different sources of uncertainty.

4. NEW NEUROIMAGING EXPERIMENT ON SOURCE PREFERENCE

Experiment Design

This experiment involves the participation of 16 subjects recruited from universities in Hong Kong. We report further details of the subjects and fMRI image acquisition procedure in the Appendix. In each trial, we require subjects to choose between two lotteries (see Fig. 1). Each lottery consists of a bet on the trailing digit – odd or even – of the closing price on the following trading day of one of two different stocks listed on the exchange.[1]

We conduct the experiment under both gain and loss trials. In the gain trials, the subjects earn the corresponding amount of money if they win the bet and receive zero otherwise. In the loss trials, subjects earn zero if they win the bet and lose the corresponding amount of money otherwise. The payoff for each gain-oriented lottery ranges from HK$150 to HK$200 while the payoff for each loss-oriented lottery ranges from losing HK$20 to losing HK$40. The total earnings of each subject consist of adding the outcome of a randomly drawn gain-oriented lottery and a randomly drawn loss-oriented lottery, plus a HK$100 endowment. To assess subjects' degree of familiarity towards the stocks, subjects are asked to indicate their degree of familiarity from 0 to 9 for each of the 48 stocks.

Experimental Results

At the behavioral level, subjects tend to choose the more familiar source of uncertainty in the gain domain ($p<0.021$). We use general linear model

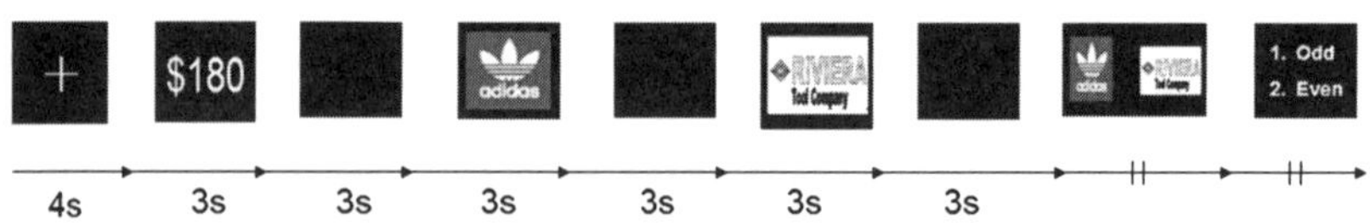

Fig. 1. Experiment Design. At the Beginning of Each Trial, a Fixation Sign is Shown to Indicate the Start of a New Trial and the Amount of the Gamble Would Appear. Then after Three Seconds, the Logos of the Two Lotteries (Stocks) are Presented Sequentially and Then Together. Subjects Indicate Their Preferences on Sources by Pressing a Left or Right Button. Afterwards, They Select the Last Digit of the Closing Price of the Chosen Stock on the Next Trading Day as Either Odd or Even by Pressing a Left or Right Button. There are 48 Trials. Half of the Trials are Gain Trails and the Reminding are Loss Trials.

analysis, with familiarity rating as a regressor, to identify neural correlates for decisions involving the choice of more familiar sources over those of less familiar sources. Regions appearing to be more active when subjects decide to bet on more familiar sources under gain-oriented lotteries included the putamen (part of the striatum; see Fig. 2), medial frontal cortex, and superior temporal gyrus (Table 1). Hsu et al. (2005) finds the striatum, implicated in reward prediction (O'Doherty et al., 2004), to be more active in the risk condition than in the ambiguity condition.[2] Hsu et al. (2005) suggests that ambiguous gambles have lower anticipated reward, thus leading to lower activation in the striatum relative to the risky gambles. The medial frontal cortex is consistently implicated in reward processing and in anticipation of risky gambles (Gehring & Willoughby, 2002). On the other hand, the middle frontal cortex and superior frontal cortex are more activated when subjects decide to bet on more familiar

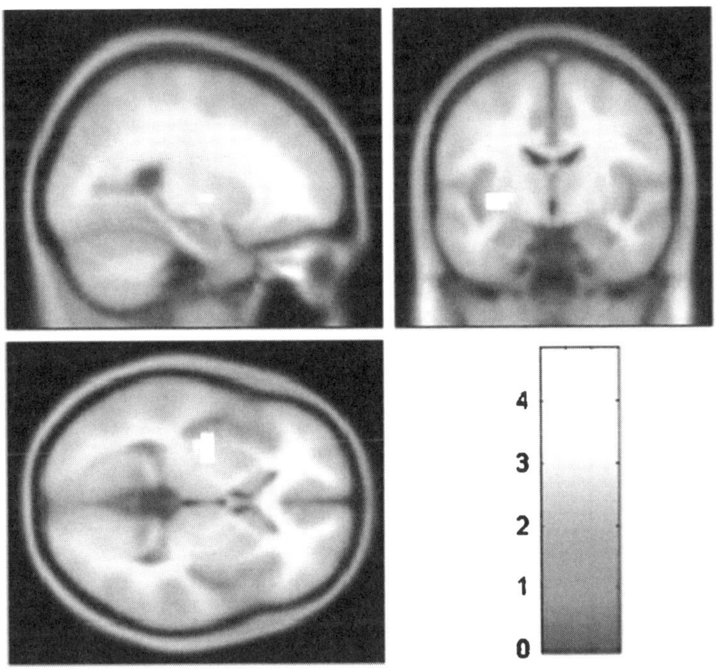

Fig. 2. Putamen Shows Higher Activation when Subjects Choose more Familiar Sources under Gain Oriented Lotteries ($P<0.005$ Uncorrected; Cluster Size $k\geqslant 9$ voxels).

Table 1. Regions Associated with Choosing a more Familiar Source under Gain-Oriented Lotteries.

Region of Activation	*X*	*Y*	*Z*	*T*-Value	*Z*-Value
Superior temporal Gyrus	−56	12	−8	5.23	3.77
Putamen	28	−12	0	4.86	3.6
Medial frontal cortex	12	−4	52	3.67	2.99
Medial frontal cortex	12	−12	60	3.24	2.72

Note: $P<0.005$ uncorrected; cluster size $k \geqslant 9$ voxels. MNI coordinates (mm) presented.

Table 2. ROI Analysis.

Region	*X*	*Y*	*Z*	*P*-Value
Familiar–Unfamiliar				
Striatum	0	−6	−6	0.03*
	9	6	6	0.01*
	−12	6	0	0.03*
Precuneus	−15	−72	51	0.01**
	12	−75	51	0.05*
	21	−84	39	0.07
Unfamiliar–Familiar				
Amygdala	−15	−15	−15	0.08
	−21	−6	−18	0.06
	33	−6	−27	0.02*
Dorsomedial prefrontal cortex	18	54	18	0.01**
	12	54	30	0.03*
	−9	48	39	0.02*
	−12	63	21	0.01**
Lateral orbitofrontal cortex	51	33	−6	0.07
	54	18	−21	0.08
	−54	36	−6	0.06
	54	27	6	0.01*

Note: *significant at the $P<0.05$ level; **significant at the $P<0.01$ level.

sources under loss-oriented lotteries. These regions have also been implicated in reward processing (Nieuwenhuis et al., 2005; Hsu et al., 2005). Intriguingly, this finding supports the hypothesis that choosing a more familiar source is more rewarding.

Region-of-Interest Analysis (ROI)

We conduct region-of-interest analysis (ROI) on the regions reported by Hsu et al. (2005), who find that the striatum is associated with risky decisions while the amygdala, dorsomedial prefrontal cortex, and lateral orbitofrontal cortex are associated with ambiguity. In the analysis of these five regions, we define the ROIs by drawing spheres of 10 mm radius centering on the peaks of activation in each of these regions. We further test the activation patterns in the familiar–unfamiliar and unfamiliar–familiar conditions and investigate whether they are similar to those in the risk–ambiguity and ambiguity–risk conditions. Most of the ROIs are significant at the p-value <0.05 level (See Table 2 for results). These findings support the hypothesis that people have distinct attitudes towards risks arising from different sources and brain activation in the familiar–unfamiliar and unfamiliar–familiar contrasts are similar to the brain activation of the risk–ambiguity and ambiguity–risk contrasts.

5. CONCLUSION

This chapter reports the first neuroimaging study of source preference in relation to ambiguity aversion. Our odd–even experimental design offers the advantage of being able to induce the same "unambiguous" probability of half for each lottery. This enables us to discriminate between the source preference approach (Chew & Sagi, 2008) and models based on multiple priors, such as α-maxmin as well as those based on non-additive probabilities, such as Choquet expected utility and cumulative prospect theory.

The behavioral result of our neuroimaging experiment shows that subjects tend to choose the more familiar source of uncertainty despite both lotteries (sources) delivering the same outcomes with equal probability. Regions that are more activated when subjects choose to bet on more familiar sources include the putamen, part of the striatum, which Hsu et al. (2005) finds to be more activated in the risky relative to the ambiguity condition. We confirm this result in a ROI analysis on the finding of Hsu et al. (2005).

It will be valuable to pursue follow up research towards understanding the neural mechanisms of source preference which encompasses a broad range of observed risk taking behavior, such as home market bias in financial markets, brand preference in marketing, the distinction between risk taking and gambling in casinos, and policy making involving social and natural risks. More generally, this study suggests that decision theory can offer a powerful tool for designing neuroeconomics experiments leading to greater understanding of neural mechanisms involved in decision-making. The methodology of neuroeconomics can in turn help discriminate among competing models of decision-making and contribute to their further theoretical development.

NOTES

1. Our odd-even design inducing the same "unambiguous" probability of one-half for each subject exemplifies Machina's (2004) "almost-objective" events which he showed to induce unanimously agree-upon revealed likelihoods.

2. Hsu et al. (2005) find caudate (part of dorsal striatum) to be more active in the risk condition than in the ambiguity condition. Both caudate (part of dorsal striatum) and putamen, involved in reward processing, are part of the striatum. See O'Doherty et al. (2004) for a discussion on the difference between the two regions in reward processing.

ACKNOWLEDGMENTS

We thank Richard Ebstein, Nicholas Hon, Tanjim Hossain, Hsu Ming, Li Geng, Li Jian, Read Montague, Ngooi Chiu Ai, Ryo Okui, Jacob Sagi, Xu Cui, Edward Yang, Rami Zwick as well as seminar participants at the Asia Pacific Meeting of Economic Science Association in Osaka (February 2007) and in Singapore (February 2008). We gratefully acknowledge Eric Set, Annie Tang, Xue Fei, and Zhu Xingtian for valuable research assistance, and the financial support of the Research Grants Council of Hong Kong.

REFERENCES

Bechara, A. (2001). Neurobiology of decision-making: Risk and reward. *Seminars in Clinical Neuropsychiatry*, *6*(3), 205–216.

Bernoulli, D. (1738/1954). Exposition of a new theory on the measurement of risk. *Econometrica*, *22*(1), 23–36.

Borch, K. (1969). A note on uncertainty and indifference curves. *Review of Economic Studies*, *36*(1), 1–4.

Bossaerts, P., Ghirardato, P., Guarneschelli, S., & Zame, W. R. (2007). *Ambiguity in asset markets: Theory and experiment*. Working paper, Division of The Humanities and Social Sciences, California Institute of Technology.

Camerer, C., & Weber, M. (1992). Recent developments in modeling preferences: Uncertainty and ambiguity. *Journal of Risk and Uncertainty*, *5*(4), 325–370.

Chew, S. H., Karni, E., & Safra, Z. (1987). Risk aversion in the theory of expected utility with rank dependent probabilities. *Journal of Economic Theory*, *42*(2), 370–381.

Chew, S. H., Li, K. K., Chark, C. H., & Zhong, S. F. (2008). *Evidence on preference towards sources of uncertainty from lab and field experiments, work-in-progress*. Department of Economics, Hong Kong University of Science and Technology.

Chew, S. H., & Sagi, J. S. (2006). Event exchangeability: Probabilistic sophistication without continuity or monotonicity. *Econometrica*, *74*(3), 771–786.

Chew, S. H., & Sagi, J. S. (2008). Small worlds: Modeling attitudes toward sources of uncertainty. *Journal of Economic Theory*, *139*(1), 1–24.

Chew, S. H., & Wakker, P. (1996). The comonotonic sure-thing principle. *Journal of Risk and Uncertainty*, *12*, 5–27.

Chua, P., Krams, M., Toni, I., Passingham, R., & Dolan, R. (1999). A functional anatomy of anticipatory anxiety. *NeuroImage*, *9*(6), 563–571.

De Finetti, B. (1937). Foresight, its logical laws, its subjective sources. In: H. E. Kyburg & H. E. Smokler (Eds), *Studies in subjective probability*. New York: Ann. Inst. Henri Poincaré Wiley.

Ellsberg, D. (1961). Risk, ambiguity, and the savage axioms. *Quarterly Journal of Economics*, *75*(4), 643–669.

Fox, C. R., & Tversky, A. (1995). Ambiguity aversion and comparative ignorance. *Quarterly Journal of Economics*, *110*(3), 585–603.

Gehring, W. J., & Willoughby, A. R. (2002). The medial frontal cortex and the rapid processing of monetary gains and losses. *Science*, *295*, 2279–2282.

Ghirardato, P., Maccheroni, F., & Marinacci, M. (2004). Differentiating ambiguity and ambiguity attitude. *Journal of Economic Theory*, *118*(2), 133–173.

Gilboa, I., & Schmeidler, D. (1989). Maxmin expected utility with non-unique prior. *Journal of Mathematical Economics*, *18*(2), 141–153.

Green, J. R., & Jullien, B. (1988). Ordinal independence in nonlinear utility theory. *Journal of Risk and Uncertainty*, *1*, 32.

Halevy, Y. (2007). Ellsberg revisited: An experimental study. *Econometrica*, *75*(2), 503–536.

Hsu, M., Bhatt, M., Adolphs, R., Tranel, D., & Camerer, C. F. (2005). Neural systems responding to degrees of uncertainty in human decision-making. *Science*, *310*, 1680–1683.

Huettel, S. A., Song, A. W., & McCarthy, G. (2005). Decisions under uncertainty: Probabilistic context influences activity of prefrontal and parietal cortices. *Journal of Neuroscience*, *25*, 3304–3311.

Huettel, S. A., Stowe, C. J., Gordon, E. M., Warner, B. T., & Platt, M. L. (2006). Neural signatures of economic preferences for risk and ambiguity. *Neuron*, *49*(5), 765–775.

Keynes, J. M. (1921). *A treatise on probability*. London: Macmillan.

Knight, F. H. (1921). *Risk, uncertainty and profit*. Boston: Houghton Mifflin Company.

Knutson, B., Taylor, J., Kaufman, M., Peterson, R., & Glover, G. (2005). Distributed neural representation of expected value. *Journal of Neuroscience*, *25*(19), 4806–4812.

Kuhnen, C. M., & Knutson, B. (2005). The neural basis of financial risk taking. *Neuron*, *47*(5), 763–770.

Levy, I., Rustichini, A., & Glimcher, P. (2007). *Neural correlates of subjective value under risky and ambiguous decision-making*. Society for neuroeconomics annual meeting, September, Salt Lake City, Utah.

Machina, M., & Schmeidler, D. (1992). A more robust definition of subjective probability. *Econometrica*, *60*(4), 745–780.

Markowitz, H. (1952). Portfolio selection. *Journal of Finance*, *7*(1), 77–91.

Mazziotta, J. C., Toga, A. W., Evans, A., Fox, P., & Lancaster, J. (1995). A probabilistic atlas of the human brain: Theory and rationale for its development. The International Consortium for Brain Mapping (ICBM). *Neuroimage*, *2*(2), 89–101.

Nieuwenhuis, S., Heslenfeld, D. J., Alting von Geusau, N. J., Mars, R. B., Holroyd, C. B., & Yeung, N. (2005). Activity in human reward-sensitive brain areas is strongly context dependent. *NeuroImage*, *25*(4), 1302–1309.

O'Doherty, J., Dayan, P., Schultz, J., Deichmann, R., Friston, K., & Dolan, R. J. (2004). Dissociable roles of ventral and dorsal striatum in instrumental conditioning. *Science*, *304*, 452–454.

Preuschoff, K., & Bossaerts, P. (2008). *Modeling decision making under ambiguity*. Poster I–68, Computation and Systems Neuroscience, Salt Lake City, Utah.

Preuschoff, K., Bossaerts, P., & Quartz, S. R. (2006). Neural differentiation of expected reward and risk in human subcortical structures. *Neuron*, *51*(3), 381–390.

Quiggin, J. (1982). A theory of anticipated utility. *Journal of Economic Behavior and Organization*, *3*(4), 323–343.

Quiggin, J., & Wakker, P. (1994). The axiomatic basis of anticipated utility: A clarification. *Journal of Economic Theory*, *64*(2), 486–499.

Ramsey, F. P. (1931). Truth and probability. In: R. B. Braithwaite (Ed.), *The foundations of mathematics and other logical essays* (pp. 156–198). London: Routledge.

Rothschild, M., & Stiglitz, J. E. (1970). Increasing risk: I. A definition. *Journal of Economic Theory*, *September*(2), 243–255.

Rustichini, A., Dickhaut, J., Ghirardato, P., Smith, K., & Pardo, J. V. (2005). A brain imaging study of the choice procedure. *Games and Economic Behavior*, *52*(2), 257–282.

Savage, L. J. (1954). *The foundations of statistics*. New York: Wiley.

Schmeidler, D. (1989). Subjective probability and expected utility without additivity. *Econometrica*, *57*(3), 571–587.

Smith, K., Dickhaut, J., McCabe, K., & Pardo, J. V. (2002). Neuronal substrates for choice under ambiguity, risk, gains, and losses. *Management Science*, *48*(6), 711–718.

Tversky, A., & Kahneman, D. (1992). Advances in prospect theory: Cumulative representation of uncertainty. *Journal of Risk and Uncertainty*, *5*(4), 297–323.

von Neumann, J., & Morgenstern, O. (1947). *Theory of games and economic behavior*. Princeton: University Press.

APPENDIX

fMRI Acquisition

fMRI was performed on a Philips Achiva 3T whole body MRI at the Jockey Club MRI Engineering Centre, Hong Kong with an 8 channel quadrature birdcage head coil. A sagittal spin echo localizer image was acquired initially. fMRI was performed in the transverse plane, parallel to the anterior–posterior commisura (AC-PC) line. A 35-slice set of fMRI images was acquired with the following scan parameters: TR = 2,000 ms; TE = 30 ms; flip angle = 90°; matrix = 64 × 64; field of view = 22 cm × 22 cm; slice thickness = 4.0 mm, without inter-slice gap. Anatomical whole brain MRI was acquired using a T1-weighted turbo spin echo (TSE) sequence with TR 2,000 ms and TE 10 ms with IR delay 800 ms. Around 700 fMRI volume images, depending on subjects' response time, were collected during each run. The first four fMRI volume images of each run were discarded to insure steady state magnetization.

Data Processing and Analysis

Post-processing of fMRI data was done using Statistical Parametric Map (SPM2) software package (Wellcome Department of Cognitive Neurology, Institute of Neurology, Queen Square, UK), running on Matlab (Version 7.0.0; Math Works Inc., Natick, MA, USA). Each fMRI image volume was automatically realigned to the first image of the time series to correct for head movements during the fMRI acquisition. The time series volumes were then registered to the brain template adopted by the International Consortium for Brain Mapping (ICBM) (Mazziotta, Toga, Evans, Fox, & Lancaster, 1995); spatial normalization into Montreal Neurological Institutes coordinates (resampled 4 mm × 4 mm × 4 mm). The spatially normalized EPI volumes were smoothed by an 8 mm full-width-half-maximum Gaussian kernel. Physiological noise was filtered using a window function that corresponds to a homodynamic impulse response function (HRF). Statistical analysis was conducted at two levels. Individual task-related activation was evaluated. To make inferences at a group level, individual data were summarized and incorporated into a random effects model.

Subjects

Sixteen right-handed undergraduate students were recruited from universities in Hong Kong. Each participant underwent fMRI scanning while performing 48 trials (not including 2 practice trials) of the experimental task illustrated in Fig. 1. Informed consent was obtained using a consent form approved by the human subjects committee at HKUST. Subjects were briefed on the (Chinese) instructions before entering the scanner. It was known that at the end of the experiment, one trial from each of the two treatments would be chosen at random, and the subject's choice on that trial would determine her pay. The earning is the total from the two randomly-chosen choices plus HK$100 endowment.

NEUROECONOMICS OF DECISION-MAKING IN THE AGING BRAIN: THE EXAMPLE OF LONG-TERM CARE

Ming Hsu, Hung-Tai Lin and Paul E. McNamara

ABSTRACT

Purpose – *Long-term care (LTC) services assist people with limitations in the ability to perform activities of daily living (ADLs) as a result of chronic illness or disabilities. We discuss possible behavioral explanations for the under-purchasing of LTC insurance, as well as the current state of knowledge on the neural mechanisms behind these behavioral factors.*

Findings/approach – *Ideas from behavioral economics are discussed, including risk-seeking over losses, ambiguity-preferring over losses, hyperbolic discounting, and the effect of the aging process on the underlying neural mechanisms supporting these decisions. We further emphasize the role of age, as aging is a highly heterogeneous process. It is associated with changes in both brain tissue as well as cognitive abilities, and both are characterized by large individual differences. Therefore, understanding the neural mechanisms is vital to understanding this heterogeneity and identifying possible methods of interventions.*

Neuroeconomics
Advances in Health Economics and Health Services Research, Volume 20, 203–225

ISSN: 0731-2199/doi:10.1016/S0731-2199(08)20009-9

Research implications – *LTC financing and insurance is a looming issue in the next 10–20 years. It is important to understand the process by which people make decisions about LTC insurance, heterogeneity in decision processes across individuals, and how these decisions interact with changes in policy and private LTC insurance markets.*

Originality/value of the chapter – *By providing an overview of the current state of knowledge in behavioral economics of LTC insurance and the neuroscience of aging, this chapter provides some new directions in the emerging area of neuroeconomics of aging.*

INTRODUCTION

Long-term care (LTC) is a collection of services that assist people with limitations in the ability to perform activities of daily living (ADL) as a result of chronic illness or disabilities. The estimated lifetime risk of entering a nursing home ranges from 31 to 50%, with an average annual cost of nursing home care of $50,000 in 1998 dollars (Mulvey & Stucki, 1999). Total annual LTC expenditures in the United States total about $100 billion, approximately 10% of the entire US health expenditure.

LTC's burden on private and public finances is substantial. About 40% are paid for out-of-pocket (McNamara & Lee, 2004). The remaining percentage is borne by the taxpayer, primarily in the form of the Medicaid program (Congressional Budge Office, 2004). This, combined with the increasing life expectancy of population, is placing tremendous burden on the federal budget. LTC expenditure is estimated, in constant 2,000 dollars, to double by 2025 and increase five-fold by 2045 (American Association of Homes and Services for the Aging, 2006). Current estimates of the financial sustainability of the Medicaid program put the date of insolvency at around 20 years, in large part due to the high costs of LTC (Marron, 2006).

Under standard life-cycle models of saving, individuals smooth their consumption or expenditure to keep the marginal utility of money constant over time (Browning & Crossley, 2001). Thus, without any LTC financing plan, once individuals need LTC services at some point during their lifetime, their expected lifetime utility will fall since then.[1] The reason is that they have to modify their expected consumption bundle through relocating their consumption and savings to make up for the greater financial impact of needing LTC on their lifetime consumption plan. Contrary to the predictions of the standard model, and despite the substantial portion paid out-of-pocket, only about 10% of the elderly in the US have private LTC insurance (Congressional Budge Office, 2004). Such policies typically promise to pay up to a specified amount per day for nursing home and home health care services for policyholders who develop chronic impairments. Annual premiums average $1,000–2,000 if the policy is purchased at age 65, and considerably more if purchased later in life. Table 1 summarizes the cost of a typical LTC insurance plan (State Farm Insurance, 2006).

As is clear from the earlier example, to effectively plan for LTC insurance, the decision maker needs, at the least, to be able to trade off between present and future consumption. This requires taking into account risk attitude, time preference, and forecast income, and consumption before and during retirement. This is clearly a nontrivial task and perhaps it is unsurprising that individuals behave sub-optimally.

There are a variety of reasons why people do not purchase LTC insurance. The most commonly invoked explanation in the past has been that the elderly are misinformed (Task Force on Long Term Health Care Policies, 1987). This explanation is less relevant today than in previous decades. For example, the awareness of private LTC insurance as an option increased from 38% in 1995 to 63% in 1999 (American Association of Homes and Services for the Aging, 2006). Another explanation invokes the existence of Medicaid as a provider of service of last resort, which serves effectively to "crowd out" private LTC insurance (Marron, 2006). This is clearly an important factor. Preliminary figures estimate that Medicaid

Table 1. Benefits and Annual Premium of a State Farm Series #97059 Policy for the State of Illinois.

	Buy Today	Buy in 10 Years	Buy in 20 Years
		(Costs below Adjusted to Keep Pace with Inflation)	
	Age 55	65	75
Daily benefit	125	200	325
Annual premium	1,370	3,646	14,277
Daily benefit at age 85 with inflation protection	540	531	529
Total benefit dollars at age 85	985,943	968,454	966,138
Total premium to age 85	41,100	72,920	142,773

crowds out private insurance purchase for over half of households (Brown & Finkelstein, 2004b).

One explanation that has been convincingly ruled out as a primary cause of under-purchasing of LTC insurance is imperfection on the supply-side of the LTC insurance market. There are a number of causes for supply-side imperfection, including transactions costs, imperfect competition, and asymmetric information. Existence of such imperfection could lead to either higher than actuarially fair pricing or less than comprehensive coverage.[2] It was found, however, that supply-side imperfection explains a small share of the under-insurance. Using a dataset that included approximate two-thirds of industry-wide sales, Brown and Finkelstein found that, in contrast to limited coverage, there are widely available policies that will cover about 90% of the expected present value of expenditures for a 65-year-old (Brown & Finkelstein, 2004a). Moreover, they found the existence of *better* than actuarially fair prices for women;[3] yet insurance rate for elderly women is similarly low as men.

WEAK DEMAND FOR LTC INSURANCE: THREE BEHAVIORAL EXPLANATIONS

Given the considerable evidence that consumers violate predictions of the standard models, as well as the considerably difficult choices that consumers face, we turn to behavioral factors that may lie behind the departure from the standard models. Behavioral models have been influential in areas such as retirement planning and saving (Laibson, 1997; Thaler & Benartzi, 2004), insurance (Hogarth & Kunreuther, 1989), and more recently in the annuities market (Brown, Kling, Mullainathan, & Wrobel, 2008). Here we note three stylized facts that apply to LTCI: (i) outcomes are clearly stated in the loss domain, (ii) the probability of the disability is ambiguous,[4] and (iii) disability can occur many years in the future.

We will discuss each in turn, but first we will review some of the basic knowledge of cognitive and neural changes that are associated with aging. There are several reasons why an understanding of the neurobiological basis of decision-making is relevant here. Practically, age is associated with an inevitable reduction in brain tissue, as well as decline in various cognitive abilities (Fig. 1). As LTCI is a decision that impacts overwhelmingly those in late-middle age to old age, this may either ameliorate or exacerbate preexisting behavioral biases (as an example, the brochure in Table 1 gives

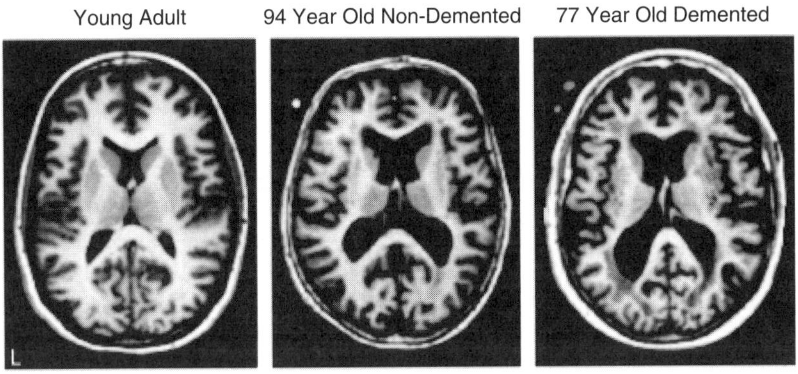

Fig. 1. Brain Differences between Young and Old, with and without Dementia (Reprinted from Buckner et al., 2004, with permission from Elsevier).

examples of outcomes for 55-, 65-, and 75-years-old). More generally, using neuroscientific data may augment the predictive capabilities of standard economic models (Glimcher & Rustichini, 2004), as well as provide guidance for policy changes in investment for future generations (Heckman, 2007).

Age-Related Changes in the Brain

Perhaps the most striking feature of age-related changes is the heterogeneity of the aging process. This is a theme that will be repeated throughout the chapter. In terms of cognitive abilities or neural degeneration, there may be little difference between a low functioning 65-year-old and high functioning 85-year-old. That is, physical age can be a poor proxy of cognitive and neural aging. In general, aging is associated with both brain volume decrease and ventricular expansion (Raz, 2005). For example, in a review of five studies on older adults with mean ages 70–81, the median annual rate of expansion of the ventricles was 4.25% (2.90–5.56%). This is as compared to the rates of younger adults, which were an order of magnitude smaller (0.43%) (Raz, 2005). This includes reduction in gray matter in dopaminergic regions such as the striatum, as well as prefrontal cortices and the insula (Bäckman & Farde, 2005; Raz, 2004, 2005), regions that are critically involved in decision-making, as we shall see later in the chapter. However, there is substantial variability in effects of aging *within* the brain (Raz, 2005). That is, whereas there is comparatively minor decrease in gray matter

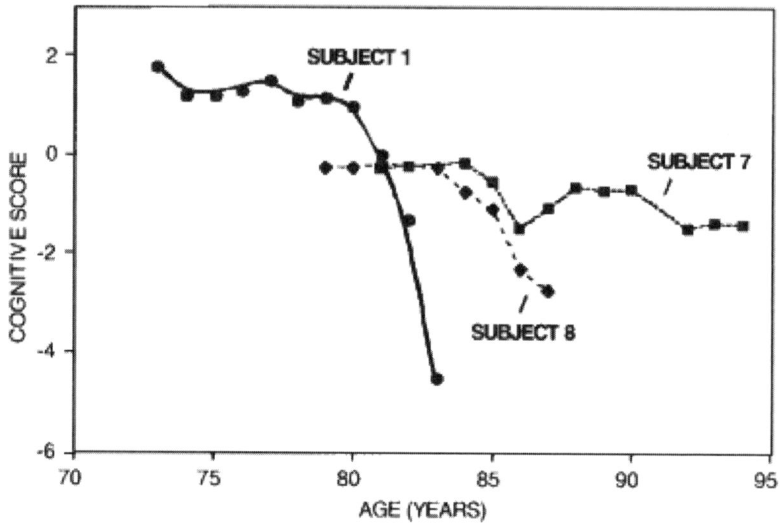

Fig. 2. Example of Longitudinal Cognitive Function in Three Individuals. *Note:* Dramatic Declines in Cognitive Functioning at Different Times for Subjects 1 and 8, and Intact Functioning in Subject 7 at an Extremely Advanced Age (Reprinted from Buckner, 2004, with permission from Elsevier).

in the visual cortex, there is substantial degradation in prefrontal cortices (for survey, see Raz, 2005) (Fig. 2).

Given the known profound effects of aging on cognitive abilities, it is surprising that the search for aging-related changes in economic decision-making has so far found mixed results. One of the earlier studies by Kovalchik, Camerer, Grether, Plott, and Allman (2005) compared a group of healthy elderly individuals (ages 70–95) to a group of Caltech undergraduates. They found little difference between the two groups across a variety of different decision tasks in terms of (1) overconfidence, (2) Iowa Gambling Task (IGT), (3) endowment effect, and (4) strategic thinking (*p*-beauty contest). Other studies, however, find substantial differences. We shall return to this point further in later portions of the chapter.

Losses

Unlike savings and investments, LTC deals clearly with outcomes in the loss domain. It is well known in behavioral economics that decision-makers tend to be risk-seeking under losses – a finding that has underpinned the development of prospect theory (Kahneman & Tversky, 1979; Tversky & Kahneman, 1992). This result has been confirmed in laboratory experiments (Cohen, Jaffray, & Said, 1985) and field data (Odean, 1998), with outcomes in health states (Verhoef, Dehaan, & Vandaal, 1994) and insurance contexts (Hogarth & Kunreuther, 1989).

Fig. 3 shows a hypothetic utility function in prospect theory. Note that the utility function is concave over gains and convex over losses. This corresponds to risk aversion for gains and risk-seeking for losses. Finally, losses have been found to be weighted more relative to gains, implying that the loss aversion coefficient $\lambda > 1$.

To see why risk-seeking behavior would result in under-insuring, note that an agent is risk-seeking if she prefers a gamble to the expected value of the gamble. That is, $\sum_{i \in S} p_i u(x_i) > u(\sum_{i \in S} p_i x_i)$, where p_i and x_i denote the probability and outcome in state i, respectively. For example, suppose that the agent will be healthy at age 80 with probability .75, but in need of LTC with probability of .25, which would cost her $10,000. Since she is risk-seeking, she will reject an actuarially fair premium of (present value) $2,500. Moreover, no insurance company can feasibly provide insurance to this agent, as it would generate negative profit in expectation.

In addition, there is good evidence that individuals exhibit patterns of preference in line with prospect theory when valuing health decisions and life durations (Verhoef et al., 1994; Bleichrodt & Pinto, 2005). Consistent with prospect theory, individuals' utility for living appears to be dependent on the reference point of the individual. Finally, there is much evidence that people behave inconsistently with expected utility theory in insurance markets. First, many people do not purchase insurance voluntarily

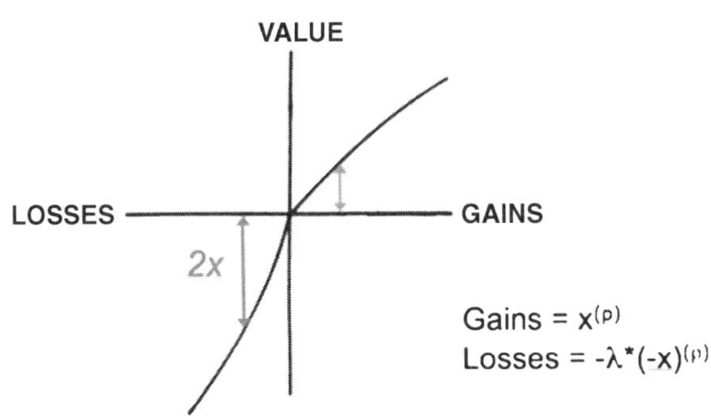

Fig. 3. A Utility Function under Prospect Theory.

(e.g., most states require mandatory automobile insurance). Second, econometric tests of field data rejects expected utility in favor of prospect theory, both in terms of non-nested model selection criterion and out-of-sample prediction (Marquis & Holmer, 1996). Finally, a crucial piece of evidence lies in the observation that people overwhelmingly reject what is called "probabilistic" insurance when it is offered to them at an actuarially fair price. This behavior violates expected utility theory, but can easily be explained by prospect theory (Camerer, 2001).

Recent neuroeconomic evidence shows that the amygdala is activated when choices are framed in terms of losses, as opposed to gains (De Martino, Kumaran, Seymour, & Dolan, 2006), suggesting a role for emotions in this overweighting. Failure to value gains and losses correctly has been found in patients with orbitofrontal and amygdala patients, mostly notably through the IGT (Bechara, Damasio, & Damasio, 2000; Bechara, Tranel, Damasio, & Damasio, 1996).

Furthermore, it is known that activity in the striatum and OFC is correlated with level of reward (Knutson, Adams, Fong, & Hommer, 2001; O'Doherty, Critchley, Deichmann, & Dolan, 2003), and the role of the insula in encoding for the valence of the stimulus (O'Doherty et al., 2003). It is now a widely accepted view that dopamine and dopaminergic regions – including the dorsal and ventral striatum, as well as the orbitofrontal cortex – are critical in different aspects of reward evaluation and reward (O'Doherty et al., 2004; Schultz, 2000, 2006). These regions undergo varying degrees of degeneration in aging humans. Parkinson's disease, for example, is characterized by the loss of pigmented dopaminergic cells in the substantia nigra. Understanding the neural mechanisms, therefore, is crucial given the prevalence and heterogeneity of such degeneration inherent in the aging process. Tom, Fox, Trepel, and Poldrack (2007) find that activation of the ventral striatum corresponds to both gains and losses. Whereas activation of the ventral striatum is positively correlated with the magnitude of the gains, it is negatively correlated with the magnitude of the losses (Fig. 4A). Importantly, differential response between gains and losses in the ventral striatum is highly correlated with behavioral measure of loss aversion (Fig. 4B).

Samanez-Larkin et al. (2007) conducted a rare study on age-related responses to gains and losses. In the study, 12 young and 12 older subjects were administrated the monetary incentive delay (MID) task. Unlike most behavioral economics studies, which focus on choice, the MID task is primarily focused on reward anticipation. In the MID task, subjects are given a cue that signals the amount of money one can gain or avoid to lose. Subjects

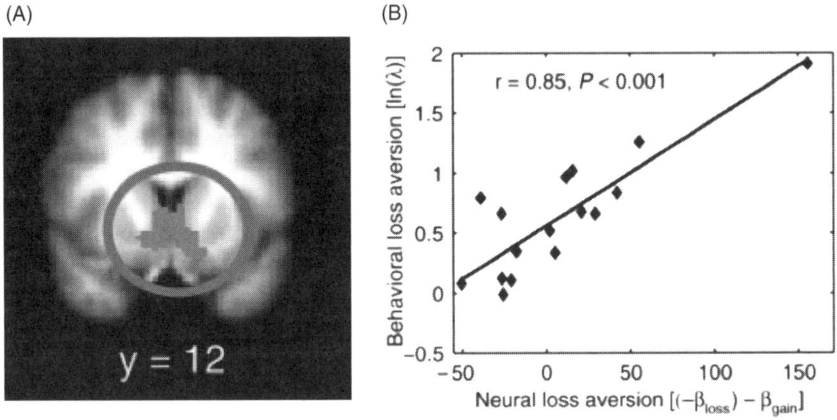

Fig. 4. (A) Conjunction Analysis of Ventral Striatum Activation with Respect to Response to Losses as well as Gains, (B) Differential Magnitude of Activation to Losses Minus Gains is Highly Correlated with Behavioral Loss Aversion (From Tom et al., 2007, reprinted with permission from AAAS).

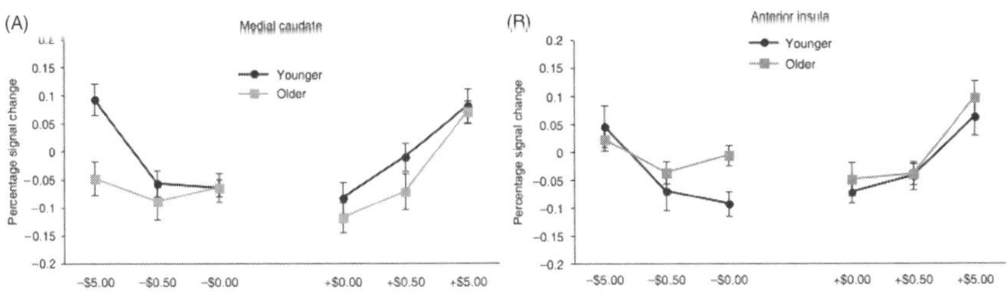

Fig. 5. BOLD Activation between Young and Old in (A) Medial Caudate and (B) Anterior Insula (Reprinted by permission from Macmillan Publishers Ltd: Samanez-Larkin et al., 2007).

win if they are able to press a button in reaction to a target quickly enough. Uncertainty is determined through calibration to the reaction time of the subject. This provides a straightforward method of assessing the neural correlates of reward anticipation in the absence of choice (Fig. 5).

Intriguingly, Samanez-Larkin et al. found a dissociation between neural responses to gain and loss in the caudate nucleus and the insula cortex. Whereas there were no differences between neural responses in the gain domain between young and older subjects, older subjects were found to have decreased activation in the loss domain relative to the young subjects. Due to the lack of a choice paradigm in the MID task, it is unclear how, or even whether, the neural changes will be reflected in choice behavior. Several intriguing possibilities exist. First, decreasing sensitivity to losses in these regions may lead to less risk-seeking behavior in the domain of losses. In addition, if the difference affects the relative weighting of losses to gains, this could also lead to lowered loss aversion. Finally, it is also possible that other regions may compensate for decreasing sensitivity in losses in these regions. Given the heterogeneity in the aging process, it will be important to include behavioral measures in future experiments to assess the impact of these neural changes on evaluation of losses.

Ambiguous Probabilities

In most real-life decisions, probabilities are vague and based on limited information. For example, a 65-year-old woman is unlikely to know the precise probability that she will need LTC at age 80. This is known in economics and decision theory as "ambiguity" (Ellsberg, 1961).

Fig. 6 illustrates the difference between risk and ambiguity. The deck on the left has a known proportion of red and black cards, and is said to be "risky"; the deck on the right has an unknown proportion of red and black cards, is said to be "ambiguous." Work in behavioral economics has shown that a substantial proportion of people are ambiguity-averse for gains and ambiguity-seeking for losses (for review, see Camerer & Weber, 1992).

Unlike risk-seeking behavior, which is modeled in expected utility theory as convexity of the utility function, ambiguity-seeking (averse) behavior is a violation of SEU (Ellsberg, 1961). A convenient form of representing

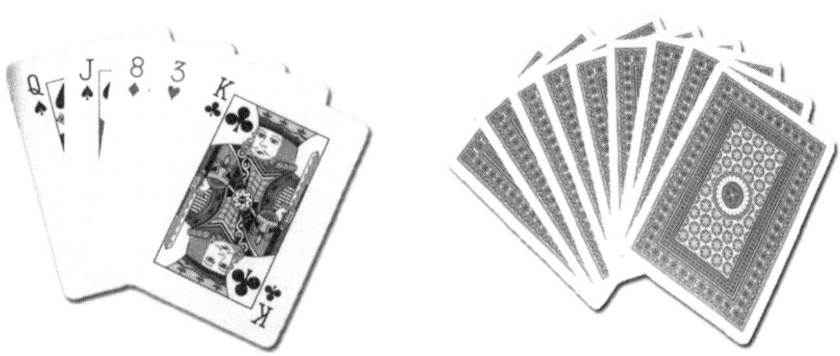

Fig. 6. The Deck on the Left is "Risky"; the Deck on the Right is "Ambiguous."

ambiguity attitudes is the α-maxmin model (Mukerji, 2003). In this model, agents are assumed to have set ordered priors over ambiguity, and take a linear combination of utilities under the best and worst case scenarios. For example, if an agent believes that the probability she will require LTC (cost $10,000) is in the interval [0.25, 0.75], her α-maxmin expected utility would be $\alpha(0.25 \times 10,000) + (1 - \alpha)(0.75 \times 10,000)$. If the agent is perfectly ambiguity-seeking, $\alpha = 1$ and she will only buy actuarially fair insurance if the actual probability of requiring LTC were $p<0.25$.

The application of ambiguous probability to insurance markets have been investigated by, among others, Hogarth and Kunreuther (1989). Hogarth and Kunreuther elicited willingness to pay from economically sophisticated subjects, including professional actuaries, under conditions of ambiguity and risk. They found that, except for small probabilities ($p = 0.01$), subjects were willing to pay *less* to insure against states with unknown probabilities (ambiguity), compared to those with known probabilities (risky) (see Table 2).

Work in neuroeconomics has elucidated the neural correlates and causal mechanisms of decision-making under ambiguity (Hsu, Bhatt, Adolphs, Tranel, & Camerer, 2005; Huettel, Stowe, Gordon, Warner, & Platt, 2006). This work has implicated the role of the amygdala, lateral OFC, and dorsal striatum in decision-making under ambiguity. Specifically, the amygdala and lateral OFC appear to signal ambiguity, while the dorsal striatum encodes a lower reward value for ambiguous gambles, compared to risky gambles (Hsu et al., 2005).

The role of the striatum is, therefore, a potentially important distinction between the behavioral effects of ambiguity versus those of loss framing. It suggests that while reward value is lowered for decisions under ambiguity, it is not under the loss frame. This is consistent with preliminary data suggesting that loss aversion can be reduced by cognitive regulation strategies (Sokol-Hessner, Hsu, Delgado, Camerer, & Phelps, in progress.); however, this has generally not been the case for ambiguity (Raiffa, 1961).

Table 2. Median Hypothetical Willingness to Pay to Insure Against a Possible Loss of $100,000.

Probability Levels		Risk
.01	1,500	1,000
.35	35,000	35,000
.65	45,000	65,000
.90	60,000	82,500

Source: Adapted from Hogarth and Kunreuther, 1989.

Finally, it was shown in Hsu et al. (2005) that patients with OFC lesions were abnormally ambiguity-neutral as well as risk-neutral over gains. As all three regions are part of the dopaminergic pathway, this raises the counter-intuitive hypothesis that those with dopaminergic system degeneration may actually purchase *more* insurance, relative to healthy comparison subjects.

Subjects were given gambles with known or unknown probabilities, and chose between picking the gamble or a sure amount that carried no risk (see Fig. 7). The top-panel conditions are called ambiguous due to the fact that the subject is missing relevant information that is available in the risk conditions (bottom-panel).

In the Card-Deck treatment, ambiguity is not knowing the exact proportion of reds and blues in the deck, whereas risk is knowing the number of cards (indicated by numbers above each deck). In the Knowledge treatment, ambiguity is knowing less about the uncertain events (e.g., Tajikistan) relative to risk (e.g., New York City).

Subjects always choose between betting on one of the two options on the left side or taking the certain payoff on the right. The stakes in the gambles, certain payoff, and the ratio of red and blues (risk condition of Card-Deck

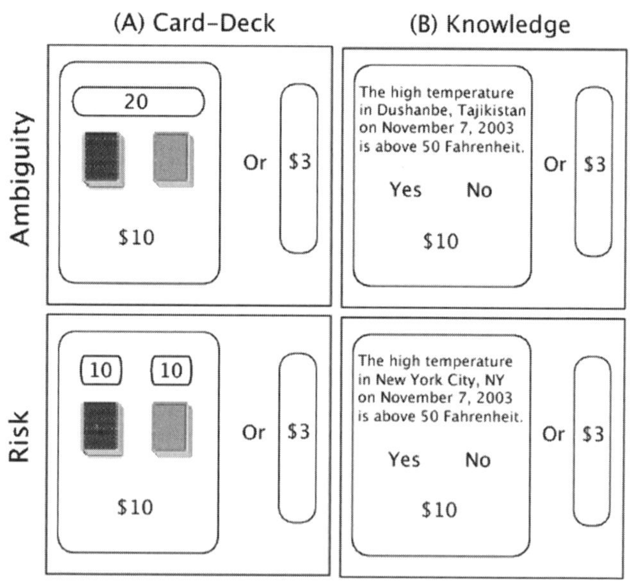

Fig. 7. Sample Screens from the Hsu et al. (A) Card-Deck Treatment, and (B) Knowledge Treatment.

treatment only) all varied during the course of the experiment. This enabled us to estimate subjects' risk and ambiguity attitudes from their choices.

The results of this imaging study implicated the role of the amygdala, lateral OFC, and dorsal striatum in decision-making under ambiguity. Specifically, it was hypothesized that the amygdala and lateral OFC signal ambiguity, while the dorsal striatum encodes a lower reward value for ambiguous gambles, compared to risky gambles (Hsu et al., 2005).

The latter is shown in Fig. 8. A random effects analysis strongly implicated the dorsal striatum as being more strongly activated during risk than ambiguity trials (Fig. 8A). This is consistent with the well-established finding that the dorsal striatum is involved in reward processing and anticipation (e.g., Schultz, Tremblay, & Hollerman, 2000; Knutson et al., 2001). This is further supported by results showing that the same dorsal striatal areas were significantly correlated with the expected value of the subjects' choices (Fig. 8C). In addition, the laterality of these activations is consistent with the fact that language processing tends to occur in the left brain, while more abstract mathematical processing tends to occur in the right brain.

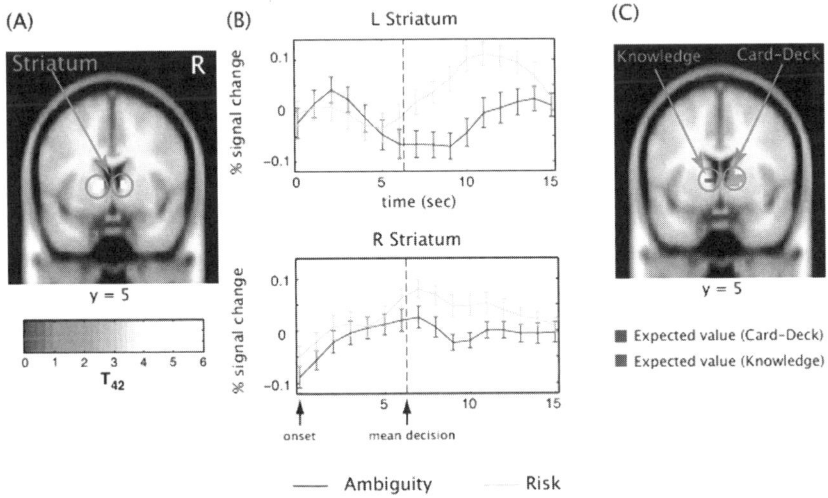

Fig. 8. (A) Greater Activation in Dorsal Striatum under Risk than Ambiguity ($p<0.001$, $k > 10$) and (B) Mean Time Courses (Time Synched to Trial Onset, Dashed Vertical Lines are Mean Decision Times; Error Bars are SEM; $n = 16$). (C) Activity in These Same Regions Also Show Correlation with Expected Value of Choices ($p<0.005$, $k > 10$).

To confirm the hypothesis that the lateral OFC is necessary for ambiguity aversion over gains, we, in collaboration with Daniel Tranel at the University of Iowa, conducted behavioral experiments similar to the Card-Deck task above using a lesion method. Twelve neurological subjects with focal brain lesions were partitioned into those whose lesions included the focus of OFC activation revealed in the fMRI study ($n = 5$) and a comparison group whose lesions in the temporal lobe did not overlap with any of our fMRI foci ($n = 7$). The two groups had equivalent IQ, mathematical ability, and performance on other background tasks as well as decision tasks. Parametric analysis using behavioral choice data from the patients confirmed the hypothesis that the lateral OFC is necessary for ambiguity aversion over gains. In particular, frontal patients are risk- and ambiguity-neutral. In contrast, the behavior of frontal patients was significantly averse to both risk and ambiguity.

To date, no known work has been done on the effects of aging on ambiguity attitude. There does exist tasks, however, that incorporate some aspects of ambiguity. These include in particular the IGT (Bechara et al., 2000; Bechara et al., 1996). In the standard IGT, subjects can choose from four decks of cards with varying schedules of gains and losses. Since the subjects do not know the distribution of gains and losses at the beginning of the experiment, the decks are *ambiguous* at the start and become *risky* towards the end of the experiment through learning.

Two studies have used the IGT to study decision-making and aging. As noted earlier, Kovalchik et al. (2005) compared a group of healthy elderly individuals (ages 70–95) to a group of Caltech undergraduates. The IGT was one of the tasks included in the paper. They find no significant differences between the two groups. On the other hand, a recent study by Denburg et al. (2007) did find significant differences between young and elderly subjects in the IGT. More importantly, they found the difference was driven mainly by an increase in the number of impaired individuals in the elderly group, rather than a global increase in the mean. Specifically, whereas only three participants out of 40 were significantly sub-optimal in the young subjects, 14 out of 40 were significantly sub-optimal in the elderly group (Fig. 9).

As is clear from our comparison of Kovalchik et al. and Denburg et al., behavioral effects of aging are not uniformly distributed in the elderly population. This underscores the point that aging itself is a heterogeneous process (Cabeza, Nyberg, & Park, 2005) and serves as an ideal illustration of the utility of combining different measures from a variety of disciplines. Imaging experiments can help elucidate this heterogeneity by looking at

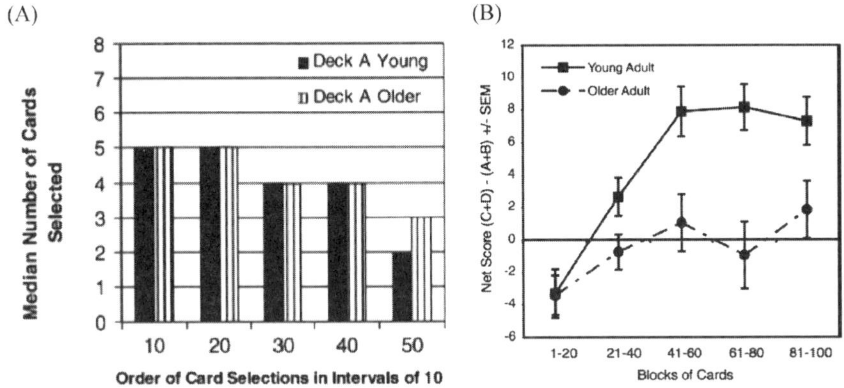

Fig. 9. Comparison of Two Studies on IGT Behavior in Aging Populations. (A) Kovalchik et al. Study Showing No Significant Difference between Young and Older Subjects. Abscissa is Median Number of Disadvantageous Cards Chosen. That is, Lower is Better. (B) Denburg et al. Study Showing Significant Difference between Young and Older Subjects. Abscissa is Difference between Advantageous and Disadvantageous Cards Chosen. That is, Higher is Better.

whether differential degeneration in regions such as the caudate and orbitofrontal cortex, implicated in Hsu et al., is driving individual differences found in Denburg et al. and Kovalchik et al.

Hyperbolic Discounting

The third stylized fact about long-term insurance is self-evident – the need for LTC can occur many years in the future. Moreover, insurance companies often require a period time, ranging from 30 to 90 days, before payment can begin (American Association of Homes and Services for the Aging, 2006). The perception and valuation of time, therefore, is critical to understanding behavior. Fortunately, time discounting has been extensively studied in both theory (Laibson, 1997) and experiments with both human (McClure, Laibson, Loewenstein, & Cohen, 2004) and non-human organisms (Mazur, 1987). This literature emphasizes the fact that organisms have a preference for immediate rewards. The theoretical literature has provided us with conveniently parameterized functional forms to capture the time inconsistencies (Laibson, 1997).

A comparison of the functional forms is given in Fig. 10: the standard time-consistent exponential discount function (assuming that $\delta = 0.97$), the

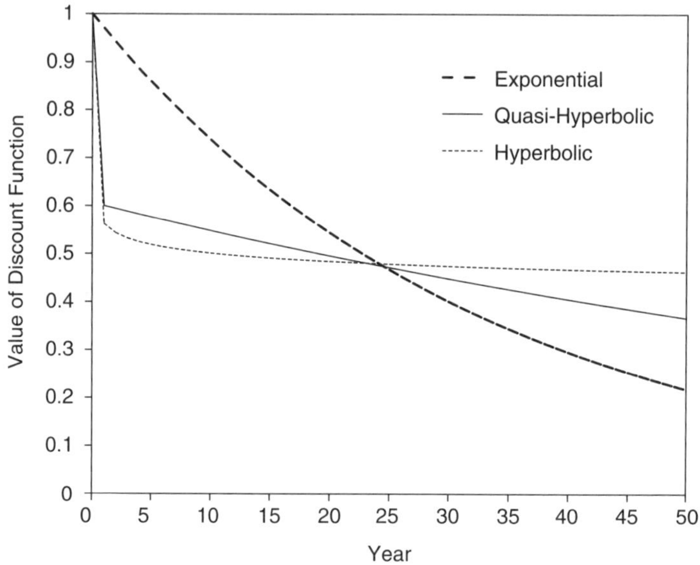

Fig. 10. Commonly Used Discount Functions.

generalized hyperbolic discount function (assuming that $\alpha = 10^5$ and $\gamma = 5 \times 10^3$), and the quasi-hyperbolic discount function (assuming that $\beta = 0.6$, $\delta = 0.99$). Note that both hyperbolic and quasi-hyperbolic discount functions underweight the immediate future much lower than does the exponential discount function.

To see how a quasi-hyperbolic agent will demand less insurance than that of a time-consistent (exponential) agent, note that the quasi-hyperbolic agent's utility function from present to future consumption is $u(c_t) + \beta\sum_{i=1}^{T-t}\delta^i u(c_{t+i})$ The exponential case can be treated as a special case with the constraint $\beta = 1$. A hyperbolic discounter would then value a loss of x dollars in t years as $\beta\delta^t u(c_t|x)$, whereas an exponential discounter would value this at $\delta^t u(c_t|x)$. Since $\beta < 1$ by assumption, the hyperbolic discounter will value the future consumption less in comparison, and hence will be willing to pay a lower premium to insure against the risks.[5]

Much work in economics, in particular, has focused on the distortionary effects of hyperbolic discounting on savings behavior as well as insurance (see Laibson, 1997). The results show considerable support for the hypothesis of hyperbolic discounting, and thus time inconsistency, in people's choices. In the case of financial choices, hyperbolic discounting results in over-consumption and under-saving (O'Donoghue & Rabin, 1999).

Applying neuroimaging to intertemporal decisions, McClure et al. found the ventral striatum to be differentially activated in immediate versus future rewards. Moreover, they hypothesized two competing systems involved in such decisions – a limbic system associated with immediate rewards, and a fronto-parietal system, including dorsolateral prefrontal and lateral intraparietal regions, with delayed rewards (McClure et al., 2004). They posited that the limbic region is associated with "immediacy-seeking," and the fronto-parietal system is a "rational" system (Fig. 11).

Although not viewed as directly involved in reward processing, dorsolateral prefrontal, temporal and parietal regions are known to be involved in working memory and executive function (Fabiani & Wee, 2001; Kramer, Fabiani, & Colcombe, 2006). Executive function, as it is commonly conceived, consists of two aspects: an evaluative aspect, related

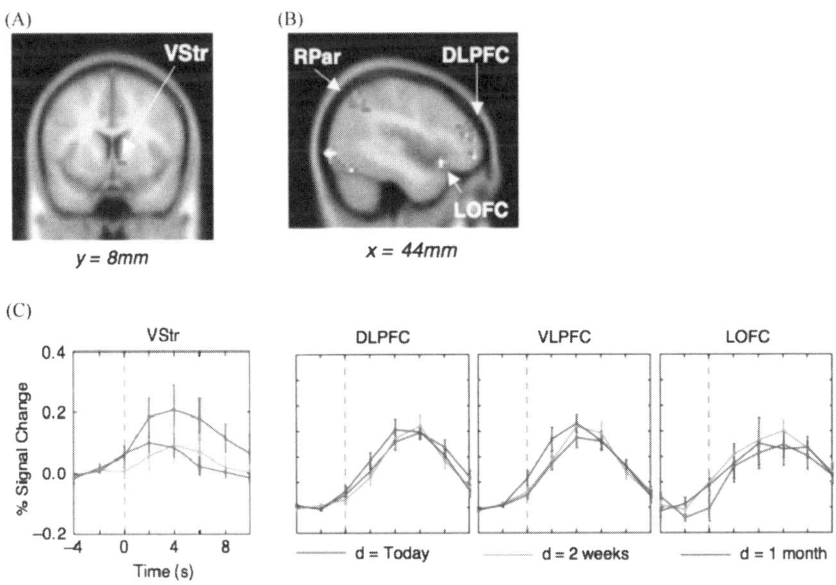

Fig. 11. (A) Ventral Striatum is Preferentially Activated for Choices when Money is Available Immediately, (B) Regions that are Activated by Choice but Independent of Delay Duration. (C) Hemodynamic Responses of Activations in (A) and (B) (From McClure et al., 2004, reprinted with permission from AAAS).

to forming, maintaining, and updating appropriate models of the environment (which may be carried out through various types of memory processes) and an action-oriented aspect, which is instead involved with the coordination of other cognitive functions, including perception, attention, and action. This coordination presumably takes place over time and is reflected in future behavior, so that when performed appropriately it can lead to successful adaptation to changing task demands.

In general, there are also disproportionate changes across the adult lifespan in the brain structures subtending these functions. Further, these structural changes appear to parallel the age-specific declines in executive control and a subset of memory processes that are supported in large part by prefrontal, parietal, and temporal regions of the brain (Robbins et al., 1998; Schretlen et al., 2000) (Fig. 12).

Compared to the previous two topics mentioned, the effect of age on time discounting is relatively well informed by existing data. The seminal study of Green, Fry, and Myerson (1994) suggested that old adults discounted the future less steeply than children, who were the most steep, and young adults, who were intermediate. More recently, it was suggested that discounting has an inverse-U relationship with age, such that there is a tendency to discount more as one reaches extreme old age (Read & Read, 2004). However, it is unknown whether this is due to brain degeneration, possibly in regions

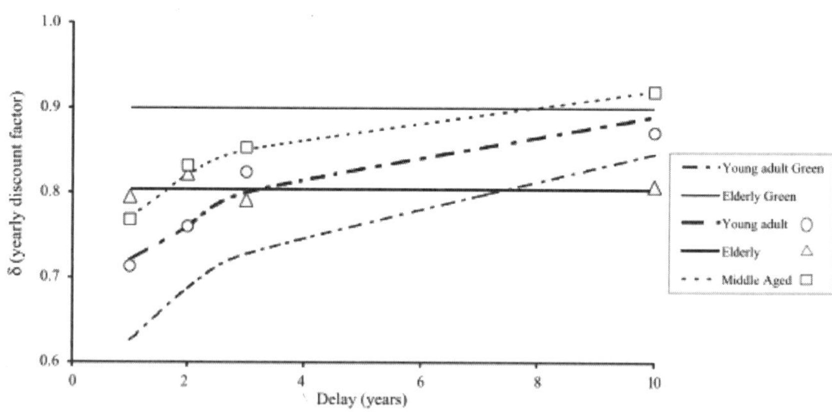

Fig. 12. Comparison of Discount Factor Across Time in Different Populations (Reprinted from Read & Read, 2004, with permission from Elsevier).

involved in cognitive control such as the anterior cingulated, or to a rational response to end of life forecasts.

CONCLUSION

LTC financing and insurance is a looming issue in the next 10–20 years. It provides a concrete example of the type of decisions that neuroeconomics is seeking to understand by taking into account the role played by psychological and biological factors in observed behaviors. In addition, answers to these questions may yield insights that could help shape public policies regarding the regulation, organization and structure of LTC insurance markets and programs.

More broadly, on the demographic level, older people hold a substantial portion of society's wealth, owing to the fact that wealth tends to accumulate with age. Social and economic mobility, however, tends to decrease in age, as human capital accumulation is generally diminishing in age. These factors contribute to the importance of both individual planning and national policy towards issues of financial decision-making and planning in aging (Peters, Finucane, MacGregor, & Slovic, 2000). In addition, the demographic shift currently experienced by much of the developed world is turning many policy issues involving aging from "important" to "urgent."

Finally, structural and cognitive changes in the brain itself provide unique challenges but also valuable opportunities for studying decision-making, which so far has overwhelmingly focused on samples of healthy young adults. Studying neural contributions to aging introduces issues that are not present, or at least not as pronounced, in current studies that include mostly college-age adults.

This chapter provides three behavioral anomalies that may underlie some of the glaring violations of standard theory in the LTC market. There is overwhelming evidence of brain changes in the aging process, including many of the regions shown earlier to be critical to reward learning and decision-making. Therefore, in the face of potentially both cognitive and neurological decline, standard measures of welfare through revealed preference may be highly problematic. Nevertheless the existing evidence regarding effects of aging on decision-making is often contradictory. Many of these contradictions reflect the preliminary nature of current knowledge on the underlying biological processes, but they also point to the difficulty and complexity of the issues associated with aging noted earlier in the chapter. Future studies are needed to untangle these difficult but important questions.

NOTES

1. However, higher risk of long-term care needs may not disrupt planned consumption of individuals who are eligible for Medicaid. For Medicaid beneficiaries, long-term care costs will be covered without further depletion of assets and income. Therefore, the impact of long-term care on lifetime consumption smoothing decisions of Medicaid eligibility will be minimal due to the fact that their limited economic resources can continue to be devoted to their own or their dependent's consumption.

2. This is called "quantity rationing" in the economics literature, which serves to sort out agents by their preferences, given imperfect information about the agents' types.

3. Brown and Finkelstein estimated a load of −0.04 cents on the dollar for women. That is, those with insurance will get back $1.04 in expected present discounted value benefit for every dollar paid out (Brown & Finkelstein, 2004a). In comparison, acute health insurance policies have typical loads of .06–.10 (Newhouse, 2002).

4. That is, it is unlikely people can estimate the precise probabilities of becoming disabled or needing long-term care.

5. Note that unlike in the case of risk or ambiguity seeking behavior, it is possible for an insurer to sell an actuarially fair policy. This will occur if the insurer is sufficiently patient relative to the insured.

REFERENCES

American Association of Homes and Services for the Aging. (2006). *Financing long-term care: A framework for America.* Washington, DC: American Association of Homes and Services for the Aging.

Bäckman, L., & Farde, L. (2005). The role of dopamine systems in cognitive aging. In: R. Cabeza, L. Nyberg & D. C. Park (Eds), *Cognitive neuroscience of aging: Linking cognitive and cerebral aging.* Oxford, New York: Oxford University Press.

Bechara, A., Damasio, H., & Damasio, A. R. (2000). Emotion, decision making and the orbitofrontal cortex. *Cerebral Cortex*, *10*(3), 295–307.

Bechara, A., Tranel, D., Damasio, H., & Damasio, A. R. (1996). Failure to respond autonomically to anticipated future outcomes following damage to prefrontal cortex. *Cerebral Cortex*, *6*(2), 215–225.

Bleichrodt, H., & Pinto, J. L. (2005). The validity of qalys under non-expected utility. *The Economic Journal*, *115*(503), 533–550.

Brown, J., & Finkelstein, A. (2004a). *Supply or demand: Why is the market for long-term care insurance so small?* National Bureau of Economic Research, Inc. Working Paper.

Brown, J. R., & Finkelstein, A. (2004b). *The interaction of public and private insurance: Medicaid and the long-term care insurance market*. Working Paper no. 10989.

Brown, J. R., Kling, J. R., Mullainathan, S., & Wrobel, M. V. (2008). *Why don't people insure late life consumption: A framing explanation of the under-annuitization puzzle*. National Bureau of Economic Research, Inc. Working Paper.

Browning, M., & Crossley, T. F. (2001). The life-cycle model of consumption and saving. *Journal of Economic Perspectives*, *15*(3), 3–22.

Buckner, R., Head, D., Parker, J., Fotenos, A., Marcus, D., Morris, J., & Snyder, A. (2004). A unified approach for morphometric and functional data analysis in young, old, and demented adults using automated atlas-based head size normalization: Reliability and validation against manual measurement of total intracranial volume. *NeuroImage*, *23*(2), 724–738.

Buckner, R. L. (2004). Three principles for cognitive aging research: Multiple causes and sequelae, variance in expression and response, and the need for integrative theory. In: R. Cabeza, L. Nyberg & D. Park (Eds), *Cognitive neuroscience of aging*. New York: Oxford University Press.

Cabeza, R., Nyberg, L., & Park, D. C. (2005). *Cognitive neuroscience of aging: Linking cognitive and cerebral aging*. Oxford, New York: Oxford University Press.

Camerer, C., & Weber, M. (1992). Recent developments in modeling preferences – Uncertainty and ambiguity. *Journal of Risk and Uncertainty*, *5*(4), 325–370.

Camerer, C. F. (2001). Prospect theory in the wild: Evidence from the field. In: D. Kahneman & A. Tversky (Eds), *Choice, values, and frames*. Cambridge: Cambridge University Press.

Cohen, M., Jaffray, J. Y., & Said, T. (1985). Individual behavior under risk and under uncertainty: An experimental study. *Theory and Decision*, *18*(2), 203–228.

Congressional Budget Office. (2004). *Financing long-term care for the elderly*. Washington, DC: Congressional Budget Office.

De Martino, B., Kumaran, D., Seymour, B., & Dolan, R. J. (2006). Frames, biases, and rational decision-making in the human brain. *Science*, *313*(5787), 684–687.

Denburg, N. L., Cole, C. A., Hernandez, M., Yamada, T. H., Tranel, D., Bechara, A., & Wallace, R. B. (2007). The orbitofrontal cortex, real-world decision making, and normal aging. *Annals of the New York Academy of Sciences*, *1121*(1), 480–498.

Ellsberg, D. (1961). Risk, ambiguity, and the savage axioms. *Quarterly Journal of Economics*, *75*(4), 643–669.

Fabiani, M., & Wee, E. (2001). Age-related changes in working memory function: A review. In: C. Nelson & M. Luciana (Eds), *Handbook of developmental cognitive neuroscience*. Cambridge, MA: MIT Press.

Glimcher, P. W., & Rustichini, A. (2004). Neuroeconomics: The consilience of brain and decision. *Science*, *306*(5695), 447–452.

Green, L., Fry, A. F., & Myerson, J. (1994). Discounting of delayed rewards: A life-span comparison. *Psychological Science*, *5*(1), 33–36.

Heckman, J. J. (2007). The economics, technology, and neuroscience of human capability formation. *Proceedings of the National Academy of Sciences, USA*, *104*(33), 13250–13255.

Hogarth, R. M., & Kunreuther, H. (1989). Risk, ambiguity, and insurance. *Journal of Risk and Uncertainty*, *2*(1), 5–35.

Hsu, M., Bhatt, M., Adolphs, R., Tranel, D., & Camerer, C. F. (2005). Neural systems responding to degrees of uncertainty in human decision-making. *Science*, *310*(5754), 1680–1683.

Huettel, S. A., Stowe, C. J., Gordon, E. M., Warner, B. T., & Platt, M. L. (2006). Neural signatures of economic preferences for risk and ambiguity. *Neuron*, *49*(5), 765–775.

Kahneman, D., & Tversky, A. (1979). Prospect theory – Analysis of decision under risk. *Econometrica*, *47*(2), 263–291.

Knutson, B., Adams, C. M., Fong, G. W., & Hommer, D. (2001). Anticipation of increasing monetary reward selectively recruits nucleus accumbens. *Journal of Neuroscience*, *21*(16), 159RC.

Kovalchik, S., Camerer, C. F., Grether, D. M., Plott, C. R., & Allman, J. M. (2005). Aging and decision making: A comparison between neurologically healthy elderly and young individuals. *Journal of Economic Behavior and Organization*, *58*(1), 79–94.

Kramer, A. F., Fabiani, M., & Colcombe, S. (2006). Contributions of cognitive neuroscience to the understanding of behavior and aging. In: J. E. Birren & K. W. Schaie (Eds), *Handbook of the psychology of aging*. New York, NY: Academic Press.

Laibson, D. (1997). Golden eggs and hyperbolic discounting. *Quarterly Journal of Economics*, *112*(2), 443–477.

Marquis, M. S., & Holmer, M. R. (1996). Alternative models of choice under uncertainty and demand for health insurance. *The Review of Economics and Statistics*, *78*(3), 421–427.

Marron, D. B. (2006). *Medicaid spending growth and options for controlling costs*. Washington, DC: Congressional Budget Office.

Mazur, J. E. (1987). An adjusting procedure for studying delayed reinforcement. In: M. L. Commons, J. E. Mazur, J. A. Nevin & H. Rachlin (Eds), *Quantitative analyses of behaviour: The effect of delay and of intervening events on reinforcement value*. Hillsdale, NJ: Lawrence Erlbaum.

McClure, S. M., Laibson, D. I., Loewenstein, G., & Cohen, J. D. (2004). Separate neural systems value immediate and delayed monetary rewards. *Science*, *306*(5695), 503–507.

McNamara, P. E., & Lee, N. (2004). Long-term care insurance policy dropping in the U.S. from 1996 to 2000: Evidence and implications for long-term care financing. *Geneva Papers on Risk and Insurance – Issues and Practice*, *29*(4), 640–651.

Mukerji, S. (2003). Risk, ambiguity and decision. *The Economic Journal*, *113*(485), F187–F188.

Mulvey, J., & Stucki, B. (1999). Retirement planning for baby boomers: The role of long-term care insurance. *Journal of Financial Service Professionals*, *53*(5), 53–58.

Newhouse, J. P. (2002). *Pricing the priceless: A health care conundrum*. Cambridge, MA: MIT Press.

Odean, T. (1998). Are investors reluctant to realize their losses? *The Journal of finance*, *53*(5), 1775–1798.

O'Doherty, J., Critchley, H., Deichmann, R., & Dolan, R. J. (2003). Dissociating valence of outcome from behavioral control in human orbital and ventral prefrontal cortices. *Journal of Neuroscience*, *23*(21), 7931–7939.

O'Doherty, J., Dayan, P., Schultz, J., Deichmann, R., Friston, K., & Dolan, R. J. (2004). Dissociable roles of ventral and dorsal striatum in instrumental conditioning. *Science*, *304*(5669), 452–454.

O'Donoghue, T., & Rabin, M. (1999). Doing it now or later. *American Economic Review*, *89*(1), 103–124.

Peters, E., Finucane, M. L., MacGregor, D. G., & Slovic, P. (2000). The bearable lightness of aging: Judgment and decision processes in older adults. In: Commission on Behavioral and Social Sciences and Education (Ed.), *The aging mind: Opportunities in cognitive research*. Washington, DC: National Academy of Sciences.

Raiffa, H. (1961). Risk, ambiguity, and the savage axioms – Comment. *Quarterly Journal of Economics*, *75*(4), 690–699.

Raz, N. (2004). The aging brain: Structural changes and their implications for cognitive aging. In: R. A. Dixon, L. Bäckman & L.-G. Nilsson (Eds), *New frontiers in cognitive aging*. Oxford, New York: Oxford University Press.

Raz, N. (2005). The aging brain observed in vivo: Differential changes and their modifiers. In: R. Cabeza, L. Nyberg & D. C. Park (Eds), *Cognitive neuroscience of aging: Linking cognitive and cerebral aging*. Oxford, NY: Oxford University Press.

Read, D., & Read, N. L. (2004). Time discounting over the lifespan. *Organizational Behavior and Human Decision Processes*, *94*(1), 22–32.

Robbins, T. W., James, M., Owen, A. M., Sahakian, B. J., Lawrence, A. D., McInnes, L., & Rabbitt, P. M. A. (1998). A study of performance on tests from the CANTAB battery sensitive to frontal lobe dysfunction in a large sample of normal volunteers: Implications for theories of executive functioning and cognitive aging. *Journal of the International Neuropsychological Society*, *4*(5), 474–490.

Samanez-Larkin, G. R., Gibbs, S. E. B., Khanna, K., Nielsen, L., Carstensen, L. L., & Knutson, B. (2007). Anticipation of monetary gain but not loss in healthy older adults. *Nature Neuroscience*, *10*(6), 787–791.

Schretlen, D., Pearlson, G. D., Anthony, J. C., Aylward, E. H., Augustine, A. M., Davis, A., & Barta, P. (2000). Elucidating the contributions of processing speed, executive ability, and frontal lobe volume to normal age-related differences in fluid intelligence. *Journal of the International Neuropsychological Society*, *6*(1), 52–61.

Schultz, W. (2000). Multiple reward signals in the brain. *Nature Reviews Neuroscience*, *1*(3), 199–207.

Schultz, W. (2006). Behavioral theories and the neurophysiology of reward. *Annual Review of Psychology*, *57*, 87–115.

Schultz, W., Tremblay, L., & Hollerman, J. R. (2000). Reward processing in primate orbitofrontal cortex and basal ganglia. *Cerebral Cortex*, *10*(3), 272–283.

Sokol-Hessner, P., Hsu, M., Delgado, M. R., Camerer, C., & Phelps, E. A. (In progress). Intentional cognitive strategies reduce individuals' loss aversion. *Proceedings of the National Academy of Sciences*.

State Farm Insurance. (2006). *Long-term care insurance* [PDF Brochure]. State Farm 2006 [cited 2006]. Available at http://www.statefarm.com/_pdf/ltc/ZH_23558.pdf

Task Force on Long Term Health Care Policies. (1987). *Report to the congress and the secretary*. Washington, DC: Government Printing Office.

Thaler, R. H., & Benartzi, S. (2004). Save More Tomorrow (TM): Using behavioral economics to increase employee saving. *Journal of Political Economy*, *112*(1), S164–S587.

Tom, S. M., Fox, C. R., Trepel, C., & Poldrack, R. A. (2007). The neural basis of loss aversion in decision-making under risk. *Science*, *315*(5811), 515–518.

Tversky, A., & Kahneman, D. (1992). Advances in prospect-theory-cumulative representation of uncertainty. *Journal of Risk and Uncertainty*, *5*(4), 297–323.

Verhoef, L. C. G., Dehaan, A. F. J., & Vandaal, W. A. J. (1994). Risk attitude in gambles with years of life – Empirical support for prospect-theory. *Medical Decision Making*, *14*(2), 194–200.

HEALTH ECONOMIC CHOICES IN OLD AGE: INTERDISCIPLINARY PERSPECTIVES ON ECONOMIC DECISIONS AND THE AGING MIND

Lisbeth Nielsen and John W. R. Phillips

ABSTRACT

Purpose – *This chapter offers an integrative review of psychological and neurobiological differences between younger and older adults that might impact economic behavior. Focusing on key health economic challenges facing the elderly, it offers perspectives on how these psychological and neurobiological factors may influence decision-making over the life course and considers future interdisciplinary research directions.*

Methodology/approach – *We review relevant literature from three domains that are essential for developing a comprehensive science of decision-making and economic behavior in aging (psychology, neuroscience, and economics), consider implications for prescription drug coverage and long-term care (LTC) insurance, and highlight future research directions.*

Findings – *Older adults face many complex economic decisions that directly affect their health and well-being, including LTC insurance, prescription drug plans, and end of life care. Economic research suggests*

Neuroeconomics
Advances in Health Economics and Health Services Research, Volume 20, 227–270

ISSN: 0731-2199/doi:10.1016/S0731-2199(08)20010-5

that many older Americans are not making cost-effective and economically rational decisions. While economic models provide insight into some of the financial incentives associated with these decisions, they typically do not consider the roles of cognition and affect in decision-making. Research has established that older age is associated with predictable declines in many cognitive functions and evidence is accumulating that distinct social motives and affect-processing profiles emerge in older age. It is unknown how these age differences impact the economic behaviors of older people and implies opportunities for path-breaking interdisciplinary research.

Originality/value of the chapter – *Our chapter looks to develop interdisciplinary research to better understand the causes and consequences of age-related changes in economic decision-making and guide interventions to improve public programs and overall social welfare.*

The past century has seen unprecedented increases in life expectancy. In less than 50 years, there will be more than 90 million Americans age 65 and older. And while many people are living longer, older individuals typically experience declines in physical and cognitive function and reductions in financial and social assets (due to retirement, relocation, and death or disability among close social network members) that impact their life quality. At the same time, they continue to face complex decisions related to maintaining financial viability post-retirement and managing healthcare needs. In the health domain alone, decisions range from the selection of insurance plans, treatment protocols, and care providers in the near term, to planning for future needs related to long-term and end of life care. These decisions can have tremendous consequences for physical health, functional capacity, and psychological and economic well-being. They can be both cognitively and emotionally challenging and evoke multiple – and sometimes conflicting – motives.

Provisions for long-term care (LTC) needs, for example, can make the difference between "aging in place" or placement in a nursing home. Moreover, these consequences often impact family members whose well-being may also be of concern to the older adult. The very abundance of options faced by the typical decision maker can – at any age – adversely affect people's abilities to absorb, process, and weigh information, and may undermine the ability make satisfactory choices (Schwartz, 2004). Consider, for example, that the number of Medicare Part D prescription drug plans (with different formularies, monthly premiums, and co-pays) available in the average state in 2006 was greater than 40 (Heiss, McFadden, & Winter, 2007). These observations highlight the need for a greater understanding of how age-related changes in psychological processes influence decision-making at different life stages, particularly in middle-to-late adulthood when many critical health-related decisions are made. We currently have only a limited understanding of how life course changes in cognition, emotion, and motivation impact decision-making. We know even less about age-related changes in the neurobiological systems associated with decision processes. What we do know is that now and in the foreseeable future, individual choice will play a central role in determining whether and how well older adults are insured for both everyday and catastrophic health care needs.

PSYCHOLOGICAL AGING AND DECISION-MAKING

Psychological research on decision-making focuses on the processes and mechanisms that drive people's choices among competing alternatives. Competent decision-making requires the exercise of cognitive abilities in order to gather relevant information, identify a set of options, understand, remember and integrate relevant information, consider possible consequences, judge their likelihood, and make comparisons or trade-offs between possible outcomes (Peters, Finucane, MacGregor, & Slovic, 2001). Optimal decision-making also requires the appropriate integration of emotionally relevant information about values and preferences into these calculations; this includes the ability to accurately forecast future preferences when planning ahead and the appropriate weighting of social information (e.g., whom to trust, whose interests need to be taken into account, etc.).

While a number of differences between younger and older adults in cognitive and emotional function have been documented in the literature, there is only limited understanding of how these differences impact decision-making in older adults. With aging, declines in working memory, attention, and some executive abilities may tax cognitive capacity needed to make decisions. At the same time, improvements in other domains such as increased knowledge (Park et al., 2002) and better ability to regulate emotional states (Carstensen & Charles, 1998) and solve emotionally charged problems (Blanchard-Fields, Janke, & Camp, 1995) may facilitate decision-making. An active area of research concerns the extent to which age-related changes in emotion – and to some extent cognition – are attributable to changes in motivation due to changing concerns and interests with age (Carstensen, 2006) or to underlying age-related changes in the neural substrates subserving these functions (Cacioppo, Berntson, Bechara, Tranel, & Hawkley, in press). Very likely, both factors play a role. Below, we review what is known about age differences and age-related changes in cognitive and emotional function, and discuss how health economic decisions may be impacted by these changes.

Cognitive Aging

It is important to appreciate that not all cognitive challenges associated with decision-making are age-related, and that not all of cognition shows age-related decline. Nonetheless, it is widely accepted that normal aging is associated with declines in so-called "fluid" cognitive skills. These skills involve the active manipulation and maintenance of information and pose demands on increasingly limited physical, temporal, and cognitive resources, over which older adults must selectively allocate (Salthouse, 1996; Verhaeghen & Salthouse, 1997). Cross-sectional studies reveal marked age differences in fluid cognitive abilities emerging in early adulthood (Salthouse, 1996; Park et al., 2002). Longitudinal studies, on the other hand, reveal more subtle age differences (related to cohort and generational effects) and a generally later onset of decline (but decline nonetheless) than might be inferred from cross-sectional comparisons (Schaie, 2005). Specifically, age-related declines in episodic memory, working memory, speed of processing, reasoning, and spatial ability have been observed in many studies. Reduced efficiency in memory processes – the encoding, maintenance, and retrieval of factual information – is perhaps the most studied aspect of age-related cognitive decline (Dobbs & Rule, 1989; Johnson, Hashtroudi, & Lindsay, 1993; Briggs, Raz, & Marks, 1999; Grady, 2000; Salthouse, 2003; Ferrer, Salthouse, Stewart, & Schwartz, 2004). Other work has focused on declines in older adults' ability to inhibit irrelevant information (Hasher & Zacks, 1988) and on a general age-related decline in speed of cognitive processing. This general slowing of cognitive processing is hypothesized to underlie a host of cognitive deficits (Salthouse, 1996). Working memory and inhibition are part of a cluster of so-called "executive functions" – a set of high level cognitive control processes involving conflict monitoring, goal initiation and inhibition, and planning. Declines in any of these processes could compromise decision-making, insofar as good choices require the ability to prioritize goals, keep multiple options in mind, disregard irrelevant information, and perform efficient (sometimes rapid) comparisons and calculations of costs and benefits.

Whether executive decline represents a distinct form of cognitive impairment in aging remains a matter of debate (Schretlen et al, 2000; Salthouse, 2003, 2005). Recent functional and structural neuroimaging studies suggest that distinct behavioral and neural profiles may characterize healthy vs. abnormal cognitive aging. Normal aging seems to impact frontal-striatal systems involved in executive control functions, which are compromised in older adults when attentional or processing demands are high. In contrast, the neurobiological deficits associated with cognitive impairment and Alzheimer's disease primarily involve medial temporal lobe regions that are important for memory encoding, consolidation, and retrieval (Hedden & Gabrieli, 2005; Buckner, 2004). Many older adults will go on to develop dementia or other neurological disorders of aging that severely impact cognitive function. It is currently estimated that 13.9% of adults over 70 in the United States have some form of dementia (Plassman et al., 2007). Thus, the overall impact of declining cognition on decision-making among older people represents a serious challenge for our aging population.

Counterbalancing this bleak outlook is additional research showing that some aspects of cognitive function are preserved or even improved in neurologically healthy older adults. So-called "crystallized" abilities, such as world knowledge and domain-specific expertise, continue to improve into midlife (Park et al., 2002; Roring & Charness, 2007). Indeed, in several financial decision-making domains, peak decision capacity seems to be somewhere in the early to mid-50s (Agarwal, Driscoll, Gabaix, & Laibson, 2008). Cognitive studies suggest that cultivated expertise may be protective of cognitive decline within the proficient domain, likely involving the increased integrity of knowledge structures and/or more flexible use of heuristics to maintain performance (Salthouse, 1990; Mireles & Charness, 2002; see Kramer, Bherer, Colcombe, Dong, & Greenough, 2004, for a review).

Moreover, not everyone shows the same rate of decline in fluid cognitive abilities with age. Likewise, some observed age differences in cognitive performance may reflect contextual constraints or motivational differences between younger and older research participants (Rahhal, Colcombe, & Hasher, 2001; Hess, 2005; Lupien, Maheu, Tu, Fiocco, & Schramek, 2007). Education appears to be an important buffer (Albert, Jones, & Savage, 1995; Chodosh, Reuben, Albert, & Seeman, 2002; Fritsch et al., 2007), and there is evidence that individuals possessing a greater sense of mastery and control over their own lives (Miller & Lachman, 2000) or a higher social economic status (Singh-Manoux, Richards, & Marmot, 2005) have healthier cognitive profiles. There is also a growing body of work suggesting that maintenance of physical fitness, social engagement, and cognitive activity in adulthood may buffer against or delay age-related cognitive decline (Kramer et al., 2004).

Decisions are Cognitively Complex

Certainly not all cognitive challenges that undermine competent decision-making are age-related. Deficits in health literacy, "the degree to which individuals have the capacity to obtain, process, and understand basic information and services needed to make appropriate decisions regarding their health," (Ratzan & Parker, 2000) are widespread in the population and have been linked to poor adherence to therapies, limited ability to engage in shared health decision-making, and higher health care costs (IOM, 2004).

Consider complex decisions regarding making provisions for future health care needs. In addition to well-functioning cognitive capacities, complete "rationality" in such contexts would require the ability to frame future health states appropriately, weighing their impact on various facets of well-being, and accurately estimating the amount of time left in life as well as the social, economic, and time costs of specific choices. Maximizing utility over alternatives is further complicated by the need to make trade-offs among time, money, subjective well-being, and objective health states, especially when not all characteristics of these states are known or fully appreciated, and no common currency for these trade-offs exists. Moreover, decisions in some health domains can be both risky (outcomes are uncertain but have known probabilities) and ambiguous (outcomes are uncertain and probabilities of outcomes are unknown) (Huettel, Stowe, Gordon, Warner, & Platt, 2006). In these cases, even the health professionals on whom we rely for information and advice are often unable to accurately assess the probability of distinct outcomes. This leaves the decision maker at a disadvantage with respect to both how to value specific states and how to assess their likelihood. Faced with such limited information, individuals (of any age) may hold inaccurate, incomplete, or even conflicting beliefs about benefits and costs of particular medical procedures or approaches to care.

Additionally, extensive research in young adults has shown that people tend to use fallible heuristics when assessing probabilities – possibly to minimize cognitive effort (Tversky & Kahneman, 1973, 1974). They are also notoriously susceptible to framing effects (Tversky & Kahneman, 1981; Slovic, 1995) and remarkably inaccurate in forecasting their own future feelings and preferences (Wilson & Gilbert, 2003; Loewenstein, 2005). Recent studies have demonstrated the challenge of anticipating the feelings and preferences of someone in a different health state from one's own (so-called "empathy gaps") (Loewenstein, 2005). Healthy people evaluate health states associated with illnesses and disabilities differently from people actually experiencing those states; they fail to appreciate the importance of adaptation to changes in health status and tend to focus narrowly on specific negative aspects of a condition (Ubel, Loewenstein, & Jepson, 2003). Unsettlingly, recent research suggests that even within individuals, changing health states may be associated with changing values regarding treatment options at the end of life (Fried, O'Leary, Van Ness, & Fraenkel, 2007). In such cases, the limits of both rational deliberation and intuition are tested, and from the perspective of decision science there is no clear optimal approach (Ubel & Loewenstein, 1997), except, perhaps, to be committed to continuing to revise choice as information and values become clearer and to view decision-making as a process rather than a discrete event (Prochaska & Velicer, 1997).

These factors (multiple options, uncertainty, reliance on heuristics, susceptibility to framing effects, forecasting errors and empathy gaps, and changing preferences over time) suggest that decision-making in the healthcare domain can test the limits of rationality. Particularly when selecting insurance plans, care providers, and treatment options in anticipation of long-term needs (e.g., planning for long-term or end of life care), decision makers face the challenge of applying subjective value to health states they are not currently experiencing and about which they have limited information. When cognition is compromised, domains are novel, and contingencies are unknown, these challenges are exacerbated. Often people choose to avoid decisions altogether and rely on others to make choices for them, resulting in asymmetric information that might lead to suboptimal outcomes. This tendency seems to be more common in older adults (see Mather, 2004, for a review). For example, in one study, more older than younger adults indicated that they would defer to their physician when making a medical treatment decision (Curley, Eraker, & Yates, 1984). People may avoid decisions for a variety of reasons. Yates and Patalano (1999) suggest that for older adults, perceptions of declining skill, conservation of effort, or deference to expertise may be among the primary motivators. But Mather (2004) argues that much decision avoidance may be in the service of emotion regulation, especially when decisions themselves elicit conflict or distress. Indeed, when decisions become too complex, people often let their feelings be their guide.

Emotional Aging

Given the complexity of information and the life-or-death nature of many health-related choices, it is not surprising that making decisions about health care and end of life matters is an emotionally charged process. Imagined experiences of future health states or problems with healthcare providers can evoke complex and sometimes mixed emotions. The cognitive challenges associated with choices under uncertainty can themselves elicit frustration, anxiety, and a desire to avoid the decision altogether. Moreover, decisions about future care often require balancing individual preferences and goals with those of one's loved ones. This adds an additional layer of emotional complexity to the decision process. Many health conditions require the day-to-day maintenance of good health through preventive behavior and compliance with medical prescriptions, necessitating not one but a series of repeated decisions played out over time. Each of these decisions may require the delay of immediate gratification (smoking, fatty foods) in order to protect the interests of one's future self, whose needs and preferences can be estimated only roughly. The emotional self-regulation requirements of these choices may be especially taxing. Are older people emotionally equipped for these multiple challenges?

Psychological research on emotional aging indicates that in contrast to a general profile of age-related decline in fluid cognitive abilities, older adults exhibit remarkable preservation in the patterns of expression, subjective experience, and physiological change associated with emotion, with the exception of a general age-related decline in the magnitude of cardiovascular responses to emotional stimuli (Cacioppo, Berntson, Kelin, & Poehlmann, 1997; Levenson, Carstensen, Friesen, & Ekman, 1991; Levenson, Carstensen, & Gottman, 1994; Tsai, Levenson, & Carstensen, 2000). Moreover, evidence from a number of laboratories suggests that older adults possess a preserved or even enhanced ability to regulate their emotional states. For example, older adults experience a decrease in the number and duration of negative emotional experiences (Carstensen, Pasupathi, Mayr, & Nesselraode, 2000), as well as an increase in positive experiences relative to younger adults (Mroczek & Kolarz, 1998), at least until very old age. These findings are consistent with older adults' self-reports of being able to effectively regulate their emotions (Gross et al., 1997; Lawton, Kleban, Rajagopal, & Dean, 1992) and control the experience and expression of anger (Phillips, Henry, Hosie, & Milne, 2006). Older adults retain the ability to voluntary regulate (suppress and amplify) emotion experience and physiology (Kunzman, Kupperbusch, & Levenson, 2005) and demonstrate information processing patterns (assessed by electrophysiological recording) that suggest greater prefrontal control over negative information processing, consistent with evidence that the prefrontal cortex serves an important role in emotion regulation (Williams et al., 2006).

Emotional complexity – the ability to appreciate more facets of emotion and to experience mixed emotions – may also be enhanced with advancing age. For example, middle aged and older adults generate more complex emotional descriptions than their younger counterparts (Labouvie-Vief, DeVoe, & Bulka, 1989, Labouvie-Vief, Diehl, Jain, & Zhang, 2007; Charles, 2005). The co-occurrence of positive and negative emotions is enhanced in some older adults and is associated with stress resilience (Ong, Bergeman, Bisconti, & Wallace, 2006). Similarly, a greater appreciation of emotional factors has been thought to underlie different approaches to problem solving that emerge in older age. For example, during emotionally charged everyday problem-solving, older adults attend to emotional factors to a greater extent than younger adults and tend to choose solutions that maintain relationships rather than arouse conflict (Blanchard-Fields et al., 1995; Blanchard-Fields, Chen, & Norris, 1997; Blanchard-Fields, Mienaltowski, & Seay, 2007; Birditt & Fingerman, 2005).

Aging and Motivation

Carstensen and colleagues (Carstensen, Isaacowitz, & Charles, 1999; Carstensen, 2006; Charles & Carstensen, 2007) have proposed socioemotional selectivity theory (SST) as a conceptual framework for understanding these findings related to emotional function in older age. The core of SST is the notion that chronological age is associated with a shift in time perspective – a growing appreciation of the limited time left in life – that leads to changes in motivation. Given these temporal limitations, older adults come to prioritize emotionally meaningful goals over more instrumental goals. This increased focus on emotional meaning enhances the use of strategies favoring the regulation of emotional states and maintenance of close relationships. Numerous studies have demonstrated that older adults, relative to younger adults, are more likely to prefer emotionally meaningful relationships and states of emotional equilibrium (see Carstensen, 2006, for a review). The postulates of SST are consistent with work on interpersonal problem-solving (cited earlier) and with studies in older married couples demonstrating more supportive behaviors and positive evaluations of spouses, even when engaged in interpersonal conflict (Carstensen, Gottman, & Levenson, 1995; Henry, Berg, Smith, & Florsheim, 2007).

Recent extensions of SST have focused on the information processing mechanisms that underlie older adults' changing profile of emotional states and preferences. Several studies provide evidence of a positivity effect, whereby older adults preferentially attend to and recall relatively more positive and less negative information than their younger counterparts (see Mather & Carstensen, 2005; Carstensen & Mikels, 2005, for reviews). This is a departure from the so-called "negativity bias" that characterizes the young (Rozin & Royzman, 2001). Studies demonstrating a reduction in the positivity effect under cognitive load (Knight et al., 2007) and showing that this effect is only evident in older adults who score high on measures of cognitive control (Mather & Knight, 2005) suggest that the positivity effect may result from effortful emotion regulation that calls upon frontally mediated executive control processes. The evidence for a "positivity effect" in emotional information processing with aging is mixed (see Murphy & Isaacowitz, 2008, for a recent meta-analysis). However, recent work has found significant age differences in the processing of negative and positive incentives and decision-relevant information, consistent with an age-related positivity effect. Scholars have also begun to explore the neurobiological correlates of these age differences (reviewed later).

Not all aspects of emotional processing are preserved in older age. Recently, more attention is being focused on individual differences in lifespan emotional development, making clear that while some people may demonstrate the resilient profiles characterized by SST, others may be susceptible to increased emotional distress (Cacioppo, Hughes, Waite, Hawkley, & Thisted, 2006; Teachman, 2006; Urry et al., 2006; Ong et al., 2006). In addition, there is evidence of general age-related decline in emotional perception. Accurate recognition of emotional facial, vocal, bodily, and contextual cues is compromised with advancing age (Isaacowitz et al., 2007; Sullivan, Ruffman, & Hutton, 2007; Ruffman, Henry, Livingstone, & Phillips, 2008). Thus, despite a greater focus on and appreciation of emotional information in aging, access to important emotional information in social contexts may be impaired in older adults (Slessor, Phillips, & Bull, 2007). These declines in appreciation of important social cues may put older adults at a disadvantage in decision contexts that require them to gather information from other people.

DECISION-MAKING: AT THE INTERFACE OF COGNITION AND EMOTION

Major questions addressed by current research in the psychology of aging concern whether and how the combined effects of cognitive decline, motivational shifts, and emotional changes impact decision-making as people age. Though there have been some suggestions in the literature of systematic effects of aging on decision-making, such as an increase in risk aversion (Wallach & Kogan, 1961; Okun, 1976), a tendency to seek less information (Johnson, 1990; Meyer, Russon, & Talbot, 1995), and a tendency to rely on experts (Curley et al., 1984), findings have been somewhat inconsistent. Likewise, the empirical research on these topics has been limited (see Yates & Patalano, 1999; Sanfey & Hastie, 2000; Peters et al., 2001; Mather, 2004, for reviews). Reduced cognitive capacity has often been invoked in explanations of decision-making deficits in older people. Yet several studies have found that older adults show preserved or even enhanced decision-making abilities. There is also little evidence to support lay impressions of more impulsive, risky behavior in youth and more cautious, less risky behavior in older age (see Mather, 2004, for a review). Some have suggested that older adults, due to extensive experience, reliance on affective information, and/or to the need to compensate for cognitive decline, may rely more on heuristics in decision-making rather than engaging in effortful analytic processing (Yates & Patalano, 1999; Peters et al., 2001). However, the impact of any such processing changes on the quality of decisions made by older adults is unknown. Heuristics, for example, can either aid decision-making (as when expertise in a domain facilitates quick decision-making) or undermine it (e.g., when dealing with novel material in an unfamiliar domain) (Peters et al., 2001).

Affective Influences on Older Adults Decision-Making

Research in the past two decades has considerably advanced our appreciation that decision-making relies not only on cognition (reasoning and analytic processes), but that emotion (or *affect*) also plays a central role (Isen, 1993; Damasio, 1994; Mellers, Schwartz, & Ritov, 1997; Loewenstein, Weber, Hsee, & Welch, 2001; Kahneman, 2003; Slovic, Finucane, Peters, & MacGregor, 2004; Löckenhoff & Carstensen, 2004). Decisions are made and evaluated with reference to the subjective value scheme of the decision maker and the subjective utility of the anticipated outcome. The process of valuation is emotionally laden, and values can be influenced both by features of the decision context and by an individual's motivational dispositions or current emotional state. Relatively little attention has yet been paid to these topics in the study of decision-making in normal aging. For example, the value changes that accompany changing time horizons may cause older adults to frame decisions differently, attend to different information, or experience different decision-related emotions. In decisions that involve time trade-offs, things like attitudes toward risk, valuations of future payoffs, and choices of decision strategies are likely to differ as a function of anticipated time remaining in life or in good health. Decisions about medical care are also likely to vary, depending on how this assessment influences goals related to survival, life quality, and the concern for the well-being of and quality of time spent with family and other social network members.

Recent studies indicate that older and younger adults may process positive and negative decision-relevant information differently, possibly impacting how preferences are constructed and how potential outcomes are evaluated. For example, Löckenhoff and Carstensen (2007) explored age differences in information-seeking and recall in a laboratory instantiation of a health care decision-making task. They found that older adults, compared to younger adults, reviewed and recalled more positive than negative information about healthcare options presented in a decision matrix, consistent with an age-related positivity effect. Notably, these age differences were eliminated when older adults were explicitly instructed to gather as much information as possible about options (Löckenhoff & Carstensen, 2007), suggesting that the initially observed age differences were motivated by goals to focus on the positive (or avoid the negative), rather than due to underlying cognitive or emotional changes. Mather and Johnson (2000) demonstrated that in retrospect, older adults are more likely than young people to view their past choices in a more positive light. This is another – possibly strategic – way of minimizing regret and managing post-decision emotions.

Older adults also appear to process information about gains and losses differently. Several monetary tasks have been used to study differences in decision-making and reward processing behaviors of younger and older adults. One is the Iowa Gambling Task (IGT) (Bechara, Damasio, Tranel, & Damasio, 1997), in which participants must make a series of financially consequential choices among four decks of cards, for which the payoffs are unknown and must be learned by trial and error. Two of the decks are disadvantageous (gains are high, but are accompanied by occasional large losses that eventually eliminate gains, resulting in overall loss if these decks are consistently selected), and two are advantageous (gains are small, but occasional losses are small as well, resulting in an overall gain if these decks are consistently selected). Studies comparing younger and older adults on the IGT have been somewhat equivocal, with several studies reporting no differences in outcomes between the younger and older (high functioning) adults (e.g., MacPherson, Phillips, & Della Sala, 2002; Lamar & Resnick, 2004; Kovalchik, Camerer, Grether, Plott, & Allman, 2005; Wood, Busemeyer, Koling, Cox, & Davis, 2005; Denburg, Recknor, Bechara, & Tranel, 2006), and others revealing impairments in some older individuals (Denburg, Tranel, & Bechara, 2005; Isella et al., 2008). Two studies in which older and younger participants performed equally well provide evidence that older adults, in contrast to younger adults, are more sensitive to gain information than loss information. Specifically, Wood et al. (2005) modeled decision-making on the IGT using parameters including attention weights for losses and wins, and found that older adults generally gave equal weight to gain and loss information from previous trials, while younger adults focused primarily on loss information when planning future card selections. Older adults also showed a greater recency effect and more rapid forgetting.

In another study, Denburg et al. (2006) found that older adults responded physiologically (with skin conductance responses (SCRs) – an index of autonomic arousal) to anticipated gains but not to anticipated losses when preparing to make card choices in the task, a pattern that is reversed in younger adults in other studies using the IGT. Moreover, older adults who showed anticipatory SCRs to advantageous choices performed better on the IGT than those who did not (Denburg et al., 2006). In both of these studies, outcomes for younger and older participants did not differ significantly; the difference appeared to lie in information processing strategies employed, particularly with respect to affective (gain/loss) information.

Research employing the Monetary Incentive Delay (MID) Task (Knutson, Fong, Bennett, Adams, & Hommer, 2003) has also revealed age differences in the processing of incentives as a function of their affective valence (loss vs. gains). The MID task is a computerized speeded reaction time task in which participants must respond quickly to cued targets signifying potential gains or losses in order to gain or avoid losing money. In a recent neuroimaging study (Samanez-Larkin et al., 2007), similar patterns of neural activation were observed in younger and older participants during anticipation of monetary gains (increased ventral striatal activation in both groups), suggesting preservation of normal reward processing functions in older adults. However, during the anticipation of monetary losses, significant age differences were observed. Younger adults showed increased insular and medial caudate activation to impending losses, but older participants did not. In related behavioral findings using the MID task, Nielsen, Knutson, & Carstensen (2008) found that when anticipating a loss, older adults do not experience the same increase in negative emotion expressed by younger adults when anticipating a loss, and – as an apparent consequence – older adults' experiences of avoiding losses are less emotionally charged.

Samanez-Larkin, Hollon, Carstensen, & Knutson (2008) recently demonstrated that, regardless of age, reduced insula activation during loss anticipation in the MID task is a predictor of poorer performance on a loss avoidance task 8–10 months later. It is unknown whether reduced insular activation is a stable characteristic of individuals, or whether insular activation during loss anticipation declines with age. If the latter is the case, this might have implications for older adults' ability to make choices in environments where they need to learn new information about loss and gain contingencies.

The coherent emerging pattern across several laboratories, using different tasks (decision matrices, IGT, and MID) and incorporating behavioral, psychophysiological, and neuroimaging measures, suggests that older adults may process information about potential positive and negative outcomes differently from their younger counterparts. Such age differences in attention to or valuation of certain types of emotional information could have important implications for decisions involving risk assessments, long-term planning, or inter-temporal trade-offs between immediate and future consumption.

This may be particularly true when making health care or end of life decisions, in which older people implicitly must make predictions about their future preferences, physical and cognitive abilities, and emotional states, and for which accurate assessments of anticipated positive *and* negative outcomes would seem essential to good decision-making. Indeed, advance directives and discussions about preferences for future care are based on the assumption that such predictions are sound. Yet there is scant research on the abilities of older adults to accurately predict their future affective states (a phenomenon known as "affective forecasting" in the social psychological literature). Recently, Nielsen et al. (2008) reported that older adults accurately forecast their affective experiences (including their lack of anticipatory negative affect) in the MID task, and are less prone to the forecasting errors demonstrated by younger adults under that paradigm. Lachman, Röcke, Rosnick, and Ryff et al. (2008) have also documented age-related improvements in forecasts of global subjective well-being in a large, population-based sample of US adults, with older adults exhibiting more accurate perceptions over a 10-year period – what the investigators call "temporal realism" – and younger adults more susceptible to temporal illusions (Lachman et al., 2008). Together, this research suggests that affective forecasting in both the short-term (hours) and long-term (years) may be improved with older age, though the relevance of this accuracy to long-term health-related decisions remains to be explored. Nonetheless, it suggests that older adults may bring the wisdom of experience to their deliberations, potentially offsetting some processing deficits or attentional biases.

Aging, Risk-Taking, and Loss Aversion

Risky situations evoke both anticipatory emotions (e.g., hope and dread) and the anticipation of future emotions (e.g., relief and regret) that can bias and influence choices (Loewenstein et al., 2001). There is evidence that risk aversion is stronger in women and lower among individuals at higher levels of income (Hartog, Ferrer-i-Carbonell, & Jonker, 2002; Barsky, Juster, Kimball, & Shapiro, 1997). In a simple economic framework, one can consider risk aversion in the context of a comparison of the expected utility of a gamble vs. the utility of the expected value of the same gamble: a risk-averse agent will derive higher utility from the expected value of the gamble while a risk-loving agent will derive higher utility from the expected utility of the gamble (Varian, 1992). In the case of insuring against adverse outcomes, risk-averse agents will value actuarially fair insurance provided by perfectly competitive markets to the point of purchasing full insurance and the utility value of insurance will increase with risk aversion (all else equal). However, rather than being an immutable characteristic of individuals (or classes of individuals, such as women or older adults), risk behavior and its associated emotions can be impacted by situational factors, including how decisions are framed. According to prospect theory (Kahneman & Tversky, 1979), choices framed as losses tend to evoke risk-seeking (e.g., a choice between (A) 100 deaths for sure and (B) a 50% probability of number of deaths and a 50% probability of 200 deaths), while choices framed as gains evoke more conservative, risk-averse behavior (e.g., a choice between (A') 100 lives saved for sure and (B') a 50% probability of 200 lives saved and a 50% probability of no lives saved). This effect is related to the fact that people evaluate losses and gains of equal magnitude differently. That is, subjectively, losses hurt more than gains feel good, so people are motivated to take risks to avoid losses, but less so to achieve gains. Given the emerging findings of differences in attention to positive and negative information in aging, and age differences in processing information about losses and gains, one might expect age differences to emerge in standard risky gamble scenarios as a function of framing (with older adults weighing negative information or information about hypothetical negative outcomes less strongly than their younger counterparts). Moreover, it is becoming clear that risk behavior can also change as a function of the process by which perceptions of risk develop – through a description of the probabilities vs. through experience of the likelihood of outcomes (Hertwig, Barron, Weber, & Erev, 2004). Given age differences (or domain differences) in experience with learning about payoff probabilities, one might also expect age differences in risk perception, and hence risk behavior, in a variety of domains. These topics have received little attention in the literature. Several studies have found that older and younger adults are similarly affected by framing effects (Mayhorn, Fisk, & Whittle, 2002; Rönnlund, Karlsson, Laggnäs, Larsson, & Lindström 2005). Another study (Deakin, Aitken, Robbins, & Sahakian, 2004) found that older adults took fewer risks and performed worse overall than younger adults (wagering less and failing to adjust wagers to probabilities) in a betting task. As reported earlier, many studies using the IGT (thought to mimic risky decision-making in the real world) have shown strategy differences, but not performance deficits in older adults.

Incidental emotions can also influence decision behavior, including risk-taking, and there are emerging findings of age differences in how incidental emotional states or moods impact risk behavior. In one study, older adults were more likely to take risks (preferring high risk-high reward options to low risk-low reward options in hypothetical medical, career choice, and business venture scenarios) when in induced positive moods, relative to neutral and negative moods, with no similar impact of positive moods on younger adults (Chou, Lee, & Ho, 2007). Another study examined the impact of incidental laboratory-induced stress on performance of younger and older adults in a simulated driving task (Mather, Gorlick, & Kryla-Lighthall, 2008). Individuals gained points for advancing a vehicle while a green or yellow light was on, but lost points if the car was still moving when the light turned red. After a stressor, younger adults took more risks (driving under yellow light) and gained more points relative to their own non-stressed control condition, but older adults took fewer risks and lost points as a consequence. These studies suggest that there may be important age differences in how incidental emotions influence risk-taking in older adults. This is relevant to health care contexts (which can be highly stressful), as well as to marketing strategies that may be used to manipulate or influence older people's choices.

Prospect theory also offers explanations for phenomena such as the endowment effect (where people will charge more to sell something they already own than they would be willing to pay to purchase the same item), and loss aversion (a preference for avoiding losses over accruing gains).

Experienced traders with extensive market experience are less likely to exhibit the endowment effect, suggesting that market experience (which may be greater in older adults in some domains) can eliminate this bias (List, 2003). Surprisingly, there has been little systematic investigation of these phenomena over the life course. One study comparing younger and older adults found no evidence of the endowment effect and no evidence of age differences in willingness to pay vs. accept for modest consumer goods (Kovalchik et al., 2005). Another recent study (Strough, Mehta, McFall, & Schuller, 2008) offers evidence that older adults are less likely to commit the "sunk cost fallacy" – the tendency to remain invested in options one has already "sunk" resources into, even when those prior investments fail to pay off. In this study, participants were presented with hypothetical risk-free investment and non-investment analogs of the same problem: to continue watching (or not) an unsatisfying movie for which they had paid money (or not). Older adults were less likely to stick with the bad choice and were more consistent in their behavior across investment and non-investment analogs of the same problem than their younger counterparts. Strough et al. (2008) suggest that this may be due to differences in emotional goals between younger and older adults, particularly a decline in focus on negative information (losses) in older individuals, leading to less loss aversion. Meanwhile, other evidence suggests that loss aversion for consumer products increases with age, though it decreases with domain expertise (Johnson, Gachter, & Herrmann, 2006). Johnson and colleagues offer a cognitive explanation for these effects based in query theory of value construction via memory retrieval (see Johnson, Häubl, & Keinan, 2007) and related to declines in inhibitory processes in older adults, on the one hand, and superior knowledge structures in experts, on the other. Further research is needed to explore the empirical and conceptual relations among phenomena such as loss aversion, endowment effects, risk perception, loss anticipation, and positivity effects and their impacts on risky choice, preferences, and other decision behaviors in aging.

NEUROECONOMICS OF AGING

As exemplified earlier, research on decision-making and aging is advancing through the convergence of approaches within psychology, economics, and neuroscience, using both tools and theories from each of these disciplines. The emerging field of neuroeconomics (or "decision neuroscience";

O'Doherty & Bossaerts, 2008) builds on the accomplishments of cognitive and affective neuroscience, adding the rich computational models from economics and methods from behavioral economics to the mix. The hope is that by understanding how economic behaviors are instantiated at the neurobiological level, traditional theories of decision-making will be improved and transformed. A neuroeconomics *of aging* will add a life span developmental approach to the field, enriching the study of decision processes with insights from decades of research on developmental processes in psychology and neurobiology, and life cycle economic decision-making in economics.

Aging and Intertemporal Choice

Neuroimaging studies of decision-making can offer insights into the neural correlates of psychological processes. When theoretically motivated, they can also serve to test and refine psychological and economic theory. The ability of neuroeconomics research to directly shed light on economic models of relevance to aging is exemplified in a recent study of intertemporal choice (McClure, Laibson, Loewenstein, & Cohen, 2004). Studies of intertemporal choice in both psychology and economics have established that, in general, people discount future rewards, reliably preferring immediate rewards over delayed rewards of equal magnitude. Traditional economic models used to explain life cycle savings and consumption behaviors have assumed an exponential discount function with an implied stability of preferences over time, an interest in maximizing one's long-range prospects as to smooth consumption over the lifecourse, and a discounting of future rewards as a function of time. Recent alternative theories of intertemporal choice, based on behavioral economic data, suggest that individuals are biased toward preferring immediate over delayed rewards, but otherwise discount exponentially over rewards delayed in time. This is suggestive of a quasi-hyperbolic discount function (Laibson, 1997). McClure et al. (2004), using functional Magnetic Resonance Imaging (fMRI), identified two separate neural systems involved in intertemporal choice: a primarily limbic/reward system that values immediate rewards, and a separate fronto-parietal system associated with making choices regardless of time delay. This finding suggests that the brain functions in a manner more consistent with quasi-hyperbolic economic models of temporal discounting. Such findings have direct implications for economic modeling of savings behavior, retirement planning, and insurance and investment decisions that impact the well-being of middle aged and older adults. To date, however, there have been no published neuroimaging studies of intertemporal choice that explore age differences in the operation of these systems under conditions of immediate vs. delayed rewards.

However, a number of behavioral theories and several cross-sectional behavioral studies have explored these issues. Typically, impulsive behavior has been considered a characteristic of youth, and has also been associated with personality traits of sensation-seeking and self-control (Sozou & Seymour, 2003; Mischel, Shoda, & Rodriguez, 1989; Steinberg, 2004). Several lines of research suggest that there might be age differences in temporal discounting. Studies in developmental neuropsychology have documented the later development of prefrontal inhibitory mechanisms necessary for self-control, resulting in a gradual development of self-regulatory ability in childhood (Rueda, Posner, & Rothbart, 2005). In older age, several processes converge that might impact intertemporal choice. On the one hand, prefrontal brain regions typically lose volume (see later) and executive functions (including inhibition) may consequently be impaired. On the other hand, changes in time perspective associated with the awareness of the limited time remaining in life are thought to motivate older adults to focus on the present, and less that on the future (Carstensen, 2006), with likely consequences for discount rates. The limited cross-sectional data that exists on changes in time preferences over the life course tend to support the view that young children and older adults tend to discount the future more, and that discount rates decline into middle age and early old age, and then increases again at the end of the lifespan (Read & Read, 2004; Green, Myerson, Lichtman, Rosen, & Fry, 1996). Importantly, in middle age, when critical investments in one's own future and in that of one's offspring are required, a lower discount rate may be adaptive. Likewise, it is consistent with other research showing that performance in a number of economic domains peaks in middle age (Agarwal et al., 2008).

The ability to delay gratification, invest in the future, and override more impulsive tendencies for immediate gratification is essential for many economic outcomes, including development of individual human capital (education and training), retirement savings, and a host of health behaviors, including exercise and diet. The available evidence suggests that this ability develops gradually over the life course, influenced by temperament, social context, and age. However, more research is needed to accurately characterize and disentangle the separate and interactive influence of individual differences and life course changes on time preference.

Decision-Making and The Aging Brain

Neuroeconomic studies of aging face the challenge of comparing neural activations between groups (e.g., younger and older adults) whose neurobiology differs on a variety of characteristics. We turn here to a brief overview of research on neurobiological changes associated with normal aging that need to be considered. We focus on their relation to cognitive and emotional function and on areas implicated in decision processes. Evidence from studies involving patients and animals with focal brain lesions, electrophysiology in animals, and neuroimaging in humans suggest a number of brain areas involved in the multiple, complex cognitive and emotional processes involved in decision-making. These include dorsolateral prefrontal systems involved in working memory, conflict monitoring, and executive function; ventromedial and orbital frontal regions involved in the processing of information related to value; regions such as the amygdala and insula that are involved in detection and processing of emotional information; and subcortical – cortical circuits for reward processing and regulation of emotion (see Krawczyk, 2002, for a review). Age-related structural or functional changes have been documented in all of these regions, though their interpretation and the implications for psychological functioning in older age remain the subject of active investigation and theorizing in research on aging.

Brain Changes with Aging

Prefrontal Cortex

Loss of cortical volume is one of the most frequently documented brain changes associated with aging. Reductions are greatest in the prefrontal cortex, with evidence pointing to loss of both gray (Raz et al., 1997) and white matter (Salat, Kaye, & Janowsky, 1999). In the dorsolateral prefrontal cortex (DLPFC), an area involved in the online manipulation of information in memory and related executive processes, age-related declines in volume have been associated with poorer performance in these cognitive domains (Raz, Gunning-Dixon, Head, Dupuis, & Acker, 1998; Head, Raz, Gunning-Dixon, Williamson, & Acker, 2002). In the orbitofrontal cortex (OFC), an area implicated in the integration of cognitive and emotional information in decision-making (Rolls, 1999; Damasio, 1994), longitudinal and cross-sectional age-related volumetric declines, and functional changes in the OFC have recently been documented (Resnick, Lamar, & Driscoll, 2007).

Neuroimaging studies examining age differences in the neural correlates of frontally mediated cognitive functions have revealed different activation patterns in older, compared to younger, adults when age groups are equated for task performance. Differences include task-specific under-activation of some brain areas, recruitment of additional brain areas, and bilateral rather than unilateral activation in older compared to younger adults. These patterns have variously been cited as evidence of either age-related decline or of compensation and plasticity in the aging brain (see Reuter-Lorenz, 2002, for a review). In the medial prefrontal cortex, an area involved in the regulation of social and emotional behaviors (Meyer-Lindenberg & Zink, 2007), recent electrophysiological findings in older adults have been interpreted as providing evidence for preservation or improvement of regulatory activity (Williams et al., 2006). More work is needed to understand and interpret age differences in activation profiles using these various methodologies, and to extend these approaches to studies of decision-making in aging.

Several laboratories are working on these issues. Age-related impairments in stimulus-reward association learning, a core executive component of decision-making that involves the integration of affective and cognitive information, have been documented in recent behavioral and neuroimaging studies (Mell et al., 2005; Marschner et al., 2005). Marschner et al. (2005) saw reduced activation in ventrostriatal reward processing areas and increase activation in frontopolar regions associated with poorer performance in a reward association learning task in older, compared to younger adults. However, performance on the task was not equated in the two age groups, which poses challenges to interpretation. Similarly, a recent neuroimaging study of risk-taking in younger and older adults found bilateral orbital frontal activation in older adults, and deactivation in younger adults in these same regions when comparing risky vs. safe choices. However, the study also documented performance differences in the two groups (older adults less likely to pursue risky options) that make it difficult to interpret these findings (Lee, Leung, Fox, Gao, & Chan, 2008).

Cortical-Subcortical Circuits

Reward and punishment are core incentives to choice, and age-related changes in the neural systems for reward processing could impact decision-making in older adults. Studies of reward processing in non-human animals indicate an important function for an extended dopamine-modulated circuitry involving the ventral striatum and prefrontal cortex (Schultz, 2002; Rolls, 1999). Midbrain dopamine neurons project to the ventral striatum, where they are thought to modulate appetitive and consummative affective states, and to the prefrontal cortex, influencing behavioral control (Rolls, 1999; Braver et al., 2001). Recent fMRI studies in humans have implicated components of this distributed network in the anticipation of monetary rewards (Knutson, Adams, Fong, & Hommer, 2001b; Breiter, Aharon, Kahneman, Dale, & Shizgal, 2001), the response to monetary outcomes (Knutson, Fong, Adams, Varner, & Hommer, 2001a, 2001b; Breiter et al., 2001; O'Doherty et al., 2001; Elliot, Friston, & Dolan, 2000), and the resolution of value conflicts in difficult decisions (Rogers et al., 1999). In addition to age-related prefrontal changes (described earlier), normal age-related changes in this circuitry include a decline in dopamine receptors and dopamine concentrations in the neostriatum and frontal lobes (Kaasinen et al., 2000; Wong, Young, Wilson, Meltzer, & Gjedde, 1997; Barili, De Carolis, Zaccheo, & Amenta, 1998), suggesting reduced modulatory influences of striatal dopamine circuits on frontal lobe functions (Goldman-Rakic, 1996). Several recent proposals have appeared in the literature suggesting that the cognitive changes associated with aging might be related to declines in the function of these dopamine circuits in both normal aging and age-related neurologic disease (Braver et al., 2001; Lieberman, 2000). In addition, it has been proposed that these circuits are involved in many of the observed modulatory effects of positive emotion on decision-making, such as increased cognitive flexibility and effort (Ashby, Isen, & Turken, 1999). Whether these changes to brain circuitry in old age impact the emotionality of reward processing in normal aging is an important topic that is only beginning to be explored (see earlier).

Other brain areas showing age-related change include the anterior cingulate (Volkow et al., 2000; Raz et al., 1997; Jernigan et al., 1991; Vaidya, Paradiso, Boles Ponto, McCormick, & Robinson, 2007), a region involved in conflict monitoring, integration of cognitive and emotional information, and many tasks requiring cognitive or emotional control; the insular cortex (Good et al., 2001), a region involved in the representation of emotional or visceral states associated with a variety of outcomes and with risk anticipation (Kuhnen & Knutson, 2005) and rejection of unfair offers in social exchange contexts (Sanfey, Rilling, Aronson, Nystrom, & Cohen, 2003); and the amygdala, a subcortical structure that plays a significant role in social fear (Olsson & Phelps, 2007; Adolphs, Tranel, & Damasio, 1998) and in the processing and relay of emotional information to both prefrontal regions and to autonomic response systems (Phelps, 2006). Exemplifying the nascent state of the science in this area, there is evidence of both age-related preservation (Good et al. 2001) and loss of volume (Mu, Xie, Zongyao, Yaquin, & Zhang, 1999) in the amygdala. Neuroimaging studies are equally equivocal as to the functional properties of the amygdala in aging. Age differences (Mather et al., 2004) and age invariance (Wright, Wedig, Williams, Rauch, & Albert, 2006) in amygdala activation during emotion information processing have been observed. Additional work, beyond the scope of this brief review, explores age-related change in additional neurotransmitters, neuropeptides, and other chemical modulaters of brain function, including the impact on cognition of changing levels of sex hormones with age.

Investigations of age-related neural change are complicated by the challenges associated with distinguishing normal from pathological brain aging, and from factors related to the interpretation of group differences in neural activation patterns between young and older adults. However, researchers are developing standard approaches to these issues, and the literature continues to evolve as new technologies, analytical strategies, and neural and behavioral probes are developed (Samanez-Larkin & D'Esposito, 2008).

Though there has been little investigation within neuroeconomics of most decision phenomena in the context of aging, a number of competing proposals are motivating current work in this area. One intriguing possibility, suggested by socioemotional selectivity theory, is that motivational changes associated with older age may exert effects on brain function and modulate the circuitry involved in processing decision-related emotional information. Others have suggested that age-related changes in socioemotional function may be attributed to neurobiological causes (Cacioppo et al., in press). Similarly, with respect to cognition, research is needed to determine the extent to which age-related changes are associated with brain changes, changes in life experience, individual difference, or sociodemographic factors that predispose for different cognitive developmental profiles.

HEALTH AND THE ECONOMICS OF AGING

In the foregoing sections of this chapter, we have laid the foundations for understanding factors at the individual level – related to both psychological change and to change in underlying neurobiology – that might impact age-related changes in decision-making. While the psychological literature on decision-making and aging remains limited, there are exciting trends in the research that are motivating a variety of lines of investigation, with researchers beginning to bridge approaches from psychology, neuroscience, and economics to tackle important issues related to aging and economic behavior. The hope is that such approaches will yield a better understanding of both the unique decision challenges faced by older people, and how preferences change over the life course. An appreciation of both of these factors is essential for the design of appropriate decision-supportive interventions addressing the needs of older individuals. Meanwhile, it is clear that individual responsibility for decision-making does not decline with age, and the decision challenges faced by older adults (as well as by younger adults planning for their older age) in both health and financial domains require the ability to process and evaluate complex information about multiple options, often on a repeated basis. Federal social programs that insure Americans against old-age risks like poor health and longevity face unprecedented challenges. Population aging will increase fiscal pressure on the Social Security, Medicare, and Medicaid programs, but increasing health care cost growth will place added pressure on the sustainability of the Medicare and Medicaid programs. As Medicare premiums grow to address increasing costs, they erode Social Security benefits that serve as a primary source of retirement income for many older Americans. The transition from defined benefit to defined contribution pensions shifts retirement wealth risk from employers to workers and places a premium on the ability to make good financial decisions to both build a nest egg and disburse it efficiently. The growth of out-of-pocket health costs will require individuals to make difficult consumption and saving choices, including perhaps reducing health care utilization or relying on safety-net programs to fill the gaps.

To address the challenges of an aging population policymakers are informed by research that provides an understanding of the economic decisions facing the older population that can guide policy and interventions to improve well-being. Interdisciplinary approaches may prove useful in developing accurate models of behavioral processes related to complex economic decisions. Two aging-related health economics topics that highlight the potential for interdisciplinary research issues are LTC and prescription drug coverage. In the next two sections, we summarize some findings from research in these areas and follow with potential research directions. Both involve complex evaluation of multiple options, weighing the subjective and economic value of future health states and trading these off against current economic needs.

Long-Term Care Insurance

As population aging rapidly increases the number of older Americans, there will likely be an accompanying increase in the demand for services that support people who are disabled to perform activities of daily living (LTC). However, there are indications that many lack private coverage for their LTC needs – about one in 10 people, 60 and over have private LTC coverage (Brown & Finkelstein, 2007). LTC needs are unpredictable and can place significant time and money pressures on older people and their families. A large fraction of elderly people will require nursing home care at some point in their lives, and about 7% will require long nursing home stays. The risk of care is particularly large for women: Brown and Finkelstein (2007) find that a 65-year-old woman has a 44% chance of ever using nursing home care during her lifetime, compared to a 27% chance for a 65-year-old man, and women typically have longer stays (2 vs. 1.3 years on average). Further, LTC can be expensive. Nursing home care in 2003 cost an average of $181 per day for a private room and a visit by a home health aide averaged $18 per hour (CBO 2004).

The Congressional Budget Office (2004) estimates that total expenditures for paid LTC services for the elderly in 2004 total about $135 billion, or roughly $15,000 per impaired senior. The elderly can support LTC needs though personal savings (self-insure), LTC insurance, time donated by a family or other caregiver and with assistance through public programs (Medicare and Medicaid). Though estimates of the value of donated care are rough, CBO concludes that the combination of donated care and out-of-pocket payments represent over half of all expenditures on LTC, while private insurance pays only 3% of expenses (fraction increases to 4% if the estimate for donated care is excluded). The rest of the expenses are covered by Medicaid and Medicare. However, the coverage provided by public systems is contingent upon specific eligibility criteria that make these less than perfect forms of insurance.

Medicare only covers home health care expenditures and LTC for a limited period of time in skilled nursing facilities following a hospitalization to support recovery from acute illness. As a result of these limitations, Medicare represented only 15% of financing for the care of elderly nursing home residents in 2007, while Medicaid represented 56% of financing (CBO, 2004). On the other hand, Medicaid provides "free" public LTC insurance for those who meet asset and income eligibility criteria. Medicaid acts as the "payer-of-last resort" – if an individual meets the means test – and has a private insurance policy, the private policy pays first. Medicaid asset thresholds vary based on marital status, state of residence, and the types of assets held by an individual. Based on these factors, the federal threshold can range from $1,500 to over $16,000.

Though theory might provide many starting points for considering low LTC insurance coverage (Norton, 2000), Medicaid provides a logical place to start considering why few purchase LTC insurance. Research by Brown, Coe, and Finkelstein (2006) considers the potential for Medicaid coverage to crowd-out private LTC coverage. They find that more generous Medicaid asset protection is associated with less private LTC insurance coverage. However, significant changes in asset thresholds were unlikely to stimulate private insurance coverage among most of the elderly population. Brown and Finkelstein (2007) explore a number of other potential explanations for the small LTC insurance market. Though they find that the LTC policies purchased are typical not actuarially fair and do not offer comprehensive coverage, they determine that these factors are not sufficient to explain the size of the market. They find large gender differences in loads, a measure that relates value of benefits to premiums; however, the gap does not produce a meaningful difference in insurance coverage between men and women. They also show that more comprehensive policies are widely available at comparable loads to the typically purchased policies with more limited coverage. The authors suggest a number of potential explanations for the gap in loads by gender not translating into differences in coverage including other factors such as Medicaid, the role of the family, and "limited rationality." Pauly (1990) shows that the elderly may choose not to purchase private LTC insurance due to the fact that private coverage provides incentives for a reduction in informal care provided by children (which may be preferred by the elderly relative to formal care).

While there appear to be a number of reasons why individuals may not buy LTC insurance, Finkelstein, McGarry, and Sufi (2005) show that some who buy LTC insurance end up dropping their coverage. Each year, about 7% of active policies are cancelled (Society of Actuaries, 2002) and since provisions exist that protect against unintentional lapse in coverage, the cancellations appear to be intentional. Finkelstein et al. (2005) find that individuals who let their policies lapse are about one-third less likely to have a subsequent nursing home admission than those who maintain their coverage. While canceling a policy might be a rational behavior in the event that new information changes the value of coverage under the policy (say improvements in health that reduce the likelihood of requiring care), their data suggests that a large fraction of cancellations occur immediately following purchase (about 12% in the first year). It is unlikely that policyholders could learn something meaningful about improvements in their health so rapidly. Other explanations for policy cancellation include income/wealth shocks or some other revelation that the policy purchase was a mistake.

LTC represents one of the largest financial risks facing the elderly. Though research has shown that some issues related to low demand for private coverage are due to policy and market failures, some results suggest that other factors may play a meaningful role in depressing demand. The elderly may be poorly informed about what is covered by Medicare and Medicaid and the quality of that coverage. Specifically, Medicaid does not protect individual wealth and may not provide the same quality or care choices that would be provided by private LTC insurance (CBO, 2004). The complexity of these contracts and the fact that about 80% are individual as opposed to group could increase transaction costs associated with purchasing private coverage. The average age of policy purchase among those over 55 is 67, with claims typically occurring about 15 years later, suggesting that age-related non-economic factors may play a key role in outcomes. Further, if individuals become aware of their LTC risks and the quality of coverage through public programs late in life, their ability to save to cover these costs are greatly limited. Research that integrates economic and non-economic factors might address unanswered questions. Three areas of particular interest concern (1) gender disparities in loads that do not lead to gender differences in coverage; (2) the presence of plans that provide more coverage at similar cost relative to those typically purchased; and (3) lapses in coverage. Answers to these types of questions may also inform insurance plan design to provide superior LTC coverage products. To date, there has been no research that integrates psychological and economic factors that motivate these choices.

Prescription Drug Coverage in Medicare – Part D

The development of effective drug therapies since the initiation of the Medicare program in the 1960s has led to an increase in the use of prescription drugs in the care of the elderly population. However, the rising cost of prescription drugs has led some older Americans to constrain their use of effective drug therapies (Soumerai et al., 2006), with adverse consequences for health (Heisler et al., 2004). These concerns contributed to the passage of the Medicare Prescription Drug, Improvement, and Modernization Act of 2003 that included the provision of a Medicare drug benefit (Part D), offering subsidized prescription drug insurance with protection against catastrophic drug costs.

The "Standard Plan" in 2006 had an annual premium of $444 and a benefit schedule that included catastrophic coverage. Specifically, the plan has a $250 deductible, pays 75% of prescription drug bills between $250 and $2,250, and a "doughnut hole" with no additional benefits until drug bills reach $5,100. The Standard Plan then pays 95% of pharmacy bills above that "catastrophic" level. Though the provision of coverage through Part D could mitigate the impact of cost constraints on adherence, the structure of benefits could constrain the benefits of coverage. Research by Hsu et al. (2006) analyzed the health and cost implications of caps on drug coverage using data from Kaiser Permanente on Medicare Advantage beneficiaries who were at least 65-years-old in January 2003 and were enrolled in a two-tiered drug plan. The plans had a cap on annual drug costs of either $1,000 or $0 (no cap). Beneficiaries with caps had lower drug consumption and worse clinical outcomes than those with uncapped benefits, and poorer adherence to drug therapies was found among chronic disease sufferers in the capped coverage group. Overall, cost savings from the caps on drug coverage (intended to control costs) were more than offset by hospitalization and emergency care costs (see also Joyce, Goldman, Karaca-Mandic, & Zheng, 2007). Risk-averse individuals or those who expect to have expenditure that will reach the doughnut hole might prefer plans with enhanced coverage relative to the Standard plan. Private insurance firms can offer plans that provide different features than the Standard Plan, such as coverage of the deductible or donut hole. However, such plans must provide benefits that are comparable or better than those of the Standard Plan. Research by Hsu et al. (2008) show that beneficiaries have limited knowledge of coverage gaps in their drug plans that in some instances leads to economic burden.

Once eligible for Part D coverage, one must enroll within a specific period of time or face a late penalty of 1% for every month of delay. Once enrolled, beneficiaries can switch plans annually at no cost, so plan selection in any given year should relate primarily to expectations of utilization in that year as opposed to a potentially more complex forecast of long-range drug expenditures.

The effectiveness of the Part D program is linked to the ability of older Americans to navigate the system and make plan choices that provide both optimal drug benefits and clear signals to the private plan providers

(McFadden, 2007). In 2006, the average number of plans available in a State was 42.5 with a range from 17 to 52 (Heiss et al., 2007). Results from the period leading up to the introduction of the program suggested that a significant and vulnerable portion of the population had limited knowledge of the Part D program. Winter et al. (2006) found that about 40% of the Medicare population had little or no knowledge about Part D and that among vulnerable groups (low SES, low self-rated health, or low cognition) the percentage reporting little or no program knowledge was worse. However, CMS data show that by the middle of June 2006, about 92% of the roughly 36 million eligible were either enrolled in Part D or had other creditable prescription drug coverage (coverage as least as good as the Part D Standard Plan). A follow-up study conducted after the initial enrollment period by Heiss, McFadden, and Winter (2006) shows that CMS outreach to vulnerable populations resulted in coverage rates that are comparable to coverage rates in the overall population for low-income and cognitively impaired subgroups. They note however, that among the uncovered about 2 million reported using one or more prescriptions at the end of 2005, suggesting that they would benefit from Standard plan coverage under reasonable assumptions. Further, even those who reported using no prescription drugs at the end of 2005 could benefit from Standard Plan benefits given both the delayed enrollment penalty and the value of catastrophic coverage in the event of a health shock. They find that coverage rates among those reporting no prescription drug use at the end of 2005 were smaller among low-income and low-education groups.

Survey data on a sample of Part D-eligible older adults reveal that among respondents who did not enroll, 61% found the enrollment process was very complicated compared to only 34% of those who did enroll (Heiss et al., 2006). About seven in 10 of all respondents reported there were too many alternative plans to choose from, and over half of the sample reported difficulty determining whether specific medications were in a plan formulary. In a broader sample including those age 65 and older, respondents reported that they disliked the cost control features of the Part D plans (the $250 deductible and coverage gap) as well as the potential for formularies to change over time. Analysis by Heiss et al. (2007) uses longitudinal data to examine the enrollment decisions of the eligible population that did not have drug coverage from other sources. They found that economic incentives, primarily drug costs in the year prior to enrollment, provided the most explanatory power for 2006 enrollments and plan choices. However, their estimates from an intertemporal optimization model of Part D enrollment decisions suggest that even those who would not benefit from enrollment in 2006 due to particularly low drug expenditures should have enrolled anyway due to the late enrollment penalty. Only 2.5% of the sample would have rationally benefited from not enrolling in 2006 and faced the late enrollment penalty.

Another dynamic aspect of the Medicare Part D benefit is the option to switch plans (re-optimize) each year at no cost. Indeed, beneficiaries will have the opportunity to calculate their expenditures in the previous year and evaluate the benefits provided by their current plan relative to alternative plans and switch if a better plan can be identified among plan options. Heiss et al. (2007) measured respondent satisfaction with their 2006 Part D plans and found that 18% are dissatisfied with their plans and almost half report dissatisfaction with their gap coverage. Despite this, the majority did not switch plans in 2007 – only about one in 10 respondents switched plans. It is curious that so little switching occurred given the dissatisfaction with features like gap coverage, the presence of alternative plans with enhanced benefits, and costless plan switching. It also raises concerns about the long run, since plans can also change their features annually, including adding tiered systems for drug coverage. If beneficiaries do not re-evaluate their plans over time or find the dynamic aspects of plan choice too complicated, they could experience the aforementioned health consequences associated with high drug expenditures. Failure to change plans may represent another case of the status quo bias, the oft-observed tendency to stick with an original choice despite the presence of economically better options (Samuelson & Zeckhauser, 1988). This is one of a variety of decision-avoidant behaviors that people may engage in to avoid experiences of uncertainty or regret and/or to minimize transaction costs and energy expenditure (Anderson, 2003).

The Medicare Part D prescription drug benefit is a significant federal subsidy to support the health and well-being of older Americans. Research to date highlights some opportunities to consider the contribution of non-economic factors and outcomes and potential interventions designed to improve outcomes. Though recent findings show that Medicare Part D has reduced overall cost-related medication nonadherence, the program has not produced a net decrease in cost-related medication nonadherence among the sickest beneficiaries (Madden et al., 2008). These results suggest that a particularly vulnerable section of the population is having difficulty finding plan options that adequately address their needs. Early results suggest that low cognition has not led to enrollment disparities, but it is less clear whether cognition has played a role in suboptimal plan choice. The fact that beneficiaries only need to forecast needs for a year at a time and choose between a tightly regulated set of options should mitigate the size of errors. However, large numbers of plans, the ability for firms to change formularies and other plan features over time, cognitive decline, and the increasing likelihood of a health shock with age could increase both the complexity of the decision in future years and the loss associated with bad decisions. Research described in previous sections implying increases in risk aversion and a desire to stabilize emotions (and perhaps consumption) at older ages could lead beneficiaries to enhance their coverage as they age. Alternatively, decisions that require individuals to consider the implications of deteriorating health may discourage some from making changes in coverage that could improve their well-being.

CONCLUSION

In the United States, population aging represents a significant fiscal challenge to both public institutions like Medicare, Medicaid, and Social Security as well as families. The complexities of LTC coverage and prescription drug options means that individuals will face an ongoing series of increasingly complicated decisions in these domains at a time when cognitive and physical resources grow increasingly limited. Health economic research suggests that many older adults are currently not making cost-effective and economically rational decisions in these domains, amplifying the potential for costly and catastrophic outcomes. While some of these choices may be rational responses to the structure of the available markets, or represent the true preferences of individuals, others may be inadvertent consequences of age-related changes in psychological processes that place older adults at a disadvantage.

Our goal in this chapter has been to provide readers with a review of relevant literature from three domains that we believe are essential for developing a comprehensive science of decision-making and economic behavior in aging: psychology, neuroscience, and economics. Research in the psychology of aging continues to offer insights into how cognitive, emotional, and motivational changes with age impact the process of decision-making and the quality of decision outcomes in older people. Neuroscience approaches work in tandem with psychology and economics to insure that theoretical explanations of behavioral findings are both biologically and psychologically plausible. Economics of aging offers real world insights into the individual and societal costs of health economic decisions and highlights the complexities of choices faced by the growing elderly population. Behavioral economics and neuroeconomics offer additional tools and models for approaching these problems and understanding how economic decision-making changes over the life cycle.

The convergence of research approaches from these disciplines around central economic problems of aging has the potential to improve our understanding of how economic decision-making is encoded and processed in the brain, to enhance economic and computational models of decision-making, and to advance our knowledge of age differences in economic behavior. The multidisciplinary approach required for these advances is not without potential pitfalls. Key to advancement is the development of a common language for researchers across the relevant domains. Appreciation by economists of the many facets and dimensions of the emotional response and of the variety of possible affective influences on economic behavior, on the one hand, and appreciation by psychologists and neuroscientists of the details of economic models and the structure of economic institutions, on the other hand, would help to advance the science.

With support from the National Institute on Aging, research in neuroeconomics of aging is currently underway in a number of laboratories, examining the influence of age on the function of dopaminergic systems for reward processing, the behavioral and neural correlates of incentive processing, and aspects of social decision-making and inter-temporal choice in older adults. Much remains to be understood about how basic decision-making processes are impacted by advancing age and the changes in time perspective that accompany the approach of life's end. Significant advances are likely to come from the study of the co-evolution and interaction of cognitive and emotional systems for self-regulation over the lifecourse and their impacts on decision processes. Individual differences in self-regulatory abilities will likely have important implications for goal setting, goal maintenance, impulsivity and delay of gratification, emotion regulation, and conflict monitoring, with consequences for health-related decision-making carried out in both the short and long term. There remain considerable knowledge gaps concerning both how chronological age and time perspective influence decisions regarding both planning for the long term – such as investment in LTC insurance and advance directives regarding end of life care – and the immediate, everyday sorts of decisions required for health maintenance, including decisions to initiate and adhere to positive health behaviors and decisions to seek medical care and treatment. Moreover, there are multiple aspects of individuals, institutions, and social contexts that impact these choices – an area where population-based studies, longitudinal research, and cross-national comparisons have the potential to offer important insights.

In addition to topics already mentioned, future work in economic decision-making and neuroeconomics of aging has the potential to shed light on questions regarding age differences and age-related change in reward sensitivity, valuation of time, risk preferences and risk behaviors, tolerance of uncertainty and ambiguity, reliance on affective vs. deliberative processes in decision-making, affective forecasting, and susceptibility to the influences of incidental affect and stress, to mention only a few. In addition, a better understanding of the social and contextual factors shaping economic behavior over the life course is needed to address questions regarding the influence of socioemotional factors on the decisions of older adults. These factors include concerns for the well-being of close others, the weighting of emotional factors over other aspects of outcomes, the influence of stereotypes and attitudes about aging on decision-making by and for older adults, and the susceptibility of older adults to social influence in decision-making. An important and intriguing question is the extent to which these age-related behavioral and brain signatures are due to motivational changes associated with age or to age-related changes in underlying neural architecture and circuitry.

Finally, a number of methodological advances would serve to advance the field of decision-making and aging. These include the development of innovative methods for measuring economic choices of relevance to middle aged and older adults in the laboratory, field, and neuroimaging environments; longitudinal research on economic behaviors and their relation to neurobiological markers of cognition and socioemotional function; assessments of the reliability of neurobiological measures of economic behaviors over the short and long term; and data on the generalizability of laboratory findings to real-world economic behaviors.

Most of the important economic decisions made in a life time are made during adulthood, and most of these decisions have tremendous implications for well-being in older age. The types of research described in this chapter can help to advance economic and psychological models of decision-making more generally and improve our understanding of the factors that promote or impede advantageous decision-making over the life course. Population aging is creating extraordinary challenges for public and private institutions as well as families. In the longer term, it is hoped that knowledge about the causes and consequences of age-related changes in economic decision-making may guide the structuring of decision-supportive interventions affecting the choices individuals make as they approach the end of life and inform policy to improve public programs and overall social welfare.

REFERENCES

Adolphs, R., Tranel, D., & Damasio, A. R. (1998). The human amygdala in social judgment. *Nature*, *393*, 470–474.

Agarwal, S., Driscoll, J. C., Gabaix, X., & Laibson, D. I. (2008). The age of reason: Financial decisions over the lifecycle. SSRN. Available at http://ssrn.com/abstract = 973790

Albert, M. S., Jones, K., & Savage, C. R. (1995). Predictors of cognitive change in older persons: MacArthur studies of successful aging. *Psychology and Aging*, *10*, 578–589.

Anderson, C. J. (2003). The psychology of doing nothing: Forms of decision avoidance result from reason and emotion. *Psychological Bulletin*, *129*, 139–167.

Ashby, F. G., Isen, A. M., & Turken, A. U. (1999). A neuropsychological theory of positive affect and its influence on cognition. *Psychological Review*, *106*(3), 529–550.

Barili, P., De Carolis, G., Zaccheo, D., & Amenta, F. (1998). Sensitivity to ageing of the limbic dopaminergic system: A review. *Mechanisms of Ageing and Development*, *106*(1–2), 57–92.

Barsky, R. B., Juster, F. T., Kimball, M. S., & Shapiro, M. D. (1997). Preference parameters and behavioral heterogeneity: And experimental approach in the health and retirement study. *The Quarterly Journal of Economics*, *112*(2), 537–579.

Bechara, A., Damasio, H., Tranel, D., & Damasio, A. R. (1997). Deciding advantageously before knowing the advantageous strategy. *Science*, *275*(5304), 1293–1295.

Birditt, K., & Fingerman, K. (2005). Do we get better at picking our battles? Age group differences in descriptions of behavioral reactions to interpersonal tensions. *Journals of Gerontology Series B: Psychological and Social Sciences*, *60*, 121–128.

Blanchard-Fields, F., Chen, Y., & Norris, L. (1997). Everyday problem-solving across the adult life span: Influence of domain specificity and cognitive appraisal. *Psychology and Aging*, *12*(4), 684–693.

Blanchard-Fields, F., Janke, H. C., & Camp, C. (1995). Age differences in problem-solving style: The role of emotional salience. *Psychology and Aging*, *10*(2), 173–180.

Blanchard-Fields, F., Mienaltowski, A., & Seay, R. B. (2007). Age differences in everyday problem-solving effectiveness: Older adults select more effective strategies for interpersonal problems. *Journal of Gerontology Series B: Psychological Sciences and Social Sciences*, *62*, 61–64.

Braver, T. S., Barch, D. M., Keys, B. A., Carter, C., Cohen, J. D., Kaye, J. A., Janowsky, J. S., Taylor, S. F., Yesavage, J. A., Mumenthaler, M. S., Jagust, W. J., & Reed, B. R. (2001). Context processing in older adults: Evidence for a theory relating cognitive control to neurobiology in healthy aging. *Journal of Experimental Psychology: General*, *130*(4), 746–763.

Breiter, H. C., Aharon, I., Kahneman, D., Dale, A., & Shizgal, P. (2001). Functional imaging of neural responses to expectancy and experience of monetary gains and losses. *Neuron*, *30*, 619–639.

Briggs, S. D., Raz, N., & Marks, W. (1999). Age-related deficits in generation and manipulation of mental images: I. The role of sensorimotor speed and working memory. *Psychology and Aging*, *14*(3), 427–435.

Brown, J., & Finkelstein, A. (2007). Why is the market for long-term care insurance so small? *Journal of Public Economics*, *91*(10), 1967–1991.

Brown, J. R., Coe, N. B., & Finkelstein, A. (2006). *Medicaid crowd-out of private long-term care insurance demand: Evidence from the Health and Retirement Survey*. National Bureau of Economic Research Working Paper no. 12536, Cambridge, MA.

Buckner, R. L. (2004). Memory and executive function in aging and AD: Multiple factors that cause decline and reserve factors that compensate. *Neuron*, *44*, 195–208.

Cacioppo, J. T., Berntson, G. G., Bechara, A., Tranel, D., & Hawkley, L. C. (in press). Could an aging brain contribute to subjective well-being? The value added by a social neuroscience perspective. In: A. Tadorov, S. T. Fiske, & D. Prentice (Eds), *Social neuroscience: Toward understanding the underpinnings of the social mind*. New York, NY: Oxford University Press.

Cacioppo, J. T., Berntson, G. G., Kelin, D. J., & Poehlmann, K. M. (1997). Psychophysiology of emotion across the lifespan. In: K. W. Schaie & M. P. Lawton (Eds), *Annual review of gerontology and geriatrics: Volume 17. Focus on emotion and adult development* (pp. 27–74). New York: Springer.

Cacioppo, J. T., Hughes, M. E., Waite, L. J., Hawkley, L. C., & Thisted, R. A. (2006). Loneliness as a specific risk factor for depressive symptoms: Cross-sectional and longitudinal analyses. *Psychology and Aging*, *21*(1), 140–151.

Carstensen, L. L. (2006). The influence of a sense of time on human development. *Science*, *312*, 1913–1915.

Carstensen, L. L., & Charles, S. T. (1998). Emotion in the second half of life. *Current Directions in Psychological Science*, *7*(5), 144–149.

Carstensen, L. L., Gottman, J. M., & Levenson, R. W. (1995). Emotional behavior in long-term marriage. *Psychology Aging*, *10*(1), 140–149.

Carstensen, L. L., Isaacowitz, D. M., & Charles, S. T. (1999). Taking time seriously: A theory of socioemotional selectivity. *American Psychologist*, *54*(3), 165–181.

Carstensen, L. L., & Mikels, J. A. (2005). At the intersection of emotion and cognition: Aging and the positivity effect. *Current Directions in Psychological Science*, *14*(3), 117–121.

Carstensen, L. L., Pasupathi, M., Mayr, U., & Nesselraode, J. R. (2000). Emotional experience in everyday life across the adult life span. *Journal of Personality and Social Psychology*, *79*(4), 644–655.

Charles, S. T. (2005). Viewing injustice: Greater emotion heterogeneity with age. *Psychology and Aging*, *20*(1), 159–164.

Charles, S. T., & Carstensen, L. L. (2007). Emotion regulation and aging. In: J. J. Gross (Ed.), *Handbook of emotion regulation*. New York: Guilford Press.

Chodosh, J., Reuben, D. B., Albert, M. S., & Seeman, T. E. (2002). Predicting cognitive impairment in high-functioning community-dwelling older persons: MacArthur studies of successful aging. *Journal of the American Geriatrics Society*, *50*(6), 1051–1060.

Chou, K. L., Lee, T. M., & Ho, A. H. (2007). Does mood state change risk-taking tendency in older adults? *Psychology Aging*, *22*(2), 310–318.

Congressional Budget Office. (2004). *Financing long-term care for the elderly*. Washington, DC: Congressional Budget Office Papers.

Curley, S. P., Eraker, S. A., & Yates, J. F. (1984). An investigation of patients' reactions to therapeutic uncertainty. *Medical Decision-making*, *4*, 501–511.

Damasio, A. R. (1994). *Descartes' error: Emotion, reason and the human brain*. New York, NY: G. P. Putnam's Sons.

Deakin, J., Aitken, M., Robbins, T., & Sahakian, B. J. (2004). Risk-taking during decision-making in normal volunteers changes with age. *Journal of the International Neuropsychological Society*, *10*, 590–598.

Denburg, N. L., Recknor, E. C., Bechara, A., & Tranel, D. (2006). Psychophysiological anticipation of positive outcomes promotes advantageous decision-making in normal older persons. *International Journal of Psychophysiology*, *61*, 19–25.

Denburg, N. L., Tranel, D., & Bechara, A. (2005). The ability to decide advantageously declines prematurely in some normal older persons. *Neuropsychologia*, *43*(7), 1099–1106.

Dobbs, A. R., & Rule, B. G. (1989). Adult age differences in working memory. *Psychology and Aging*, *4*(4), 500–503.

Elliot, R., Friston, K. J., & Dolan, R. J. (2000). Dissociable neural responses in human reward systems. *The Journal of Neuroscience*, *20*(16), 6159–6165.

Ferrer, E., Salthouse, T. A., Stewart, W. F., & Schwartz, B. S. (2004). Modeling age and retest processes in longitudinal studies of cognitive abilities. *Psychology Aging*, *19*(2), 243–259.

Finkelstein, A., McGarry, K., & Sufi, A. (2005). Dynamic inefficiencies in insurance markets: Evidence from long-term care insurance. *American Economic Review (Papers and Proceedings)*, *95*(2), 224–228.

Fried, T. R., O'Leary, J., Van Ness, P., & Fraenkel, L. (2007). Inconsistency over time in the preferences of older persons with advanced illness for life-sustaining treatment. *Journal of the American Geriatric Society*, *55*(7), 1007–1014.

Fritsch, T., McClendon, M. J., Smyth, K. A., Lerner, A. J., Friedland, R. P., & Larsen, J. D. (2007). Cognitive functioning in healthy aging: The role of reserve and lifestyle factors early in life. *The Gerontologist*, *47*, 307–322.

Goldman-Rakic, P. S. (1996). Regional and cellular fractionation of working memory. *Proceedings of the National Academy of Sciences, USA*, *3*(24), 13473–13480.

Good, C. D., Johnsrude, I. S., Ashburner, J., Henson, R. N. A., Friston, K. J., & Frackowiak, R. S. J. (2001). A voxel-based morphometric study of ageing in 465 normal adult human brains. *NeuroImage*, *14*, 21–36.

Grady, C. L. (2000). Functional brain imaging and age-related changes in cognition. *Biological Psychology*, *54*, 259–281.

Green, L., Myerson, J., Lichtman, D., Rosen, S., & Fry, A. (1996). Temporal discounting in choice between delayed rewards: The role of age and income. *Psychology and Aging*, *11*(1), 79–84.

Gross, J. J., Carstensen, L. L., Pasupathi, M., Tsai, J., Gotestam Skorpen, C., & Hus, A. Y. C. (1997). Emotion and aging: Experience, expression, and control. *Psychology and Aging*, *12*, 590–599.

Hartog, J., Ferrer-i-Carbonell, A., & Jonker, N. (2002). Linking measured risk aversion to individual characteristic. *Kyklos*, *55*, 3–26.

Hasher, L., & Zacks, R. T. (1988). Working memory, comprehension, and aging: A review and a new view. In: G. H. Bower (Ed.), *The psychology of learning and motivation: Advances in research and theory* (Vol. 22, pp. 193–225). San Diego, CA: Academic Press.

Head, D., Raz, N., Gunning-Dixon, F., Williamson, A., & Acker, J. D. (2002). Age-related differences in the course of cognitive skill acquisition: The role of regional cortical shrinkage and cognitive resources. *Psychology and Aging*, *17*(1), 72–84.

Hedden, T., & Gabrieli, J. D. (2005). Healthy and pathological processes in adult development: New evidence from neuroimaging of the aging brain. *Current Opinion in Neurology*, *18*, 740–747.

Heisler, M., Langa, K. M., Eby, E. L., Fendrick, A. M., Kabeto, M. U., & Piette, J. D. (2004). The health effects of restricting prescription medication use because of cost. *Medical Care*, *42*(7), 626–634.

Heiss, F., McFadden, D., & Winter, J. (2006). *Who failed to enroll in Medicare Part D, and why? Early results*. Health Affairs Data Watch, August, w344–w354.

Heiss, F., McFadden, D., & Winter, J. (2007). *Mind the gap! Consumer perceptions and choices of Medicare Part D prescription drug plans*. National Bureau of Economic Research Working Paper no. 13627, Cambridge, MA.

Henry, N. J., Berg, C. A., Smith, T. W., & Florsheim, P. (2007). Positive and negative characteristics of marital interaction and their association with marital satisfaction in middle-aged and older couples. *Psychology Aging*, *22*(3), 428–441.

Hertwig, R., Barron, G., Weber, E. U., & Erev, I. (2004). Decisions from experience and the effect of rare events on risky choice. *Psychological Science*, *15*, 534–539.

Hess, T. M. (2005). Memory and aging in context. *Psychology Bulletin*, *131*(3), 383–406.

Hsu, J., Fung, V., Price, M., Huang, J., Brand, R., Hui, R., Fireman, B., & Newhouse, J. (2008). Medicare beneficiaries' knowledge of part d prescription drug program benefits and responses to drug costs. *The New England Journal of Medicine*, *299*(16), 1929–1936.

Hsu, J., Price, M., Huang, J., Brand, R., Fung, V., Hui, R., Fireman, B., Newhouse, J., & Selby, J. (2006). Unintended consequences of caps on Medicare drug benefits. *The New England Journal of Medicine*, *354*(22), 2349–2359.

Huettel, S. A., Stowe, C. J., Gordon, E. M., Warner, B. T., & Platt, M. L. (2006). Neural signatures of economic preferences for risk and ambiguity. *Neuron*, *49*, 765–775.

Institute of Medicine. (2004). Health literacy: A prescription to end confusion. In: L. Nielsen-Bohlman, A. M. Panzer & D. A. Kindig (Eds), *Committee on Health Literacy, Board on Neuroscience and Behavioral Health*. Washington, DC: National Academies Press.

Isaacowitz, D. M., Löckenhoff, C. E., Lane, R. D., Wright, R., Sechrest, L., Riedel, R., & Costa, P. T. (2007). Age differences in recognition of emotion in lexical stimuli and facial expressions. *Psychology Aging*, *22*(1), 147–159.

Isella, V., Mapelli, C., Morielli, N., Pelati, O., Franceschi, M., & Appollonio, I. M. (2008). Age-related quantitative and qualitative changes in decision making ability. *Behavioral Neurology*, *19*, 59–63.

Isen, A. M. (1993). Positive affect and decision-making. In: M. Lewis & J. M. Haviland (Eds), *Handbook of emotions*. New York, NY: The Guilford Press.

Jernigan, T. L., Archibald, S. L., Berhow, M. T., Sowell, E. R., Foster, D. S., & Hesselink, J. R. (1991). Cerebral structure on MRI, Part I: Localization of age-related changes. *Biological Psychiatry*, *29*, 55–67.

Johnson, E. J., Gachter, S., & Herrmann, A. (2006). *Exploring the nature of loss aversion*. University of Nottingham Centre for Decision Research and Experimental Economics (CeDEx). Discussion Paper no. 2006-02. Available at http://www.nottingham.ac.uk/economics/cedex/papers/2006-02.pdf

Johnson, E. J., Häubl, G. G., & Keinan, A. (2007). Aspects of endowment: A query theory of value construction. *Journal of Experimental Psychology: Learning, Memory, and Cognition*, *33*, 461–474.

Johnson, M. K., Hashtroudi, S., & Lindsay, D. S. (1993). Source monitoring. *Psychological Bulletin*, *114*(1), 3–28.

Johnson, M. M. S. (1990). Age differences in decision-making: A process methodology for examining strategic information processing. *Journal of Gerontology*, *45*(2), 75–78.

Joyce, G. F., Goldman, D. P., Karaca-Mandic, P., & Zheng, Y. (2007). Pharmacy benefit caps and the chronically ill. *Health Affairs*, *26*(5), 1333–1344.

Kaasinen, V., Vilkmanb, H., Hietalac, J., Någrend, K., Heleniuse, H., Olssonf, H., Fardef, L., & Rinne, J. O. (2000). Age-related dopamine D2/D3 receptor loss in extrastriatal regions of the human brain. *Neurobiology of Aging*, *21*, 683–688.

Kahneman, D. (2003). A perspective on judgment and choice: Mapping bounded rationality. *American Psychologist*, *58*(9), 697–720.

Kahneman, D., & Tversky, A. (1979). Prospect theory: An analysis of decision under risk. *Econometrica*, *47*(2), 263–292.

Knight, M., Seymour, T. L., Gaunt, J. T., Baker, C., Nesmith, K., & Mather, M. (2007). Aging and goal-directed emotional attention: Distraction reverses emotional biases. *Emotion*, *7*(4), 705–714.

Knutson, B., Adams, C. M., Fong, G. W., & Hommer, D. (2001b). Anticipation of increasing monetary reward selectively recruits nucleus accumbens. *The Journal of Neuroscience*, *21*, 5472–5476.

Knutson, B., Fong, G. W., Adams, C. M., Varner, J. L., & Hommer, D. (2001a). Dissociation of reward anticipation and outcome with event-related fMRI. *Neuroreport*, *12*(17), 3683–3687.

Knutson, B., Fong, G. W., Bennett, S. M., Adams, C. M., & Hommer, D. (2003). A region of mesial prefrontal cortex tracks monetarily rewarding outcomes: Characterization with rapid event-related fMRI. *NeuroImage*, *18*, 263–272.

Kovalchik, S., Camerer, C., Grether, D. M., Plott, C. R., & Allman, J. M. (2005). Aging and decision making: A comparison between neurologically healthy elderly and young individuals. *Journal of Economic Behavior & Organization*, *58*, 79–94.

Kramer, A. F., Bherer, L., Colcombe, S. J., Dong, W., & Greenough, W. T. (2004). Environmental influences on cognitive and brain plasticity during aging. *Journals of Gerontology Series A: Biological Sciences and Medical Sciences*, *59*(9), M940–M957.

Krawczyk, D. C. (2002). Contributions of the prefrontal cortex to the neural basis of human decision-making. *Neuroscience Biobehavioral Reviews*, *26*(6), 631–664.

Kuhnen, C. M., & Knutson, B. (2005). The neural basis of financial risk-taking. *Neuron*, *47*, 763–770.

Kunzman, U., Kupperbusch, C. S., & Levenson, R. W. (2005). Behavioral inhibition and amplification during emotional arousal: A comparison of two age groups. *Psychology and Aging*, *20*, 144–158.

Labouvie-Vief, G., DeVoe, M., & Bulka, D. (1989). Speaking about feelings: Conceptions of emotion across the life span. *Psychology and Aging*, *4*, 425–437.

Labouvie-Vief, G., Diehl, M., Jain, E., & Zhang, F. (2007). Six-year change in affect optimization and affect complexity across the adult life span: A further examination. *Psychology and Aging*, *22*, 738–751.

Lachman, M. E., Röcke, C., Rosnick, C., & Ryff, C. D. (2008). Realism and illusion in Americans' temporal views of their life satisfaction: Age differences in reconstructing the past and anticipating the future. *Psychological Science*, *19*(9), forthcoming.

Laibson, D. I. (1997). Golden eggs and hyperbolic discounting. *Quarterly Journal of Economics*, *62*, 443–477.

Lamar, M., & Resnick, S. M. (2004). Aging and prefrontal functions: Dissociating orbitofrontal and dorsolateral abilities. *Neurobiology of Aging*, *25*, 553–558.

Lawton, M. P., Kleban, M. H., Rajagopal, D., & Dean, J. (1992). Dimensions of affective experience in three age groups. *Psychology and Aging*, *7*, 171–184.

Lee, T. M. C., Leung, A. W. S., Fox, T. T., Gao, J.-H., & Chan, C. C. H. (2008). Age-related differences in neural activities during risk-taking as revealed by functional MRI. *Social Cognitive and Affective Neuroscience*, *3*, 7–15.

Levenson, R. W., Carstensen, L. L., Friesen, W. V., & Ekman, P. (1991). Emotion, physiology, and expression in old age. *Psychology and Aging*, *6*(1), 28–35.

Levenson, R. W., Carstensen, L. L., & Gottman, J. M. (1994). Influence of age and gender on affect, physiology, and their interrelations: A study of long-term marriages. *Journal of Personality and Social Psychology*, *67*(1), 56–68.

Lieberman, M. D. (2000). Intuition: A social cognitive neuroscience approach. *Psychological Bulletin*, *126*, 109–137.

List, J. A. (2003). Does market experience eliminate market anomalies? *Quarterly Journal of Economics*, *118*, 41–71.

Löckenhoff, C. E., & Carstensen, L. L. (2004). Socioemotional selectivity theory, aging, and health: The increasingly delicate balance between regulating emotions and making tough choices. *Journal of Personality*, *72*, 1395–1424.

Löckenhoff, C. E., & Carstensen, L. L. (2007). Aging, emotion, and health-related decision strategies: Motivational manipulations can reduce age differences. *Psychology of Aging*, *22*, 134–146.

Loewenstein, G. F. (2005). Hot–cold empathy gaps and medical decision-making. *Health Psychology*, *24*(4), S49–S56.

Loewenstein, G. F., Weber, E. U., Hsee, C. K., & Welch, N. (2001). Risk as feelings. *Psychology Bulletin*, *127*(2), 267–286.

Lupien, S. J., Maheu, F., Tu, M., Fiocco, A., & Schramek, T. E. (2007). The effects of stress and stress hormones on human cognition: Implications for the field of brain and cognition. *Brain Cognition*, *65*(3), 209–237.

MacPherson, S. E., Phillips, L. H., & Della Sala, S. (2002). Age, executive function and social decision-making: A dorsolateralprefronatal theory of cognitive aging. *Psychology and Aging*, *17*, 598–609.

Madden, J. M., Graves, A. J., Zhang, F., Adams, A. S., Briesacher, B. A., Ross-Degnan, D., Gurwitz, J. H., Pierre-Jacques, M., Safran, D. G., Adler, G. S., & Soumerai, S. B. (2008). Cost-related medication nonadherence and spending on basic needs following implementation of Medicare Part D. *Journal of the American Medical Association*, *299*(6), 1922–1928.

Marschner, A., Mell, T., Wartenburger, I., Villringer, A., Reischies, F. M., & Heekeren, H. R. (2005). Reward-based decision-making and aging. *Brain Research Bulletin*, *67*(5), 382–390.

Mather, M. (2004). A review of decision-making processes: Weighing the risks and benefits of aging. In: L. L. Carstensen & C. R. Hartel (Eds), *When I'm 64* (pp. 145–173). Washington, DC: National Academy of Sciences.

Mather, M., Canli, T., English, T., Whitfield, S., Wais, P., Ochsner, K., Gabrieli, J. D. E., & Carstensen, L. L. (2004). Amygdala responses to emotionally valenced stimuli in older and younger adults. *Psychological Science*, *15*, 259–263.

Mather, M., & Carstensen, L. L. (2005). Aging and motivated cognition: The positivity effect in attention and memory. *Trends in Cognitive Science*, *9*, 496–502.

Mather, M., Gorlick, M., & Kryla-Lighthall, N. (2008). To brake or accelerate when the light turns yellow? Age differences in how stress affects risk-taking in a driving game. Poster presented at Social and Affective Neuroscience 2008, Boston, MA.

Mather, M., & Johnson, M. K. (2000). Choice-supportive source monitoring: Do our decisions seem better to us as we age? *Psychology and Aging*, *15*, 596–606.

Mather, M., & Knight, M. (2005). Goal-directed memory: The role of cognitive control in older adults' emotional memory. *Psychology and Aging*, *20*, 554–570.

Mayhorn, C. B., Fisk, A. D., & Whittle, J. D. (2002). Decisions, decisions: Analysis of age, cohort, and time of testing on framing of risky decision options. *Human Factors*, *44*(4), 515–521.

McClure, S. M., Laibson, D., Loewenstein, G., & Cohen, J. D. (2004). Separate neural systems value immediate and delayed monetary rewards. *Science*, *306*(5695), 503–507.

McFadden, D. (2007). A dog's breakfast. *Wall Street Journal*, Commentary, February 16, A15.

Mell, T., Heekeren, H. R., Marschner, A., Wartenburger, I., Villringer, A., & Reischies, F. M. (2005). Effect of aging on stimulus–reward association learning. *Neuropsychologia*, *43*(4), 554–563.

Mellers, B., Schwartz, A., & Ritov, I. (1997). Emotion-based choice. *Journal of Experimental Psychology: General*, *128*(3), 332–345.

Meyer, B. J. F., Russon, C., & Talbot, A. (1995). Discourse comprehension and problem-solving: Decision about the treatment of breast cancer by women across the life span. *Psychology and Aging*, *10*(1), 84–103.

Meyer-Lindenberg, A., & Zink, C. F. (2007). Imaging genetics for neuropsychiatric disorders. *Child and Adolescent Psychiatric Clinics of North America*, *16*(3), 581–597.

Miller, L. S., & Lachman, M. E. (2000). Cognitive performance and the role of health and control beliefs in midlife. *Aging Neuropsychology and Cognition*, *7*, 69–85.

Mireles, D. E., & Charness, N. (2002). Computational explorations of the influence of structured knowledge on age-related cognitive decline. *Psychology Aging*, *17*(2), 245–259.

Mischel, W., Shoda, Y., & Rodriguez, M. L. (1989). Delay of gratification in children. *Science*, *244*, 933–938.

Mroczek, D. K., & Kolarz, C. M. (1998). The effect of age on positive and negative affect: A developmental perspective on happiness. *Journal of Personality and Social Psychology*, *75*(5), 1333–1349.

Mu, Q., Xie, J., Zongyao, W., Yaquin, W., & Zhang, S. (1999). A quantitative MR study of the hippocampal formation, the amygdala, and the temporal horn of the lateral ventricle in healthy subjects 40 to 90 years of age. *American Journal of Neuroradiology*, *20*, 207–211.

Murphy, N., & Isaacowitz, D. (2008). Preferences for emotional information in older and younger adults: A meta-analysis of memory and attention tasks. *Psychology and Aging*, *23*(2), 263–286.

Nielsen, L., Knutson, B., & Carstensen, L. L. (2008). Affect dynamics, affective forecasting and aging. *Emotion*, *8*(3), 318–330.

Norton, E. (2000). Long-term care. In: A. J. Culyer & J. P. Newhouse (Eds), *Handbook of health economics* (Vol. 1, pp. 955–994). Amsterdam, The Netherlands: Elsevier Science.

Okun, M. A. (1976). Age and cautiousness in decision. *Human Development*, *19*, 220–233.

Olsson, A., & Phelps, E. A. (2007). Social learning of fear. *Nature Neuroscience*, *10*, 1095–1102.

Ong, A. D., Bergeman, C. S., Bisconti, T. L., & Wallace, K. A. (2006). Psychological resilience, positive emotions, and successful adaptation to stress in later life. *Journal of Personality and Social Psychology*, *91*(4), 730–749.

O'Doherty, J., Kringelbach, M. L., Rolls, E. T., Hornak, J., & Andrews, C. (2001). Abstract reward and punishment representation in the human orbitofrontal cortex. *Nature Neuroscience*, *4*(1), 95–102.

O'Doherty, J. P., & Bossaerts, P. (2008). Toward a mechanistic understanding of human decision-making: Contributions of functional neuroimaging. *Current Directions in Psychological Science*, *17*, 119–123.

Park, D. C., Lautenschlager, G., Hedden, T., Davidson, N. S., Smith, A. D., & Smith, P. K. (2002). Models of visuospatial and verbal memory across the adult life span. *Psychology Aging*, *17*, 299–320.

Pauly, M. V. (1990). The rational nonpurchase of long-term care insurance. *The Journal of Political Economy*, *98*(1), 153–168.

Peters, E., Finucane, M. L., MacGregor, D. G., & Slovic, P. (2001). The unbearable lightness of aging: Judgment and decision processes in older adults. In: P. C. Stern & L. L. Carstensen (Eds), *The aging mind: Opportunities in cognitive research* (pp. 144–165). Washington, DC: National Academy of Sciences.

Phelps, E. A. (2006). Emotion and cognition: Insights from studies of the human amygdala. *Annual Review of Psychology*, *57*, 27–53.

Phillips, L. H., Henry, J. D., Hosie, J. A., & Milne, A. B. (2006). Age, anger regulation and well-being. *Aging and Mental Health*, *10*(3), 250–256.

Plassman, B. L., Langa, K. M., Fisher, G. G., Heeringa, S. G., Weir, D. R., Ofstedal, M. B., Burke, J. R., Hurd, M. D., Potter, G. G., Rodgers, W. L., Steffens, D. C., Willis, R. J., & Wallace, R. B. (2007). Prevalence of dementia in the United States: The aging, demographics, and memory study. *Neuroepidemiology*, *29*(1–2), 125–132.

Prochaska, J. O., & Velicer, W. F. (1997). The transtheoretical model of health behavior change. *American Journal of Health Promotion*, *12*, 38–48.

Rahhal, T. A., Colcombe, S. J., & Hasher, L. (2001). Instructional manipulations and age differences in memory: Now you see them, now you don't. *Psychology Aging*, *16*(4), 697–706.

Ratzan, S. C., & Parker, R. M. (2000). Introduction. In: C. R. Selden, M. Zorn, S. C. Ratzan, & R. M. Parker (eds), *National Library of Medicine Current Bibliographies in Medicine: Health Literacy, NLM Pub. No. CBM 2000-1, U.S.* Bethesda, MD: Department of Health and Human Services, National Institutes of Health. Available at http://www.nlm.nih.gov/archive//20061214/pubs/cbm/hliteracy.html#15

Raz, N., Gunning, F. M., Head, D., Dupuis, J. H., McQuain, J., Briggs, S. D., Loken, W. J., Thornton, A. E., & Acker, J. D. (1997). Selective aging of the human cerebral cortex observed in vivo: Differential vulnerability of the prefrontal gray matter. *Cerebral Cortex*, *7*(3), 268–282.

Raz, N., Gunning-Dixon, F. M., Head, D., Dupuis, J. H., & Acker, J. D. (1998). Neuroanatomical correlates of cognitive aging: Evidence from structural magnetic resonance imaging. *Neuropsychology*, *12*(1), 95–114.

Read, D., & Read, N. L. (2004). Time discounting over the lifespan. *Organizational Behavior and Human Decision Processes*, *94*(1), 22–32.

Resnick, S. M., Lamar, M., & Driscoll, I. (2007). Vulnerability of the orbitofrontal cortex to age-associated structural and functional brain changes. *Annals of the New York Academy of Sciences*, *1121*, 562–575.

Reuter-Lorenz, P. (2002). New visions of the aging mind and brain. *Trends in Cognitive Sciences*, *6*(9), 394–400.

Rogers, R. D., Owen, A. M., Middleton, H. C., Williams, E. J., Pickard, J. D., Sahakian, B. J., & Robbins, T. W. (1999). Choosing between small, likely rewards and large, unlikely rewards activates inferior and orbital prefrontal cortex. *The Journal of Neuroscience*, *20*(19), 9029–9038.

Rolls, E. T. (1999). *The brain and emotion*. Oxford, UK: Oxford University Press.

Rönnlund, M., Karlsson, E., Laggnäs, E., Larsson, L., & Lindström, T. (2005). Risky decision making across three arenas of choice: Are younger and older adults differently susceptible to framing effects? *The Journal of General Psychology*, *132*(1), 81–92.

Roring, R. W., & Charness, N. (2007). A multilevel model analysis of expertise in chess across the lifespan. *Psychology and Aging*, *22*(2), 291–299.

Rozin, P., & Royzman, E. B. (2001). Negativity bias, negativity dominance, and contagion. *Personality and Social Psychology Review*, *5*, 296–320.

Rueda, M. R., Posner, M. I., & Rothbart, M. D. (2005). The development of executive attention: Contributions to the emergence of self-regulation. *Developmental Neuropsychology*, *22*(2), 573–594.

Ruffman, T., Henry, J. D., Livingstone, V., & Phillips, L. H. (2008). A meta-analytic review of emotion recognition and aging: Implications for neuropsychological models of aging. *Neuroscience and Biobehavioral Review*, *32*(4), 863–881.

Salat, D. H., Kaye, J. A., & Janowsky, J. S. (1999). Prefrontal gray and white matter volumes in healthy aging and Alzheimer disease. *Archives of Neurology*, *56*(3), 338–344.

Salthouse, T. A. (1990). Influence of experience on age difference in cognitive functioning. *Human Factors*, *32*, 551–569.

Salthouse, T. A. (1996). The processing-speed theory of adult age differences in cognition. *Psychological Review*, *103*(3), 403–428.

Salthouse, T. A. (2003). Memory aging from 18 to 80. *Alzheimer's Disease and Associated Disorders*, *17*(1), 162–167.

Salthouse, T. A. (2005). Relations between cognitive abilities and measures of executive functioning. *Neuropsychology*, *19*, 532–545.

Samanez-Larkin, G. & D'Esposito, M. (2008). Group comparisons: Imaging the aging brain. *Social Cognitive and Affective Neuroscience*, *3*(3), 290–297.

Samanez-Larkin, G. R., Gibbs, S. E. B., Nielsen, L., Khanna, K., Carstensen, L. L., & Knutson, B. (2007). Anticipation of monetary gain but not loss in healthy older adults. *Nature Neuroscience*, *10*, 787–791.

Samanez-Larkin, G. R., Hollon, N. G., Carstensen, L. L., & Knutson, B. (2008). Individual differences in insular sensitivity during loss anticipation predict avoidance learning. *Psychological Science*, *19*, 320–323.

Samuelson, W., & Zeckhauser, R. (1988). Status quo bias in decision-making. *Journal of Risk and Uncertainty*, *1*, 7–59.

Sanfey, A. G., & Hastie, R. (2000). Judgment and decision-making across the adult life span: A tutorial review of psychological research. In: D. C. Park & N. Schwarz (Eds), *Cognitive aging: A primer* (pp. 253–273). Philadelphia, PA: Psychology Press.

Sanfey, A. G., Rilling, J. K., Aronson, J. A., Nystrom, L. E., & Cohen, J. D. (2003). The neural basis of economic decision-making in the ultimatum game. *Science*, *300*(5626), 1755–1758.

Schaie, K. W. (2005). What can we learn from longitudinal studies of adult development? *Research in Human Development*, *2*(3), 133–158.

Schretlen, D., Pearlson, G. D., Anthony, J. C., Aylward, E. H., Augustine, A. M., Davis, A., & Barta, P. (2000). Elucidating the contributions of processing speed, executive ability, and frontal lobe volume to normal age-related differences in fluid intelligence. *Journal of the International Neuropsychological Society*, *6*, 52–61.

Schultz, W. (2002). Getting formal with dopamine and reward. *Neuron*, *36*, 241–263.

Schwartz, B. (2004). The tyranny of choice. *Scientific American*, *April*, 71–75.

Singh-Manoux, A., Richards, M., & Marmot, M. (2005). Socioeconomic position across the lifecourse: How does it relate to cognitive function in mid-life? *Annals of Epidemiology, 15*(8), 572–578.

Slessor, G., Phillips, L. H., & Bull, R. (2007). Exploring the specificity of age-related differences in theory of mind tasks. *Psychology and Aging, 22*(3), 639–643.

Slovic, P. (1995). The construction of preference. *American Psychologist, 50*(5), 364–371.

Slovic, P., Finucane, M. L., Peters, E., & MacGregor, D. G. (2004). Risk as analysis and risk as feelings: Some thoughts about affect, reason, risk, and rationality. *Risk Analysis, 24*(2), 311–322.

Society of Actuaries. (2002). *Long-Term Care Experience Committee Intercompany Study 1984–1999*. Schaumburg, IL: Society of Actuaries.

Soumerai, S., Pierre-Jacques, M., Zhang, F., Ross-Degnan, D., Adams, A., Gurwitz, J., Adler, G., & Safran, D. G. (2006). Cost-related medication nonadherance among the elderly and the disabled: A national survey one year before the Medicare drug benefit. *Archives of Internal Medicine, 166*, 1829–1835.

Sozou, P. D., & Seymour, R. M. (2003). Augmented discounting: Interaction between ageing and time-preference behavior. *Proceedings from the Royal Society of London, 270*, 1047–1053.

Steinberg, L. (2004). Risk-taking in adolescence: What changes, and why? *Annals of the New York Academy of Sciences, 1021*, 51–58.

Strough, J., Mehta, C. M., McFall, J. P., & Schuller, K. L. (2008). Are older adults less subject to the sunk-cost fallacy than younger adults? *Psychological Science, 19*(7), 653–659.

Sullivan, S., Ruffman, T., & Hutton, S. B. (2007). Age differences in emotion recognition skills and the visual scanning of emotion faces. *Journals of Gerontology Series B: Psychological Science and Social Science, 62*(1), 53–60.

Teachman, B. A. (2006). Aging and negative affect: The rise and fall and rise of anxiety and depression symptoms. *Psychology and Aging, 21*(1), 201–207.

Tsai, J. L., Levenson, R. W., & Carstensen, L. L. (2000). Autonomic, subjective, and expressive responses to emotional films in older and younger Chinese Americans and European Americans. *Psychology Aging, 15*(4), 684–693.

Tversky, A., & Kahneman, D. (1973). Availability: A heuristic for judging frequency and probability. *Cognitive Psychology, 5*, 207–232.

Tversky, A., & Kahneman, D. (1974). Judgment under uncertainty: Heuristics and biases. *Science, 27*(185), 1124–1131.

Tversky, A., & Kahneman, D. (1981). The framing of decisions and the psychology of choice. *Science, 211*, 453–458.

Ubel, P. A., & Loewenstein, G. (1997). The role of decision analysis in informed consent: Choosing between intuition and systematicity. *Social Science and Medicine, 44*(5), 647–656.

Ubel, P. A., Loewenstein, G., & Jepson, C. (2003). Whose quality of life? A commentary exploring discrepancies between health state evaluations of patients and the general public. *Quality of Life Research, 12*(6), 599–607.

Urry, H. L., van Reekum, C. M., Johnstone, T., Kalin, N. H., Thurow, M. E., Schaefer, H. S., Jackson, C. A., Frye, C. J., Greischar, L. L., Alexander, A. L., & Davidson, R. J. (2006). Amygdala and ventromedial prefrontal cortex are inversely coupled during regulation of negative affect and predict the diurnal pattern of cortisol secretion among older adults. *Journal of Neuroscience, 26*(16), 4415–4425.

Vaidya, J. G., Paradiso, S., Boles Ponto, L. L., McCormick, L. M., & Robinson, R. G. (2007). Aging, grey matter, and blood flow in the anterior cingulate cortex. *Neuroimage*, *37*(4), 1346–1353.

Varian, H. R. (1992). *Microeconomic analysis* (3rd ed., pp. 172–197). New York, NY: W.W. Norton and Company.

Verhaeghen, P., & Salthouse, T. A. (1997). Meta-analyses of age–cognition relations in adulthood: Estimates of linear and nonlinear age effects and structural models. *Psychological Bulletin*, *122*(3), 231–249.

Volkow, N. D., Logan, J., Fowler, J. S., Wang, G. J., Gur, R. C., Wong, C., Felder, C., Gatley, S. J., Ding, Y. S., Hitzemann, R., & Pappas, N. (2000). Association between age-related decline in brain dopamine activity and impairment in frontal and cingulate metabolism. *American Journal of Psychiatry*, *157*, 75–80.

Wallach, M. A., & Kogan, N. (1961). Aspects of judgment and decision-making: Interrelationships and changes with age. *Behavioral Science*, *6*, 23–36.

Williams, L. M., Brown, K. J., Palmer, D., Liddell, B. J., Kemp, A. H., Olivieri, G., Peduto, A., & Gordon, E. (2006). The mellow years: Neural basis of improving emotional stability over age. *Journal of Neuroscience*, *26*(24), 6422–6430.

Wilson, T., & Gilbert, D. T. (2003). Affective forecasting. *Advances in Experimental Social Psychology*, *35*, 345–411.

Winter, J., Balza, R., Caro, F., Heiss, F., Jun, B., Matzkin, R., & McFadden, D. (2006). Medicare prescription drug coverage: Consumer information and preferences. *Proceedings of the National Academy of Sciences*, *103*, 7929–7934.

Wong, D. F., Young, D., Wilson, P. D., Meltzer, C. C., & Gjedde, A. (1997). Quantification of neuroreceptors in the living human brain: III. D2-like dopamine receptors: Theory, validation, and changes during normal aging. *Journal of Cerebral Blood Flow and Metabolism*, *17*, 316–330.

Wood, S., Busemeyer, J., Koling, A., Cox, C. R., & Davis, H. (2005). Older adults as adaptive decision makers: Evidence from the Iowa Gambling Task. *Psychology and Aging*, *20*(2), 220–225.

Wright, C. I., Wedig, M. M., Williams, D., Rauch, S. L., & Albert, M. S. (2006). Novel fearful faces activate the amygdala in healthy young and elderly adults. *Neurobiology of Aging*, *27*, 361–374.

Yates, J. F., & Patalano, A. L. (1999). Decision-making and aging. In: D. C. Park, R. W. Morrell & K. Shifren (Eds), *Processing of medical information in aging patients: Cognitive and human factors perspectives* (pp. 31–54). Mahwah, NJ: Lawrence Erlbaum Associates.

CHILD HEALTH DISPARITIES, SOCIO-ECONOMIC STATUS, AND SCHOOL ENROLLMENT DECISIONS: EVIDENCE FROM GERMAN ELEMENTARY SCHOOL ENTRANCE EXAMS

Martin Salm and Daniel Schunk

ABSTRACT

Purpose – *This chapter examines the role of child health for the intergenerational transmission of human capital.*

Methodology/approach – *The chapter uses unique administrative data from German elementary school entrance examinations. The chapter considers child health conditions such as obesity, low birth weight, ear problems, eye problems, behavioral problems, asthma, and allergies. We control for socio-economic and demographic characteristics of children and their parents as well as for institutional factors such as duration of pre-school attendance.*

Findings – *We find that health conditions are more common among children of less-educated parents. We also find that health conditions have*

Neuroeconomics
Advances in Health Economics and Health Services Research, Volume 20, 271–288

ISSN: 0731-2199/doi:10.1016/S0731-2199(08)20011-7

a substantially negative impact on school readiness, and the negative impact is considerably stronger for children of less-educated parents. In total, 55% of the school readiness gap can be attributed to health factors. Specifically, 19% of the gap can be attributed to differences in the prevalence of health conditions, and 36% of the gap can be attributed to differences in the severity of the impact. Thus, policies aimed at reducing disparities in child achievement should also focus on improving the health of disadvantaged children.

Originality – *First, our study quantifies the extent to which the school readiness gap between parental education groups can be attributed to child health. Second, our data are of extraordinary quality, since they consist of a full sample of all children in one city and since they are collected during detailed examinations that were administered by government pediatricians.*

1. INTRODUCTION

Child development at an early age is an important predictor for educational achievement and labor market outcomes later in life (Currie, 2000). In this study we examine the role of child health for the intergenerational transmission of human capital. We look at the effect of child health conditions such as obesity, low birth weight, ear and eye problems, behavioral problems, asthma, and allergies on school readiness. We examine whether or not disparities in health between children of different education groups can explain differences in school readiness, and we determine what share of differences in school readiness between children of college-educated parents and children of less-educated parents can be attributed to child health conditions. For this purpose, we use unique administrative data based on German elementary school entrance exams. These exams include a detailed assessment of children's health, as well as various measures of child development. They are compulsory for all German children at age six prior to entering elementary school, and are administered by government pediatricians. Based on the examination results pediatricians issue a recommendation about whether or not a child is ready to start elementary school, and this recommendation decision is the outcome variable that we consider in this chapter.

From the previous literature it is well known that there is a strong correlation between child health and parents' socio-economic status.

Children of higher-educated parents tend to be in better health. This relationship is documented for several countries such as the United States (Case, Lubotsky, & Paxson, 2002), Canada (Currie & Stabile, 2003), and the United Kingdom (Currie, Shields, & Price, 2007). There is also a literature that links child health to cognitive development. In a study based on Peruvian data, Paxson and Schady (2007) find that health measures such as height for age and weight for age are related to language development. Kaestner and Corman (1995) find that low birth weight, stunted growth, and severe diseases are related to lower reading ability and lower math ability of children.

Currie (2005) surveys possible pathways in the relationship between child health and school readiness. Ill health can affect child development in several ways: Pain, stress, and fatigue reduce the ability to concentrate and to learn. For example, a child with an earache will find it hard to sit down and listen to a story. Illness can also crowd out other activities, if children spend a lot of time in bed, at doctors' offices, or in the hospital. Illness can also alter the relationships between parents, children, and others in ways that can negatively affect cognitive development. For example, parents who are concerned about their children's health might discourage them from exploring their surroundings. Finally, some illnesses can also have a direct negative impact on school readiness. For example, children with attention deficit disorders find it hard to concentrate over longer periods.

A negative effect of child health on school readiness does not by itself explain disparities in school readiness between socio-economic groups. However, such an effect can explain disparities in school readiness between parental education groups, if child health conditions are more common among the less-educated group (prevalence effect), or if child health conditions have a stronger negative impact on school readiness for the less-educated group (severity effect). Health conditions can have a stronger impact on school readiness if the negative consequences of the disease are less compensated through the positive effects of adequate medical treatment or parental intervention. For example, asthma attacks are one of the most common causes of hospital stays for young children, but they can mostly be avoided through medical treatment and adherence to medical guidelines (Currie, 2005).

In our study we find that health conditions such as low birth weight, ear problems, eye problems, behavioral problems, and asthma have a strong negative impact on school readiness. We also find that health conditions tend to be more prevalent among children of less-educated parents, and that health conditions have a stronger impact on school readiness for children of less-educated parents. In total, health conditions account for 54.6% of the difference in school readiness between education groups. 18.6% of the total difference can be attributed to differences in the prevalence of conditions, and 36% of the difference can be attributed to differences in the severity of the effect of health conditions on school readiness. While this study considers only a snapshot of the relationship between health conditions and social and cognitive skills at the early age of about six years, it is important to stress that experiences at this age have a strong effect on the development of brain architecture and neurochemistry (Katz & Shatz, 1996; Knudsen, Heckman, Cameron, & Shonkoff, 2006), and therefore are of highest importance for the determination of adult capacities. Thus, the striking differences that our study reveals already at early age stress the importance of investing in the early years of disadvantaged children such that the development of a wide range of adult capacities, including those that affect performance in the workplace, is further facilitated. The study continues as follows. Section 2 describes the data. Section 3 discusses the identification strategy. Section 4 presents our results, and Section 5 concludes.

2. DATA

Our analysis is based on administrative data, which we obtained from the Department of Health Services of the city of Osnabrueck. Osnabrueck is the third largest city in the German state of Lower Saxony and has about 170,000 citizens. The data cover the years from 2002 to 2005. The data have been collected during official school entrance examinations, in which government pediatricians examine various aspects of children's development as well as their health. Based on these examinations pediatricians give recommendations on whether or not children are ready to start elementary school. These examinations are compulsory for all children at the age of six years, but there are no penalties if children do not take part. In sum, almost all children go through this examination. The examination takes between 50 and 70 min. In the case of Osnabrueck, the school entrance examination has been arranged in a highly standardized manner since the year 2000 (for details see Rohling, 2002), and the scope of the recorded data has been increased considerably in 2002. From 2002 on, the data involve various medical and developmental tests, collection of data from each child's medical history (which is contained in the child's mandatory "vaccination record" (Impfpass) and in the child's mandatory "health record (Kinder-Untersuchungsheft)," as well as the completion of two questionnaires on socio-demographic information and pre-school experiences of the children, which are answered by parents.

Our data includes information on 4,977 regular school entrance examinations which took place in the years 2002–2005. We excluded from our sample observations which did not include information on parents' education, birth weight, mother's age, pre-school attendance, and parents' employment. The remaining estimation sample consists of observations on 3,814 children. Based on this sample, we defined two sub-samples based on parents' education. 1,322 children had at least one parent with a college degree. We classify them as children of highly educated parents. For the remaining 2,492 children, neither of the parents had a college degree. We classify them as children of less-educated parents.

The dependent variable is the pediatrician's school enrollment recommendation. This is the assessment of the school physician on whether or not a child is ready to start elementary school. For this recommendation, pediatricians take into account examination results on children's cognition, language ability, body coordination, and basic knowledge. The pediatrician's recommendation is not legally binding. The final decision is made by the headmaster of the admitting elementary school in cooperation with the parents. Nevertheless, this recommendation is followed in almost all cases. Children who are deemed not ready to start elementary school usually start elementary school in the following year after going through another school entrance exam. 9.6% of all children do not receive a pediatrician's recommendation to start elementary school (see Table 1). For children of college-educated parents, this share was 4.1%, while the share of children of non-college-educated parents who were deemed not ready for elementary school was 12.6%, i.e., more than three times the share for the children of college-educated parents.

Our data includes detailed information on health conditions. Information on health conditions come from three sources: medical examinations during the school entrance examination, children's official vaccination and health records, which parents are asked to bring to the exam, and information provided by parents. During the examination, pediatricians examined children's height and weight as well as their eyesight and hearing ability. Children above the 85th percentile of the body mass index (BMI) distribution in our sample are classified as overweight. Children below the 5th percentile of the weight distribution in our sample are classified as underweight. These definitions follow standard classifications from the U.S. Department of Health and Human Services (Center for Disease Control & Prevention, 2007). A binary variable that indicates ear problems takes on the value one if

Table 1. Sample Means, by Parental Education.

Variable	Full Sample	Less Education	College Education
School enrollment	0.903	0.874	0.959
	(0.294)	(0.331)	(0.196)
Overweight	0.149	0.179	0.092
	(0.356)	(0.384)	(0.289)
Underweight	0.044	0.043	0.045
	(0.205)	(0.203)	(0.208)
Low birth weight	0.056	0.062	0.043
	(0.230)	(0.242)	(0.204)
Ear problems	0.102	0.098	0.110
	(0.303)	(0.297)	(0.313)
Eye problems	0.191	0.195	0.184
	(0.393)	(0.396)	(0.388)
Behavioral problems	0.174	0.197	0.130
	(0.379)	(0.398)	(0.337)
Asthma	0.064	0.071	0.053
	(0.246)	(0.256)	(0.224)
Allergy	0.034	0.035	0.032
	(0.182)	(0.184)	(0.177)
Age in months	6.178	6.186	6.164
	(0.295)	(0.302)	(0.280)
Female	0.499	0.487	0.476
	(0.499)	(0.499)	(0.499)
Preschool 3+ years	0.808	0.769	0.881
	(0.393)	(0.421)	(0.323)
No sibling	0.205	0.212	0.190
	(0.403)	(0.409)	(0.392)
2+ siblings	0.281	0.282	0.279
	(0.449)	(0.450)	(0.448)
Two parents	0.838	0.805	0.900
	(0.368)	(0.396)	(0.298)
Missing father education	0.109	0.145	0.043
	(0.312)	(0.352)	(0.203)
Missing mother education	0.008	0.010	0.004
	(0.089)	(0.099)	(0.067)
Parent full time employed	0.815	0.768	0.905
	(0.387)	(0.422)	(0.292)
Age of mother	36.099	34.898	38.363
	(5.092)	(5.057)	(4.330)
Turkey	0.073	0.093	0.037
	(0.261)	(0.290)	(0.189)
Eastern Europe	0.112	0.131	0.076
	(0.315)	(0.337)	(0.265)
Other foreigners	0.039	0.051	0.018
	(0.195)	(0.220)	(0.133)
Observations	3,814	2,492	1,322

Note: Standard deviations in parentheses.

there are limitations in hearing ability. These include children whose hearing ability is so limited that they are classified as disabled, children who are recommended to see an ear doctor, if they are not already in treatment, and also children whose hearing deficit is not so severe as to require medical treatment. A binary variable on eye problems takes on the value one if there are limitations in visual ability. Visual exams may be taken with glasses and include a test for the ability to see in three dimensions. Children who cannot distinguish red and green colors are not classified as visually impaired. Information on birth weight comes from mandatory children's health records (Kinder-Untersuchungsheft), which parents are asked to bring to the examination. We create a binary variable for children with low birth weight according to whether weight at birth was less than 2,500 g (this follows the International Statistical Classification of Diseases and Related Health Problems, WHO, 2007).

Information on behavioral problems is elicited from three sources. Before beginning the examination, parents are asked to fill out a form, which includes questions on whether children are hyperactive or have difficulties concentrating. While their children are being examined, parents are asked to fill out another form with questions about their children's emotional problems, social behavior, hyperactivity, and other behavioral problems. Parents are reassured that their answers are not likely to influence the physicians' school enrollment recommendation. The third source of information comes from the pediatricians' observations during the examinations. From those pieces of information, we create a binary variable for the pediatricians' overall assessment of whether a child faces behavioral problems. Our definition includes both children who are referred to see a child psychiatrist as well as children with less severe behavioral problems. Information on asthma and allergies is based on information by parents. We create a binary variable for children who are affected by asthma. This definition includes both severe and less severe forms of asthma. Our definition for allergies includes allergic rhinitis and eczema. For this condition, we exclude mild cases.

Health conditions are quite common among young children in our data (see Table 1). 14.9% are overweight and 4.4% are underweight. 5.6% were born with low birth weight. 10.2% are affected by ear problems and 19.1% are affected by eye problems. 17.4% face behavioral problems. 6.4% of children have asthma and 3.4% are affected by allergies. Many health conditions are more common among children of less-educated parents than among children of highly-educated parents. This relationship holds for being overweight (17.9% vs. 9.2%), low birth weight (6.2% vs. 4.3%), eye problems (19.5% vs. 18.4%), behavioral problems (19.7% vs. 13.0%), asthma (7.1% vs. 5.3%), and other allergies (3.5% vs. 3.2%). In contrast, for being underweight and having ear problems, prevalence is not higher for children with less-educated parents. In sum, health problems tend to be far more common among children of less-educated parents. This is especially true for conditions that might be related to parental behaviors such as smoking (low birth weight, asthma) or parenting style (being overweight, behavioral problems).

Our analysis also includes information on socio-economic and demographic characteristics of children and their parents. Children's age is measured in years and months. For example, a child who is six years and six months of age is assigned an age of 6.5 years. We create dummy variables for gender (female vs. male), pre-school attendance (3+ years vs. less than 3 years), number of siblings (one sibling is omitted group), type of family (child lives with both parents vs. other types), and the age of the mother at the time of the examination. We include indicator variables for children with missing information on mother's education and on father's education, for children who have at least one parent in full-time employment, and for children with ethnic origins in Turkey, Eastern European countries, or other foreign countries. The mean age of children in our sample is 6.1 years (see Table 1). 49.9% are female and 80.8% attended pre-school for 3+ years. 20.5% have no siblings, while 28.1% have 2+ siblings. 83.8% of children live with both parents. Information on fathers' education is missing for 10.9% of the sample, and information on mothers' education for 0.8% of our sample. Information on fathers' education is often missing for children with single mothers. For 81.5% at least one parent is full-time employed. The average age of the mother at the time of the examination is 36 years. 7.3% of children are of Turkish ethnic origin, 11.2% of children have ethnic origins in Eastern European countries including Russia, and 3.9% have ethnic origins in other foreign countries.

3. IDENTIFICATION STRATEGY

We estimate a linear probability model for the effect of child health conditions on the pediatricians' school enrollment recommendations. The dependent variable is the school enrollment recommendation for child i (y_i). Explanatory variables include a vector of child health characteristics (H_i) and a vector of socio-economic and demographic characteristics (Z_i). The estimation equation is:

$$y_i = \alpha + H_i'\beta + Z_i'\gamma + \varepsilon_i$$

β and γ are vectors of estimation coefficients. α is the intercept, and ε_i an error term for child i. The coefficients β measure the association between health conditions and school readiness. One caveat concerns the question of whether these coefficients can be interpreted as a causal effect of health conditions on school readiness. These coefficients could also be driven by other factors such: an example is parenting style, if there are parenting styles that influence both the probability of health conditions and also affect school readiness in other ways than through health. In order to address such an omitted variable bias, we include a detailed list of variables Z_i into our estimation, which control for socio-economic and demographic characteristics of children and their parents. Furthermore, note that small children typically do not undertake conscientious decisions about their health in general or about (medical) prevention in particular. Therefore, it seems unlikely that causality runs in the other direction, i.e., that better cognitive development or higher school readiness has a causal impact on health conditions.

We estimate separate models for the full sample and for the two subsamples of children with highly educated parents and children with less-educated parents. As discussed earlier, children with less-educated parents are three times more likely not to be ready to start school than children with highly-educated parents. In the next step, we examine how much of the differences in school readiness can be attributed to differences in the prevalence and severity of health conditions. For this purpose we use decomposition analysis, similar to Oaxaca (1973). We first calculate the part of the difference that can be attributed to differences in the prevalence of health conditions. For this calculation we keep β, the size of the effect of health conditions on school readiness, as well as all other factors, constant between education groups. The prevalence effect can be calculated by the formula:

$$\text{prevalence\_effect} = (\overline{H}_{\text{highedu}} - \overline{H}_{\text{lowedu}})' \beta_{\text{pooled}}$$

where $\overline{H}_{\text{highedu}}$ is the vector of mean values for health conditions for the high education sample, while $\overline{H}_{\text{lowedu}}$ is the vector of mean values for health conditions for the low education sample. β_{pooled} is the vector of estimation coefficients for the reference group. Following Neumark (1988) we take estimation coefficients for the pooled sample as the reference group.

We also calculate how much of the difference in school readiness can be attributed to differences in the size of the effect of health conditions on school readiness. The size of the effect of health conditions for the high education sample is measured by the vector of estimation coefficients

β_{highedu}, while the size of this effect for the low education sample is measured by the vector of estimation coefficients β_{lowedu}. These coefficients could differ, if, for example, one group receives better medical treatment, complies more with doctor's guidelines, or is better able to compensate the negative consequences of health conditions in some other way. In order to calculate the effect of differences in coefficients, we keep the prevalence of diseases as well as all other factors constant. The severity effect can be calculated by the following formula:

$$\text{severity\_effect} = \overline{H}'_{\text{pooled}}(\beta_{\text{highedu}} - \beta_{\text{lowedu}})$$

where the vector $\overline{H}_{\text{pooled}}$ refers to the prevalence of health conditions for the pooled sample. The sum of prevalence effect and severity effect constitute the total effect of disparities in child health conditions on differences in school readiness between education groups.

4. RESULTS

Estimation results for the linear probability model are shown in Table 2. Column 1 shows results for the full sample, which includes both children of college-educated parents and of less-educated parents. We find no significant relationship between school readiness and BMI. Neither overweight children nor underweight children are less likely to be ready for school. In contrast, there is a strong link between school readiness and low birth weight. For children with a birth weight of less than 2,500 g, school readiness is reduced by 10.2% compared to children with higher birth weight. Previous studies also find a strong negative relationship between low birth weight and child development (see, e.g., Behrman & Rosenzweig, 2004). Hearing problems have a significantly negative effect on school readiness (by 5%). One possible explanation is that hearing loss can slow down language development (Currie, 2005). Poor eyesight also has a negative impact on school readiness (by 3%). Poor eyesight can have a negative impact on the ability to recognize pictures and on body coordination. Behavioral problems reduce the likelihood of children being ready for school by 17.9%. Children with behavioral disorders such as attention deficit disorder or hyperactivity have great difficulty with basic tasks such as sitting still and listening to instructions. They are not school-ready almost by definition. Asthma is also related to lower school readiness (by 5.2%). Asthma is the leading cause of children's trips to the emergency room and of children being hospitalized

Table 2. Regression Results for School Enrollment, by Parental Education.

	Full Sample (1)	Less Education (2)	College Education (3)
Overweight	−0.002	0.0007	0.006
	(0.012)	(0.016)	(0.018)
Underweight	0.020	0.022	0.016
	(0.022)	(0.031)	(0.025)
Low birth weight	−0.107**	−0.107**	−0.081**
	(0.020)	(0.026)	(0.025)
Ear problems	−0.050**	−0.094**	0.019
	(0.015)	(0.021)	(0.017)
Eye problems	−0.030**	−0.030	−0.023
	(0.011)	(0.016)	(0.013)
Behavioral problems	−0.179**	−0.193**	−0.116**
	(0.012)	(0.016)	(0.015)
Asthma	−0.052**	−0.066**	−0.001
	(0.018)	(0.024)	(0.023)
Allergy	0.058*	0.084*	0.015
	(0.025)	(0.034)	(0.029)
Age in months	0.105**	0.136**	0.056**
	(0.015)	(0.021)	(0.019)
Female	0.054**	0.061**	0.037**
	(0.009)	(0.012)	(0.010)
Pre-school 3+ years	0.112**	0.119**	0.059**
	(0.012)	(0.015)	(0.016)
No sibling	0.000	0.004	−0.011
	(0.012)	(0.016)	(0.015)
2+ siblings	−0.043**	−0.058**	−0.022
	(0.011)	(0.015)	(0.012)
Two parents	−0.031	−0.029	−0.033
	(0.017)	(0.022)	(0.022)
Education father missing	−0.066**	−0.075**	−0.002
	(0.019)	(0.024)	(0.032)
Education mother missing	−0.056	−0.078	0.077
	(0.050)	(0.062)	(0.078)
Parent full time employed	0.029*	0.014	0.044*
	(0.014)	−0.018	(0.019)
Age of mother	0.001	0.004	−0.013
	(0.010)	(0.013)	(0.015)
Age of mother^2	0.000	−0.000	0.000
	(0.000)	(0.000)	(0.000)
Turkey	0.004	0.035	−0.109**
	(0.019)	(0.024)	(0.030)
Eastern Europe	0.001	0.012	−0.034
	(0.015)	(0.020)	(0.021)

Table 2. *(Continued)*

	Full Sample (1)	Less Education (2)	College Education (3)
Other foreigners	−0.016	0.008	−0.121**
	(0.023)	(0.028)	(0.039)
Observations	3,814	2,492	1,322
R^2	0.15	0.16	0.11

Note: Standard errors in parentheses. *Significant at 5%; **Significant at 1%.

(Currie, 2005). If not controlled adequately, asthma can severely limit children's activity. However, if controlled correctly, asthma should have little or no direct effect on cognitive development (Currie, 2005). In contrast, other allergies are positively correlated with school readiness. This relationship most likely does not reflect a positive impact of allergies on school readiness, but a selection bias. In contrast to most other health variables in our data, diagnoses of allergies are not based on pediatricians' examinations, but on parents' reports, and better-informed parents are more likely to know about their children's allergies.

Among socio-economic and demographic variables, school readiness increases with age (by 10.5% per year), and girls are significantly more likely to be school-ready than boys (by 5.4%). Children who have attended pre-school for 3+ years are also more likely to be ready for school (by 11.2%). This could reflect a positive treatment effect of pre-school. It could as well reflect a selection effect, since pre-schools charge fees in Germany, and children of disadvantaged families are less likely to attend pre-school. There is no difference between children without siblings and children with one sibling, the omitted reference group. However, children with two or more siblings are less likely to be school-ready (by 4.3%). There is no advantage for children who live with both parents, but children with missing information on their father's education are less likely to be school-ready (by 6.6%). These are typically children whose mothers do not fill out questions about their children's fathers in the questionnaire from which our data are collected. Children with at least one parent in full-time employment are more likely to be ready for school (by 2.9%). After controlling for other characteristics, there is no significant relationship between school readiness and missing information on mother's education, mother's age, and country of ethnic origin.

Column 2 shows estimation results for children whose parents do not have a college degree. Estimation results are generally similar to the results for the full sample. There is no significant effect of the BMI on school readiness. Neither being overweight nor being underweight has an effect. However, school readiness is significantly reduced by low birth weight (by 10.7%), by ear problems (by 9.4%), by behavioral problems (by 19.3%), and by asthma (by 5.5%). For many health conditions, negative effects tend to be stronger for the sample with less-educated parents than for the full sample, namely for ear problems, behavioral problems, and asthma. For poor eyesight, the estimation coefficient is exactly the same as for the full sample, but is no longer statistically significant. Allergies are correlated with a higher likelihood of being ready for school. Among socio-economic and demographic characteristics, there is a significantly positive relationship between school readiness and age (by 13.6% per year of age), being female (by 6.1%) and 3+ years of pre-school attendance (by 11.9%). There is a significantly negative relationship between school readiness and having two or more siblings (by 5.8%) and with missing information on father's education (by 7.5%). The coefficients of all other variables are not significantly different from zero.

Column 3 shows estimation results for the sub-sample of children with at least one college-educated parent. These estimation results vary noticeably from results in columns 1 and 2. Again, there is no significant relationship between BMI and school readiness, and low birth weight is associated with lower school readiness (by 8.1%). However, the effect is smaller than for children of less-educated parents. There is no significant correlation between school readiness and ear problems. This finding indicates that children of college-educated parents can somehow compensate for the negative consequences of hearing loss, maybe because parents talk more with children or because of better medical treatment. For eye problems, there is also no significant effect. Behavioral problems reduce school readiness by 11.6%. Although a large effect, this coefficient is smaller than for children of less-educated parents. This finding indicates that behavioral problems are either less severe for children of college-educated parents or that these parents are better able to address these problems through parental behaviors or through obtaining medical treatment. There is no effect for asthma and for other allergies on school readiness. If asthma is well controlled, asthma attacks can be prevented, so that child development does not need to be impaired by properly treated asthma. Among socio-economic and demographic variables, school readiness is increased by higher age (10.5% per year of age), being female (by 5.4%), and pre-school attendance of 3+ years (by 5.9%). The positive coefficient for pre-school attendance is smaller for children with college-educated parents than for children of less-educated parents. Children with at least one parent in full-time employment are more likely to be school-ready (by 4.4%), while children with ethnic origins in Turkey and other foreign countries are less likely to be school-ready by 10.9% and 12.1%, respectively.

Table 3 shows results for the decomposition analysis. The total gap in school readiness between children of college-educated parents and children of less-educated parents is 8.6 percentage points. Differences in the prevalence of health conditions can explain a gap of 1.6 percentage points, and differences in the size of the effects of health conditions on school readiness can explain a gap of 3.1 percentage points. Thus, as share of the total gap, the prevalence effect amounts to 18.6% of the difference in school readiness between education groups, and the severity effect can explain 36% of the difference. In sum, 54.6% of the achievement gap between education groups can be explained by health factors. These findings suggest that health factors are very important for the intergenerational transmission of human capital. Numerous previous studies have examined the intergenerational transmission of human capital and they have typically looked at pathways such as pre-birth factors (Bjorklund, Lindahl, & Plug, 2006), income (Blau, 1999; Beck, Dearing, & McCartney, 2004), and mother's employment (Ruhm, 2004). Health has typically not been considered as an important factor in this relationship, at least not for developed countries. In a back-of-the-envelope calculation, Currie (2005) estimated that health factors might explain up to 25% of the achievement gap between white and black children in the United States at school entry. Our results suggest that the influence of health might be even stronger.

Table 3. Decomposition Analysis.

	School Enrollment
Mean: Parents with college education	0.960
Mean: Parents with less than college education	0.874
Total difference	0.086
	(100%)
Prevalence effect	0.016
	(18.60%)
Severity effect	0.031
	(36.05%)
Total health effect	0.036
	(54.65%)

5. CONCLUSION

We use unique administrative data from German elementary school entrance examinations in order to examine the role of child health for the intergenerational transmission of human capital. We look at child health conditions such as obesity, low birth weight, ear problems, eye problems, behavioral problems, asthma, and allergies. We find that health conditions are more common among children of less-educated parents. We also find that health conditions have a substantially negative impact on school readiness, and that the negative impact on school readiness is considerably stronger for children of less-educated parents. In total, 54.64% of the difference in school readiness between children of college-educated parents and children of less-educated parents can be attributed to health factors. We have decomposed these 54.6% into two effects: 18.6% can be attributed to differences in the prevalence of health conditions, and 36% can be attributed to differences in the severity of the impact. These findings suggest that health is a very important pathway for the intergenerational transmission of human capital, and that policies aimed at reducing disparities in child development should also aim at reducing disparities in health. This is likely not just a question of access to medical care. Health insurance is (almost) universal in Germany. Possible interventions could include health examinations in pre-schools and health training for pre-school teachers and parents of small children in order to enable them to better recognize and address children's health problems. Our findings for highly-educated parents suggest that common health conditions such as ear problems or asthma need not have negative consequences on child development, if they are addressed appropriately.

These findings are subject to some caveats. The first caveat concerns the interpretation of the relationship between health conditions and school readiness as a causal effect. We find that children with health conditions are less likely to be ready for school. However, such a relationship could also be explained by other factors: one such factor could be parenting style, if there are parenting styles that affect both the probability of health conditions, and also affect school readiness in other ways than through health. We try to address this possible omitted variable bias by including a detailed list of parents' characteristics in our estimation, but it is never possible to control for all relevant parental characteristics. A second caveat refers to the assessment of school readiness. School readiness is assessed by experienced pediatricians after careful examinations, but this assessment always includes a subjective component, which depends on the pediatricians' discretion.

This study has shown how the socio-economic environment and the health conditions in early life affect human cognitive and social development, and we have put particular emphasis on the complex interrelationship between child health conditions and the child's socio-economic environment. Through focusing on children, our chapter stresses the importance of the early years for the determination of capacities of cognition, and as such it is in line with a recently increasing attention of health economists to the early years and to models of parental investment instead of adult investment (Heckman, 2007). This increase in attention is further strengthened by evidence from neuroscience which shows, first, that early experiences shape the brains architecture due to increased capacity for neural plasticity, and, second, that neural circuits are built in a hierarchical way in which the development of higher level-circuits is dependent on the successful development of lower level and earlier developed circuits (Knudsen et al., 2006). In other words, many important determinants of the brain's architecture that persist into adulthood develop during childhood. We believe that further research into the mechanisms of brain development will contribute significantly to a better understanding of the complex interrelationship between health conditions, socio-economic background, and the development of social and cognitive skills. Which brain architectures that determine adult capabilities relevant for performance in the workplace are already shaped at young age? How do untreated eye or ear problems in children affect the development of these brain architectures?[1] If we enrich our existing knowledge of the neural basis of economic behavior of adults with models of brain development at early age, and add knowledge from developmental psychology and health economics, we will be better able to understand, model, and positively influence the process of human capital formation.

NOTE

1. Early findings on the relationship between the visual system and the early development of important neural circuits have already been obtained in animal research (Hensch, 2005).

ACKNOWLEDGMENTS

We are greatly obliged to the department of health services of the city of Osnabrueck and in particular to Inge Rohling, MD, for making the data available to us and for patiently answering endless questions about the data and details of school entrance examinations. We thank Axel Börsch-Supan, Hendrik Jürges, Mathis Schröder, and seminar participants at the University of Mannheim for many valuable suggestions. We also thank Michael Ingenhaag and Doerte Heger for excellent research assistance.

REFERENCES

Beck, A., Dearing, E., & McCartney, K. (2004). Incomes and outcomes in early childhood. *Journal of Human Resources*, *39*, 980–1007.

Behrman, J., & Rosenzweig, M. (2004). Returns to birthweight. *Review of Economics and Statistics*, *86*, 586–601.

Bjorklund, A., Lindahl, M., & Plug, E. (2006). The origins of intergenerational associations: Lessons from Swedish adoption data. *Quarterly Journal of Economics*, *106*, 999–1028.

Blau, D. (1999). The effect of income on child development. *Review of Economic and Statistics*, *81*, 261–276.

Case, A., Lubotsky, D., & Paxson, C. (2002). Economic status and health in childhood: The origins of the gradient. *American Economic Review*, *92*, 1308–1334.

Center for Disease Control and Prevention. (2007). U.S. Department of Health and Human Services. Accessed on May 7, 2007. Available at http://www.cdc.gov/nccdphp/dnpa/bmi/childrens_BMI/about_childrens_BMI.htm#How%20is%20BMI%20calculated

Currie, J. (2000). Child health in developed countries. In: A. Culyer & J. Newhouse (Eds), *Handbook of health economics* (Vol. 1B). Amsterdam: North Holland.

Currie, J. (2005). Health disparities and gaps in school readiness. *The Future of Children. School Readiness: Closing Racial and Ethnic Gaps*, *15*(1), 117–138.

Currie, A., Shields, M., & Price, S. (2007). Is the child health/family income gradient universal? Evidence from England. *Journal of Health Economics*, *26*, 212–232.

Currie, J., & Stabile, M. (2003). Socioeconomic status and child health: Why is the relationship stronger for older children? *American Economic Review*, *93*, 1813–1823.

Heckman, J. J. (2007). The economics, technology, and neuroscience of human capability formation. *Proceedings of the National Academy of Sciences*, *104*, 13250–13255.

Hensch, T. K. (2005). Critical period mechanisms in developing visual cortex. *Current Topics in Developmental Biology*, *69*, 215–237.

Kaestner, R., & Corman, H. (1995). *The impact of child health and family inputs on child cognitive development*. NBER Working Paper no. 5357. Cambridge, MA: National Bureau of Economic Research.

Katz, L. C., & Shatz, C. J. (1996). Synaptic activity and the construction of cortical circuits. *Science*, *274*, 1133–1138.

Knudsen, E. I., Heckman, J. J., Cameron, J. L., & Shonkoff, J. L. (2006). Economic, neurobiological and behavioral perspectives on building America's future workforce. *Proceedings of the National Academy of Sciences*, *103*, 10155–10162.

Neumark, D. (1988). Employers' discriminatory behaviour and the estimation of wage discrimination. *Journal of Human Resources*, *23*, 279–295.

Oaxaca, R. (1973). Male–female wage differentials in urban labor markets. *International Economic Review*, *14*, 693–709.

Paxson, C., & Schady, N. (2007). Cognitive development among young children in Ecuador. *Journal of Human Resources*, *42*, 49–84.

Rohling, I. (2002). *Gesundheit und Entwicklungsstand der Osnabruecker Schulanfaenger*. Stadt Osnabrück: Fachbereich Soziales und Gesundheit.

Ruhm, C. (2004). Parental employment and child cognitive development. *Journal of Human Resources*, *39*, 155–192.

World Health Organization. (2007). International Statistical Classification of Diseases and Related Health Problems – Version for 2007. Accessed on May 7, 2007. Available at http://www.who.int/classifications/apps/icd/icd10online/?gp05.htm + p05

TEMPORAL DISCOUNTING AS A MEASURE OF EXECUTIVE FUNCTION: INSIGHTS FROM THE COMPETING NEURO-BEHAVIORAL DECISION SYSTEM HYPOTHESIS OF ADDICTION

Warren K. Bickel and Richard Yi

ABSTRACT

Conceptual paper purpose – *The purpose of this chapter is to examine a new conceptual model of addiction and interpret the results from delay discounting studies in light of this new perspective.*

Methodology/approach – *To accomplish this we (1) introduce this new conceptual model, (2) briefly review executive function, including evidence for executive dysfunction among the addicted, (3) describe the unique relationship of temporal discounting to the new model and executive dysfunction, and (4) reinterpret the discounting literature in light of this new conceptual model.*

Findings – *Addicted individuals discount the future more than controls. This is consistent with greater relative activation of the impulsive system*

Neuroeconomics
Advances in Health Economics and Health Services Research, Volume 20, 289–309

ISSN: 0731-2199/doi:10.1016/S0731-2199(08)20012-9

and decreased relative activation of the executive system. It also supports the new conceptual model of addiction.

Research implications – *The new model provides a model for understanding the observations from the broader area of research in temporal discounting.*

Originality/value of chapter – *Given the view of executive function as important for the cross-temporal organization of behavior, we think that temporal discounting, the valuing of future commodities, qualifies this process to be included as an executive function.*

Decision-making is increasingly recognized as resulting from the interaction of multiple neuro-behavioral systems (Daw, Niv, & Dayan, 2005; Jentsch & Taylor, 1999; Redish & Johnson, 2007). Significant evidence from multiple sources and a variety of analytical levels suggest that an imbalance between these systems is a fundamental constituent in the process of addiction (Baler & Volkow, 2006; Bechara, 2005; Bickel et al., 2007; Everitt & Robbins, 2005; Redish & Johnson, 2007). Recently, there has been growing support for a new conceptual model of addiction where decisions often result from a competition between two regions of the brain. The competing neuro-behavioral decision systems model suggests that one region of the brain associated with executive processes is hypoactive in addiction; thus the addicted have what may be called executive dysfunction. In this chapter, we are interested in exploring the application of this new conceptual model of addiction and interpreting the results from discounting studies in light of this new perspective on executive function. To accomplish this we will (1) introduce this new conceptual understanding of addiction, (2) briefly review executive function, including evidence for executive dysfunction among the addicted, (3) describe the unique relationship of temporal discounting to the neuro-behavioral decision systems model, and (4) reinterpret the discounting literature in light of this new conceptual model.

COMPETING NEURO-BEHAVIORAL DECISION SYSTEMS AS A NEW CONCEPTUAL MODEL OF ADDICTION

The competing neuro-behavioral decision systems model hypothesizes that decision-making associated with addiction is the byproduct of competition between two brain regions and associated processes. One group of these processes, closely linked to dopamine activity, is associated with activity in evolutionarily old brain structures involved in reinforcement. These structures include the amygdala, dorsolateral striatum, nucleus accumbens, and other related structures. Conditioned-approach behavior to drug cues has been related to abnormal activity in the amygdala and ventral striatum, suggesting "exaggerated processing of the incentive value of substance-related cues (Bechara, 2005, p. 1459)." Moreover, other addiction research using imaging technology has demonstrated that the amygdala is over-responsive to reward (London, Ernst, Grant, Bonson, & Weinstein, 2000). These observations have led to the hypothesis that limbic structures associated with the mid-brain dopamine pathway are important in signaling the valence (positive or negative) of immediate outcomes (Bechara, 2005; Bechara & Damasio, 2005; McClure, Laibson, Loewenstein, & Cohen, 2004), and that the orbitofrontal cortex and ventral striatum are involved in evaluating the valence of rewards, particularly positive rewards (Padoa-Schioppa & Assad, 2006; Schoenbaum, Setlow, Saddoris, & Gallagher, 2003). Recent data suggests that negative valence may be evaluated in the insula (Knutson, Rick, Wimmer, Prelec, & Loewenstein, 2007). fMRI and other evidence suggest that these structures, which we will refer to as the *impulsive action system*, show altered responsiveness in addicts (Volkow & Fowler, 2000).

Another system that has recently been identified in the study of addiction is the prefrontal cortex (PFC; Volkow, Fowler, & Wang, 2004). The PFC is an evolutionarily younger brain region found in humans and higher mammals. It is part of the neocortex on the anterior part of the frontal lobes. Neuroimaging research has indicated decreased activity or volumetric reduction among addicts relative to controls in regions that compose the PFC (Bickel et al., 2007; Fein, Di Sclafani, & Meyerhoff, 2002; Franklin et al., 2002; Volkow & Fowler, 2000). Although a variety of other terms refer to this competing neural system, we will refer to it as the *executive* system. The executive system is thought to be involved in actions such as working toward a defined goal, prediction and expectation of outcomes, determining future consequences of current activities, and social control (Barkley, 1997).

According to competing neuro-behavioral decision systems theory, addiction, at least in part, results from a shift in balance between these two systems such that the impulsive action system (e.g., striatal and mid-brain reinforcement structures) is hyperactive, while the executive system (e.g., PFC) is hypoactive. As a result of this imbalance, emphasis is placed on immediate outcomes and consequences. The causes of decreased executive function may result from a variety of non-exclusive factors: dysfunction may predate addiction, result from the use of drugs that produce morphological changes in the brain (e.g., toxicity), and/or result from atrophy due to lack of the executive system's use consistent with use-dependent plasticity observed in the cortex (Weiller & Rijntjes, 1999).

Behavioral therapeutic efforts in addiction have focused largely on reinforcing abstinence (contingency management) and using some form of CBT. We speculate that reinforcing abstinence, which provides a more immediate consequence for short periods of drug abstinence, may harness and constrain the impulsive system. Immediate consequences to reinforce abstinence appear to operate through the impulsive system, which is sensitive to immediate reinforcement and is consistent with the short temporal horizons among the addicted. However, CBT is a therapy explicitly designed to employ cognitive processes and learning of new skills to produce change (Aharonovich, Nunes, & Hasin, 2003; Carroll, 1998); a functioning executive system may be a necessary precondition for treatment success. However, if the executive system is dysfunctional, then we might expect less than maximal results from CBT.

AN OVERVIEW OF EXECUTIVE FUNCTION

Given the central role of executive function in the competing neuro-behavioral decision-making systems hypothesis as applied to addiction, it is useful to consider executive functions in greater detail. Executive function has been defined in a variety of ways, ranging from frontal lobe functions (Struss & Benson, 1986) to defining it by its components, such as effortful and flexible organization and strategic planning (Denckla, 1994; see Barkley, 1997, for a review of the history of executive functions). Despite the range of components described previously, a central theme evident in many of these views is that the executive system permits evaluation of, and planning for, the future (Barkley, 1997; Denckla, 1994; Dennett, 1995). Recognizing that the processes that comprise executive functioning may differ in the absence of a singular definition of executive function, we will employ Barkley's proposed definition because it synthesizes and organizes the various notions into an understandable and consistent description that allows empirical understanding of other disorders (e.g., Barkley, 1997). Specifically, executive functions refer to classes of self-directed behavior that change one's future behavior and, in turn, change one's future outcomes associated with that behavior (Barkley, 1997, 2004). Note that executive function as employed here is distinct and different from other cognitive functions such as intelligence (e.g., Schuck & Crinella, 2005).

One interesting aspect of different executive function components is that they often recruit overlapping or similar brain regions (Duncan & Owen, 2000). This utilization of the same brain regions may indicate an important commonality, suggesting that the same brain regions may serve different functions in different behaviors. Alternatively, this observation may indicate that the level of specificity of our efforts to measure brain activity may be insufficient to distinguish small regional differences in activation. Indeed, the smallest unit of functional magnetic resonance imaging (fMRI) analysis is the pixel, which summarizes the activity of approximately 200,000 neurons (Smith-Churchland, 2002).

Additionally, contemporary perspectives on executive functions and PFC marshal substantial evidence supporting its development as an adaptation to environmental pressure associated with group and social living (Barkley, 2004; Geary, 2004). Non-kin reciprocal altruism and coalition formation are processes that require the exchange of goods and services now for other ones later. Clearly, memory, consideration of the future, and behavioral inhibition of the immediate response may all be necessary to engage in reciprocal altruism.

Components of Executive Function

Given that the notions of executive behaviors are still forming, we will delve deeper into executive functions to provide an understanding of contemporary thinking and our proposed conceptualization. Specifically, there have been several organizational schemas proposed for executive function. Here, we extend prior approaches and propose that executive function is composed of the following three groups (Barkley, 1997; Cicerone et al., 2005): (1) cross-temporal organization of behavior (CTOB), (2) emotional and activation regulation, and (3) metacognitive processes (MCP). Defining and measuring these functions requires that we treat them as discrete and independent, though we recognize that they may overlap and interact.

(1) *Cross-Temporal Organization of Behavior (CTOB).* CTOB refers to processes that permit consideration and planning of future circumstances. The anterior cingulate, hippocampus, and dorsolateral, prefrontal, and orbital frontal cortex are relevant to many behaviors in this group (e.g., Johnson, van der Meer, & Redish, 2007). We have

identified five component processes that may be included under this scheme: (1) attention and concentration, (2) memory (working and verbal), (3) behavioral flexibility, (4) planning, and (5) response inhibition. These processes may permit responding in favor of temporally remote goals. For example, reaching a temporally remote goal requires development of a plan to reach that goal, retention of the plan via memory, maintenance of attention on that goal without distraction by some other event, inhibition of competing responses, and modification of plans as circumstances change.

(2) *Emotional and Activation Self-Regulation (EASR)*. EASR refers to both (1) emotional processing where emotional response is needed to supplement a current behavior and is initiated by environmental cues to determine the most adaptive response (e.g., somatic marker hypothesis) and (2) initiative and energizing behavior at a level appropriate for goal attainment. Brain regions associated with these functions include the orbitofrontal cortex closely associated with the limbic nuclei involved in emotional processing and the inferior medial frontal region, such as the anterior cingulate, in activation. Studies demonstrated that an inability to incorporate emotional responding leads to suboptimal decision-making and poor capacity to generate and maintain actions (Bechara, 2005; Cicerone et al., 2005).

(3) *Metacognitive Processes (MCP)*. MCP refers to social cognition, self-awareness, and evaluation of one's behavior in relation to others. Patients with orbitofrontal damage exhibit decreased social awareness and exhibit overly familiar and inappropriate interpersonal behavior. It is suggested that such deficits are associated in part with a "lack of online behavioral monitoring" (Beer, John, Scabini, & Knight, 2006; pp. 871). A related important concept for addiction is anosognosia. Anosognosia refers to the lack of awareness that one suffers from an illness (Starkstein, Jorge, Mizrahi, & Robinson, 2006). A variety of disorders are associated with individuals denying any disorder despite frank and obvious impairment. The "denial" observed among many addicted individuals may be a form of anosognosia. Unfortunately, there is scant evidence regarding components of MCP in addiction; thus, we will not address them further.

We note that earlier research efforts used a variety of complex laboratory measures to study executive function. These measures often involve multiple executive functions and therefore lead to some confusion about the specificity of the components of executive function. For example, the Wisconsin Card

Sort Task presents a participant with numerous cards (see Wikipedia, for a more detailed description). Each card has multiple dimensions (e.g., color, shape, number), of which only one dimension is appropriate to classify a stimulus at a time. The participant is asked to sort these cards into piles and is informed if they are making the correct response. In the course of sorting the cards, the correct dimension could change. Clearly, success in this task requires a variety of functions working together. These functions include attention to the stimulus features, working memory to ensure further selection of the correct task, and response inhibition to not respond to a previously correct response. Fortunately, a variety of new laboratory measures have been developed that involve a smaller set of the components and therefore permit greater specificity of the component behaviors.

The Stop Signal task (Lappin & Eriksen, 1966) is an example of an assessment that involves a smaller set of components. Specifically, the Stop Signal task is designed to assess an individual's ability to suppress or inhibit a motor response. In this reaction time task, participants are typically asked to respond as quickly as possible (e.g., button press) to the onset of a GO signal (such as the appearance of a circle) that appears on a monitor. On a small percentage of trials, the onset of a visual or auditory STOP signal following the onset of a GO signal cues the participant to stop or inhibit the initiated GO response. By varying the duration of time between the onset of the GO and STOP signals, the assessment is able to indirectly measure the reaction time to the STOP signal. Thus, the demands on working memory are minimized (Tillman, Thorell, Brocki, & Bohlin, 2008) and the evaluation is isolated to inhibitory control.

EVIDENCE OF HYPOACTIVE EXECUTIVE FUNCTIONING AMONG ADDICTS

Growing evidence in addiction research supports evidence of executive dysfunction (e.g., deficits of planning) and decreased activity in the brain regions related to executive functioning. This information has been thoroughly reviewed (see Dom, Sabbe, Hulstijn, & van den Brink, 2005; Rogers & Robbins, 2001; Verdejo-Garcia, Lopez-Torrecillas, Gimenez, & Perez-Garcia, 2004). Here, we will briefly review a portion of the literature.

Many studies consistently demonstrate that addiction to cocaine and/or amphetamines (including methamphetamine) is associated with significant impairments in a variety of neuropsychological performances, despite periods of abstinence. Impairments associated with stimulant dependence includes all six components of CTOB: (1) attention (Ardila, Rosselli, & Strumwasser, 1991; Ersche, Clark, London, Robbins, & Sahakian, 2006; Hoff, Riordan, O'Donnell, & DeLisi, 1991; Strickland et al., 1993), (2) memory (Ardila et al., 1991; Strickland et al., 1993), (3) behavioral flexibility (Ersche et al., 2006), (4) planning (Ersche et al., 2006), (5) discounting of delayed rewards (Bornovalova, Daughters, Hernandez, Richards, & Lejuez, 2005; Coffey, Gudleski, Saladin, & Brady, 2003; Heil, Johnson, Higgins, & Bickel, 2006; Hoffman et al., 2006; Monterosso, Ehrman, Napier, O'Brien, & Childress, 2001), and (6) response inhibition (Cocaine: Fillmore & Rush, 2002; Hester & Garavan, 2004; Li, Milivojevic, Kemp, Hong, & Sinha, 2006; Verdejo-Garcia, Perales, & Perez-Garcia, 2007). Impairments also include the two components of EASR: (1) emotional self-regulation (Aguilar de Arcos, Verdejo-Garcia, Peralta-Ramirez, Sanchez-Barrera, & Perez-Garcia, 2005; Verdejo-Garcia, Bechara, Recknor, & Perez-Garcia, 2006) and (2) activation (Blum et al., 2000; Nunes, Rothenberg, Sullivan, Carpenter, & Kleber, 2006). The activation dysfunction we refer to here may overlap with depressive symptoms that derive directly from substance dependence. Furthermore, non-stimulant substance abuse appears to have similar effects: impairments in neuropsychological function is observed following chronic use of alcohol (Ratti, Bo, Giardini, & Soragna, 2002; Tuck & Jackson, 1991; Zinn, Stein, & Swartzwelder, 2004), marijuana (Karila, Vignau, Alter, & Reynaud, 2005; Solowij & Michie, 2007; Verdejo-Garcia et al., 2006), and opiates (Davis, Liddiard, & McMillan, 2002; Ornstein et al., 2000).

THE RELATIONSHIP OF TEMPORAL DISCOUNTING TO THE NEURO-BEHAVIORAL DECISION SYSTEMS MODEL

To examine the relationship of temporal discounting to the new conceptual model of addiction, we will first briefly review the findings from studies of discounting among the addicted, as well as neuroeconomic studies of temporal discounting that identify the brain regions associated with discounting.

Temporal Discounting and Addiction

A variety of studies have demonstrated both that individuals can value commodities over years, and that addicts discount the future substantially more than individuals without that disorder (Bickel & Johnson, 2003; Bickel & Marsch, 2001; Reynolds, 2006; Yi, Mitchell, & Bickel, in press). Consider as an example a study by Madden, Petry, Badger, and Bickel (1997) where the temporal discounting by opioid-dependent individuals and matched controls were compared. This study, as do most in this area, employed discounting procedures that are similar to those used in psychophysical experiments (Richards, Mitchell, de Wit, & Seiden, 1997). In psychophysical studies, participants are presented with two stimuli: a standard stimulus and another stimulus that is adjusted until the two are considered to be equivalent (Stevens, 1975).

Similarly, the procedures used by Madden et al. (1997) presented subjects with a choice between a standard larger-later reward (e.g., $1,000 delivered in one year) and an immediate reward whose magnitude was adjusted to determine the value of the immediate reward that the participant subjectively considered approximately equal to the standard reward (e.g., Green, Fry, & Myerson, 1994). This point of equivalence is referred to as the *indifference point* for that particular delay interval. Indifference points were obtained from opioid-dependent individuals and matched controls for a variety of delays (1 week to 25 years) for a hypothetical $1,000 and a hypothetical amount of heroin worth $1,000 (for the opioid-dependent individuals only). The data from this study was plotted as *indifference curves* (the best-fitting curve of indifference points plotted as a function of the delay interval) and are presented here in Fig. 1. In the upper panel are the indifference curves obtained from opioid-dependent individuals and controls when they were discounting a hypothetical $1,000. In the bottom panel are indifference curves obtained from opioid-dependent individuals when they were discounting a $1,000 of money (replotting the data from the upper panel) and a comparable amount of heroin. Greater discounting is indicated by lower indifference points (y-axis) and proximate location of the indifference curve to both axes. Opioid-dependent individuals discounted money more than controls and discounted heroin more than money.

One way to quantify the magnitude differences between these plots is to use the time frame in which the commodity loses approximately half its value. For controls, $1,000 lost half its value in approximately 5 years, while for opioid-dependent individuals, $1,000 lost half its value in approximately 6 months – a 10-fold difference. For opioid-dependent individuals, heroin lost more than half its value in the shortest time frame examined, resulting in discounting that is roughly 25-fold more than their discounting of money, and roughly 250-fold more than the discounting of money by controls. These extreme differences in discounting raise an important question: what mechanisms underlie this behavior and how might they be altered by the addiction processes?

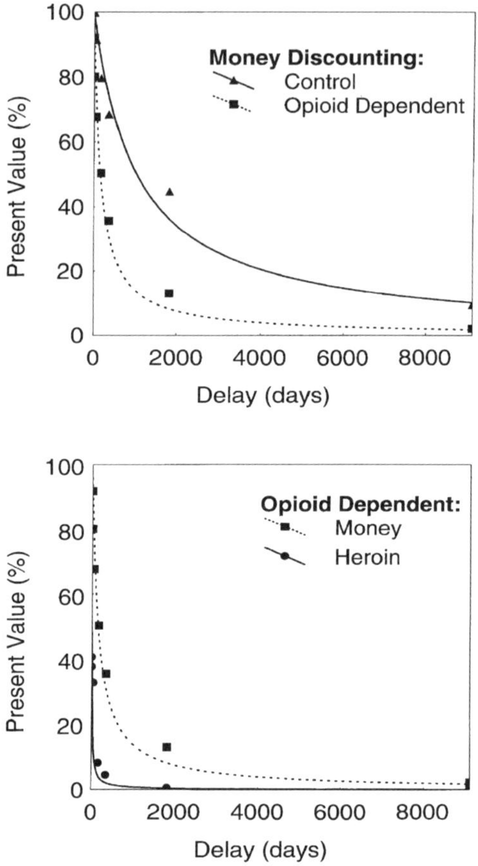

Fig. 1. Median Indifference Points as a Function of Delay for Small Immediate and Larger Later Hypothetical Heroin and Money Rewards. Upper Panel Compares the Indifference Points for the Discounting of a $1,000 for Controls and Opioid-Dependent Participants. The Lower Panel Compares the Discounting of $1,000 and $1,000 Worth of Heroin for Opioid-Dependent Participants (Madden et al., 1997).

Neuroeconomics of Discounting

A seminal paper published in *Science* reported on the neural correlates of temporal discounting in normal adult participants (McClure et al., 2004). Specifically, research participants made a series of choices between immediate and delayed choices or delayed and even more delayed (e.g., 1 month vs. 1.5 months) choices. Using event-related fMRI techniques, discounting decisions were shown to entail two separate brain regions. Specifically, choice of the immediate reward was correlated with activity in the limbic systems associated with the mid-brain dopamine systems. Choices of delayed rewards were associated with activation of portions of the PFC and parietal cortex associated with deliberative processes, cognitive control, and numerical computation. The authors stated that choices were related to the relative activation of the two brain regions, referring to interaction of these two brain regions as competitive. More specifically, when the limbic system was activated, the immediate options were favored, while greater relative activity in the cortex was related to selection of the delayed option.

In a similar study, Tanaka et al. (2004) had research participants learn about different options, including when a small immediate monetary reward was obtained or when a small immediate loss was incurred with a larger delayed monetary reward. When the immediate reward was obtained, significant activity was observed in the lateral orbital cortex and striatum, while selection of the delayed reward was associated with significant activity in dorsolateral PFC, inferior parietal cortex, dorsal rape nucleus, and cerebellum. These findings are consistent with the findings of McClure et al. (2004).

McClure, Ericson, Laibson, Loewenstein, and Cohen (2007) have systematically extended these observations by using a primary reward (juice) and substantially shorter time frame (now vs. 5 min). There results were consistent with the prior profile of results: immediate choices were associated with limbic activation, and choices for the deferred reward produced greater relative activation in the PFC and posterior parietal cortex. Moreover, relative activation predicted actual choice behavior. In contrast, Wittmann, Leland, and Paulus (2007) examined the discounting of hypothetical money and found that when the delayed option was selected, there was activation in the insular cortex, posterior cingulate, temporal gyrus, angular gyrus, inferior parietal lobule, and cuneus. However, they observed that no brain region reached significance with selection of immediate reward. They suggested that this absence of activation might be due to the hypothetical nature of the rewards.

Overall, the results of all these studies can be viewed with the lens originally proposed by McClure and colleagues (2004). They note that their results could be interpreted two ways. First, their results could be interpreted as consistent with the hypotheses that cortex and parietal brain regions are associated with inhibition of the immediate choice.

However, activation of the fronto-parietal system occurred during choices between two delayed choices and the limbic system was not activated. Thus, there was no impulse to be inhibited. Instead, the authors hypothesize that the "fronto-parietal region may project future benefits (through abstract reasoning or possibly 'simulation' with imagery), providing top-down support for responses that favor greater long-term reward and allowing them to compete effectively with limbically-mediated responses when these are present" (McClure et al., 2004, p. 507). Thus, delay discounting is a behavioral process that is correlated with both cortical and limbic activation. These regions, in turn, appear to be correlated with more impulsive responding associated with valuing of the immediate reinforcer and behavior controlled by executive functions associated with valuing of future rewards, respectively.

To conclude this section, the brain regions associated with discounting as indicated by imaging studies (reviewed above) generally indicate that when the immediate option is selected, there is greater activity in portions of the limbic region; when choices are made in favor of the delayed option, there is greater relative activity in aspects of the cortex. If these imaging observations are reliably observed, then the greater discounting that is observed in all the forms of addiction can be interpreted. That interpretation would indicate that overall, many more present-focused choices are made by the addicted than by controls. We would therefore expect greater relative activity in the limbic region and relatively less activity in the prefrontal areas, providing considerable support for the Competing Neuro-behavioral Decision Systems Hypothesis. Indeed, the concordance of the behavioral and neuroimaging data with the Competing Neuro-behavioral Decisions Systems Hypothesis suggests strongly that temporal discounting assessments provide a summary measure of the relative control of these two brain regions and therefore could be used to examine the efficacy of a treatment.

A REINTERPRETATION OF TEMPORAL DISCOUNTING

In reinterpreting the temporal discounting evidence, there are two aspects we would like to address. First, we will examine the implications of the observed discounting results to brain mechanisms identified in the new model described earlier. Second, we will interpret novel aspects of discounting (social and past discounting) from the context of executive function.

First, if we use the temporal discounting as a measure of the degree of relative control between the competing brain regions, then we could use that to interpret the results of existing studies and determine whether those observations are concordant with other independent observations. For example, discounting is shown to decrease with age (Green et al., 1994; Green & Myerson, 1996), indicating that younger children discount the most. The competing brain regions viewpoint would suggest that the younger children have a less active executive function than adults. Next, withdrawal processes associated with the cessation of drug use has been shown to increase the degree of discounting, suggesting either that withdrawal increases activity in the limbic impulsive system and/or decreases activity in the prefrontal executive systems. Additionally, evidence of the effects of longer term drug cessation show that addicts who are abstinent either approximate controls or are intermediate between currently using addicts and controls. These data suggests that there is less relative control by the impulsive brain system and relatively more by the executive system. Importantly, each one of these speculations can be tested empirically to verify if they occur.

Second, Rachlin and Jones (2008) (also, Jones & Rachlin, 2006) propose and provide supporting data for the construct of social discounting. Related to temporal discounting, social discounting refers to the reduction of the subjective value of an outcome to an "other" as a function of the social distance between the self and the other. Rachlin (2000) proposes that in an environment of reciprocity, altruism (otherwise noted as positive or unselfish social behavior) requires that the self delay gratification (in other words, exhibit low temporal discounting). This type of relationship between intertemporal and interpersonal decision-making suggests that a similar, if not the same, underlying process contributes to temporal and social discounting. The social discounting data to-date supports this notion. Moreover empirical evidence demonstrates that less discounting of the future is significantly correlated with increased likelihood of cooperation as measured with prisoner dilemma procedures (Harris & Madden, 2002; Yi, Johnson, & Bickel, 2005). This suggests the importance of executive functions in social competence and social decision-making and indicates that deficiencies in executive function may lead to decreased effectiveness in social exchange.

The evidence for an intertemporal/interpersonal connection is not limited to these observations. An extensive body of literature suggests that the regions of the brain responsible for CTOB influence social behavior. Following frontal lobe damage, previously responsible and conscientious

Phineas Gage would devise "... many plans of future operations, which are no sooner arranged than they are abandoned in turn for others appearing more feasible ..." and show "... little deference for his fellows, impatient of restraint or advice ..." (Harlow, 1868). Other case reports further suggest that lesions of the brain responsible for executive function can affect both cross-temporal and interpersonal behavior (Elsinger & Damasio, 1985; Mataro et al., 2001; Saver & Damasio, 1991; Warriner & Velikonja, 2006).

Buckner and Carroll (2007) suggest that a shared brain network is responsible for thinking about the future and taking on the perspective of another person. The commonality is that both require the cognitive act of self-projecting perspective from the immediate to some alternative, whether that perspective is of the self at a later time or of a different person. Because self-controlled (i.e., low temporal discounting) and altruistic (i.e., low social discounting) behaviors require the ability to self-project to the alternative perspective, and to the extent that self-projection is an executive function, assessment of discounting may provide an index of executive function that is relevant for cross-temporal and social behavior.

Finally, executive functioning can also be incorporated into the interpretation of results from studies of past discounting. Current evidence indicates that not only are future outcomes discounted as a function of temporal distance from the present to the future, they are also discounted as a function of temporal distance from the present to the past (i.e., past discounting). Qualitatively and quantitatively, discounting of past outcomes reveals the same features as discounting of future outcomes (Bickel, Yi, Kowal, & Gatchalian, 2008; Yi, Gatchalian, & Bickel, 2006). Furthermore, very high correlations are observed between rates of future and past discounting.

This is consistent with Buckner and Carroll's (2007) conceptualization of self-projection (an executive function). Self-projection is necessary in thinking about the future as well as thinking about the past: episodic memory requires that the individual shift perspective from the present to the past. Extensive neuropsychological testing provides support for this conceptualization. The Iowa Gambling Task is one assessment that can evaluate the ability to learn from past experiences. Participants are asked to choose from one of four decks of cards, with each card representing some gain or loss. Two of these decks are considered disadvantageous because they result in overall loss over time, while the remaining two decks result in overall gain and are considered advantageous. Studies of both temporal discounting and the Iowa Gambling Task indicate relative deficits in substance abusers (Bechara et al., 2001; Grant, Contoreggi, & London, 2000;

Petry, Bickel, & Arnett, 1998; Petry & Casarella, 1999; Reynolds, 2006) compared to controls, supporting the past/future association.

This is also consistent with Trope and Liberman's (2003) Temporal Construal Theory, which suggests that the same variables that affect the interpretation of future events also affect interpretation of past events. For instance, the mental representation of events tends to be concrete and subordinate when the events are of small future or past distance; this mental representation tends to be abstract and superordinate when the events are of large future or past distance.

CONCLUSION

Collectively, this chapter provides a synthesis of several related areas and provides a basis for interpreting a variety of diverse findings from a consistent viewpoint. Specifically, the Competing Neuro-behavioral Decisions Systems Model of Addiction is consistent both with the results of temporal discounting studies and with observed findings in addiction. The model stipulates that a hyperactive impulsive system and a hypoactive executive system underlie what we call addiction. This is consistent with a variety of neuroscience findings on addiction. Moreover, neuroscience studies of temporal discounting suggest that more immediate choices result from greater relative activation of the impulsive system and choices of more delayed options result from relative greater activation of the executive system. The observation that addicted individuals discount the future more than controls is consistent with greater relative activation of the impulsive system and decreased relative activation of the executive system, and it supports the new conceptual model of addiction. Moreover, the new model provides a basis for understanding the observations from the broader area of research in temporal discounting as we illustrated in this chapter. Lastly, given the view of executive function as important for the CTOB, we believe that temporal discounting, the valuing of future commodities, qualifies this process to be included as an executive function.

ACKNOWLEDGMENTS

This research was supported by NIDA grants R37 DA 006526-18, R01 DA 11692-09, R01 DA022386-02, R03 DA021707-01, Wilbur Mills Chair Endowment, and in part by the Arkansas Biosciences Institute, a partnership of scientists from Arkansas Children's Hospital, Arkansas State University, the University of Arkansas-Division of Agriculture, the University of Arkansas, Fayetteville, and the University of Arkansas for Medical Sciences. The Arkansas Biosciences Institute is the major research component of the Tobacco Settlement Proceeds Act of 2000.

REFERENCES

Aguilar de Arcos, F., Verdejo-Garcia, A., Peralta-Ramirez, M. I., Sanchez-Barrera, M., & Perez-Garcia, M. (2005). Experience of emotions in substance abusers exposed to images containing neutral, positive, and negative affective stimuli. *Drug and Alcohol Dependence*, *78*(2), 159–167.

Aharonovich, E., Nunes, E., & Hasin, D. (2003). Cognitive impairment, retention and abstinence among cocaine abusers in cognitive-behavioral treatment. *Drug and Alcohol Dependence*, *71*(2), 207–211.

Ardila, A., Rosselli, M., & Strumwasser, S. (1991). Neuropsychological deficits in chronic cocaine abusers. *International Journal of Neuroscience*, *57*(1–2), 73–79.

Baler, R. D., & Volkow, N. D. (2006). Drug addiction: The neurobiology of disrupted self-control. *Trends in Molecular Medicine*, *12*(12), 559–566.

Barkley, R. A. (1997). Behavioral inhibition, sustained attention, and executive functions: Constructing a unifying theory of ADHD. *Psychological Bulletin*, *121*(1), 65–94.

Barkley, R. A. (2004). Adolescents with attention-deficit/hyperactivity disorder: An overview of empirically based treatments. *Journal of Psychiatric Practice*, *10*(1), 39–56.

Bechara, A. (2005). Decision making, impulse control and loss of willpower to resist drugs: A neurocognitive perspective. *Nature Neuroscience*, *8*(11), 1458–1463.

Bechara, A., & Damasio, A. R. (2005). The somatic marker hypothesis: A neural theory of economic decision. *Games and Economic Behavior*, *52*, 336–372.

Bechara, A., Dolan, S., Denburg, N., Hindes, A., Anderson, S. W., & Nathan, P. E. (2001). Decision-making deficits, linked to a dysfunctional ventromedial prefrontal cortex, revealed in alcohol and stimulant abusers. *Neuropsychologia*, *39*(4), 376–389.

Beer, J. S., John, O. P., Scabini, D., & Knight, R. T. (2006). Orbitofrontal cortex and social behavior: Integrating self-monitoring and emotion-cognition interactions. *Journal of Cognitive Neuroscience*, *18*(6), 871–879.

Bickel, W. K., & Johnson, M. W. (2003). Junk time: Pathological behavior as the interaction of evolutionary and cultural forces. In: R. E. Vuchinich & N. Heather (Eds), *Choice, behavioural economics and addiction* (pp. 249–271). Pergamon: London.

Bickel, W. K., & Marsch, L. A. (2001). Toward a behavioral economics understanding of drug dependence: Delay discounting processes. *Addiction*, *96*, 73–86.

Bickel, W. K., Miller, M. L., Yi, R., Kowal, B. P., Lindquist, D. M., & Pitcock, J. A. (2007). Behavioral and neuroeconomics of drug addiction: Competing neural systems and temporal discounting processes. *Drug and Alcohol Dependence*, *90S*, S85–S91.

Bickel, W. K., Yi, R., Kowal, B. P., & Gatchalian, K. M. (2008). Cigarette smokers discount past and future rewards symmetrically and more than controls: Is discounting a measure of impulsivity? *Drug and Alcohol Dependence*, *96*, 256–262.

Blum, K., Braverman, E. R., Holder, J. M., Lubar, J. F., Monastra, V. J., Miller, D., Lubar, J. O., Chen, T. J., & Comings, D. E. (2000). Reward deficiency syndrome: A biogenetic model for the diagnosis and treatment of impulsive, addictive, and compulsive behaviors. *Journal of Psychoactive Drugs*, *32*(i–iv), 1–112.

Bornovalova, M. A., Daughters, S. B., Hernandez, G. D., Richards, J. B., & Lejuez, C. W. (2005). Differences in impulsivity and risk-taking propensity between primary users of crack cocaine and primary users of heroin in a residential substance-use program. *Experimental and Clinical Psychopharmacology*, *13*(4), 311–318.

Buckner, R. L., & Carroll, D. C. (2007). Self-projection and the brain. *Trends in Cognitive Sciences*, *11*(2), 49–57.

Carroll, K. M. (1998). A cognitive-behavioral approach: Treating cocaine addiction. In: *National institute on drug abuse therapy manuals for drug addiction, manual 1, national institute of drug abuse* (pp. 98–4308). Rockville, MD: NIH Publication.

Cicerone, K. D., Dahlberg, C., Malec, J. F., Langenbahn, D. M., Felicetti, T., Kneipp, S., Ellmo, W., Kalmar, K., Giacino, J. T., Harley, J. P., Laatsch, L., Morse, P. A., & Catanese, J. (2005). Evidence-based cognitive rehabilitation: Updated review of the literature from 1998 through 2002. *Archives of Physical Medicine and Rehabilitation*, *86*(8), 1681–1692.

Coffey, S. F., Gudleski, G. D., Saladin, M. E., & Brady, K. T. (2003). Impulsivity and rapid discounting of delayed hypothetical rewards in cocaine-dependent individuals. *Experimental and Clinical Psychopharmacology*, *11*(1), 18–25.

Davis, P. E., Liddiard, H., & McMillan, T. M. (2002). Neuropsychological deficits and opiate abuse. *Drug and Alcohol Dependence*, *67*(1), 105–108.

Daw, N. D., Niv, Y., & Dayan, P. (2005). Uncertainty-based competition between prefrontal and dorsolateral striatal systems for behavioral control. *Nature Neuroscience*, *8*(12), 1704–1711.

Denckla, M. B. (1994). Measurement of executive function. In: G. R. Lyon (Ed.), *Frames of reference for the assessment of learning disabilities: New views on measurement issues* (pp. 117–142). Baltimore: Paul H. Brookes Publishing.

Dennett, D. (1995). *Darwin's dangerous idea: Evolution and the meanings of life*. New York: Simon & Schuster.

Dom, G., Sabbe, B., Hulstijn, W., & van den Brink, W. (2005). Substance use disorders and the orbitofrontal cortex: Systematic review of behavioural decision-making and neuroimaging studies. *The British Journal of Psychiatry*, *187*(3), 209–220.

Duncan, J., & Owen, A. M. (2000). Common regions of the human frontal lobe recruited by diverse cognitive demands. *Trends in Neurosciences*, *23*(10), 475–483.

Elsinger, P., & Damasio, A. R. (1985). Sever disturbance of higher cognition after bilateral frontal lobe ablation: Patient EVR. *Neurology*, *35*, 1731–1741.

Ersche, K. D., Clark, L., London, M., Robbins, T. W., & Sahakian, B. J. (2006). Profile of executive and memory function associated with amphetamine and opiate dependence. *Neuropsychopharmacology*, *31*(5), 1036–1047.

Everitt, B. J., & Robbins, T. W. (2005). Neural systems of reinforcement for drug addiction: From actions to habits to compulsion. *Nature Neuroscience*, *8*(11), 1481–1489.

Fein, G., Di Sclafani, V., & Meyerhoff, D. J. (2002). Prefrontal cortical volume reduction associated with frontal cortex function deficit in 6-week abstinent crack-cocaine dependent men. *Drug and Alcohol Dependence*, *68*(1), 87–93.

Fillmore, M. T., & Rush, C. R. (2002). Impaired inhibitory control of behavior in chronic cocaine users. *Drug and Alcohol Dependence*, *66*(3), 265–273.

Franklin, T. R., Acton, P. D., Maldjian, J. A., Gray, J. D., Croft, J. R., Dackis, C. A., O'Brien, C. P., & Childress, A. R. (2002). Decreased gray matter concentration in the insular, orbitofrontal, cingulate, and temporal cortices of cocaine patients. *Biological Psychiatry*, *51*(2), 134–142.

Geary, D. C. (2004). *Origin of mind: Evolution of brain, cognition, and general intelligence.* Washington, DC: American Psychology Association Press.

Grant, S., Contoreggi, C., & London, E. D. (2000). Drug abusers show impaired performance in a laboratory test of decision making. *Neuropsychologia*, *38*(8), 1180–1187.

Green, L., Fry, A. F., & Myerson, J. (1994). Discounting of delayed rewards: A life-span comparison. *Psychological Science*, *5*, 33–36.

Green, L., & Myerson, J. (1996). Exponential versus hyperbolic discounting of delayed outcomes: Risk and waiting time. *American Zoologist*, *36*(4), 496–505.

Harlow, J. M. (1868). Recovery from the passage of an iron bar through the head. *Publications of the Massachusetts Medical Society*, *2*, 327–347.

Harris, A. C., & Madden, G. J. (2002). Delay discounting and performance on the prisoner's dilemma game. *The Psychological Record*, *52*, 429–440.

Heil, S. H., Johnson, M. W., Higgins, S. T., & Bickel, W. K. (2006). Delay discounting in currently using and currently abstinent cocaine-dependent outpatients and non-drug-using matched controls. *Addictive Behaviors*, *31*(7), 1290–1294.

Hester, R. K., & Garavan, H. (2004). Executive dysfunction in cocaine addiction: Evidence for discordant frontal, cingulated, and cerebellar activity. *Journal of Neuroscience*, *24*(49), 11017–11022.

Hoff, A. L., Riordan, H., O'Donnell, D. W., & DeLisi, L. E. (1991). Cross-sectional and longitudinal neuropsychological test findings in first episode schizophrenic patients. *Schizophrenia Research*, *5*, 197–198.

Hoffman, W. F., Moore, M., Templin, R., McFarland, B., Hitzemann, R. J., & Mitchell, S. H. (2006). Neuropsychological function and delay discounting in methamphetamine-dependent individuals. *Psychopharmacology (Berl)*, *188*(2), 162–170.

Jentsch, J. D., & Taylor, J. R. (1999). Impulsivity resulting from frontostriatal dysfunction in drug abuse: Implications for the control of behavior by reward-related stimuli. *Psychopharmacology*, *146*, 373–390.

Johnson, A., van der Meer, M. A., & Redish, A. D. (2007). Integrating hippocampus and striatum in decision-making. *Current Opinion in Neurobiology*, *17*(6), 692–697.

Jones, B., & Rachlin, H. (2006). Social discounting. *Psychological Science*, *17*(4), 283–286.

Karila, L., Vignau, J., Alter, C., & Reynaud, M. (2005). Acute and chronic cognitive disorders caused by cannabis use. *La Revue du praticien*, *55*(1), 23–26.

Knutson, B., Rick, S., Wimmer, G. E., Prelec, D., & Loewenstein, G. (2007). Neural predictors of purchases. *Neuron*, *53*(1), 147–156.

Lappin, J. S., & Eriksen, C. W. (1966). Use of a delayed signal to stop a visual reaction-time response. *Journal of Experimental Psychology*, *72*(6), 805–811.

Li, C.-S. R., Milivojevic, V., Kemp, K., Hong, K., & Sinha, R. (2006). Performance monitoring and stop signal inhibition in abstinent patients with cocaine dependence. *Drug and Alcohol Dependence*, *85*(3), 205–212.

London, E. D., Ernst, M., Grant, S., Bonson, K., & Weinstein, A. (2000). Orbitofrontal cortex and human drug abuse: Functional imaging. *Cerebral Cortex*, *10*(3), 334–342.

Madden, G. J., Petry, N. M., Badger, G. J., & Bickel, W. K. (1997). Impulsive and self-control choices in opioid-dependent patients and non-drug-using control participants:

Drug and monetary rewards. *Experimental and Clinical Psychopharmacology*, *5*(3), 256–262.

Mataro, M., Jurado, M. A., Garcia-Sanchez, C., Barraquer, L., Costa-Jussa, F. R., & Junque, C. (2001). Long-term effects of bilateral frontal brain lesion: 60 years after injury with an iron bar. *Archives of Neurology*, *58*(7), 1139–1142.

McClure, S. M., Ericson, K. M., Laibson, D. I., Loewenstein, G., & Cohen, J. D. (2007). Time discounting for primary rewards. *Journal of Neuroscience*, *27*(21), 5796–5804.

McClure, S. M., Laibson, D. I., Loewenstein, G., & Cohen, J. D. (2004). Separate neural systems value immediate and delayed monetary rewards. *Science*, *306*(5695), 503–507.

Monterosso, J., Ehrman, R., Napier, K. L., O'Brien, C. P., & Childress, A. R. (2001). Three decision-making tasks in cocaine-dependent patients: Do they measure the same construct? *Addiction*, *96*(12), 1825–1837.

Nunes, E., Rothenberg, J., Sullivan, M., Carpenter, K., & Kleber, H. (2006). Behavioral therapy to augment oral naltrexone for opioid dependence: A ceiling on effectiveness? *The American Journal of Drug and Alcohol Abuse*, *32*(4), 503–517.

Ornstein, T. J., Iddon, J. L., Baldacchino, A. M., Sahakian, B. J., London, M., Everitt, B. J., & Robbins, T. W. (2000). Profiles of cognitive dysfunction in chronic amphetamine and heroin abusers. *Neuropsychopharmacology*, *23*, 113–126.

Padoa-Schioppa, C., & Assad, J. A. (2006). Neurons in the orbitofronal cortex encode economic value. *Nature*, *441*, 223–226.

Petry, N. M., Bickel, W. K., & Arnett, M. (1998). Shortened time horizons and insensitivity to future consequences in heroin addicts. *Addiction*, *93*(5), 729–738.

Petry, N. M., & Casarella, R. (1999). Excessive discounting of delayed rewards in substance abusers with gambling problems. *Drug and Alcohol Dependence*, *56*(1), 25–32.

Rachlin, H. (2000). *The science of self-control*. Cambridge, MA: Harvard University Press.

Rachlin, H., & Jones, B. A. (2008). Social discounting and delay discounting. *Journal of Behavioral Decision Making*, *21*(1), 29–43.

Ratti, M. T., Bo, P., Giardini, A., & Soragna, D. (2002). Chronic alcoholism and the frontal lobe: Which executive functions are impaired? *Acta Neurologica Scandinavica*, *105*(4), 276–281.

Redish, A. D., & Johnson, A. (2007). A computational model of craving and obsession. *Annals of the New York Academy of Sciences*, *1104*, 324–339.

Reynolds, B. (2006). A review of delay-discounting research with humans: Relations to drug use and gambling. *Behavioural Pharmacology*, *17*(8), 651–667.

Richards, J. B., Mitchell, S. H., de Wit, H., & Seiden, L. S. (1997). Determination of discount functions in rats with an adjusting-amount procedure. *Journal of the Experimental Analysis of Behavior*, *67*(3), 353–366.

Rogers, R. D., & Robbins, T. W. (2001). Investigating the neurocognitive deficits associated with chronic drug misuse. *Current Opinion in Neurobiology*, *11*(2), 250–257.

Saver, J. L., & Damasio, A. R. (1991). Preserved access and processing of social knowledge in a patient with acquired sociopathy due to ventromedial frontal damage. *Neuropsychologia*, *29*(12), 1241–1249.

Schoenbaum, G., Setlow, B., Saddoris, M. P., & Gallagher, M. (2003). Encoding predicted outcome and acquired value in orbitofrontal cortex during cue sampling depends upon input from basolateral amygdale. *Neuron*, *39*(5), 855–867.

Schuck, S. E. B., & Crinella, F. M. (2005). Why children with ADHD do not have low IQs. *Journal of Learning Disabilities*, *38*(3), 262–280.

Smith-Churchland, P. (2002). *Brain-wise: Studies in neurophilosophy*. Cambridge, MA: MIT Press.

Solowij, N., & Michie, P. T. (2007). Cannabis and cognitive dysfunction: Parallels with endophenotypes of schizophrenia? *Journal of Psychiatry and Neuroscience*, *32*(1), 30–52.

Starkstein, S. E., Jorge, R., Mizrahi, R., & Robinson, R. G. (2006). A diagnostic formulation for anosognosia in Alzheimer's disease. *Journal of Neurology, Neurosurgery, and Psychiatry*, *77*(6), 719–725.

Stevens, S. S. (1975). *Psychophysics*. New York: Wiley.

Strickland, T. L., Mena, I., Villanueva-Meyer, J., Miller, B. L., Cummings, J., Mehringer, C. M., Satz, P., & Myers, H. (1993). Cerebral perfusion and neuropsychological consequences of chronic cocaine use. *The Journal of Neuropsychiatry and Clinical Neuroscience*, *5*(4), 419–427.

Struss, D. T., & Benson, D. F. (1986). *The frontal lobes*. New York: Raven Press.

Tanaka, S. C., Doya, K., Okada, G., Ueda, K., Okamoto, Y., & Yamawaki, S. (2004). Prediction of immediate and future rewards differentially recruits cortico-basal ganglia loops. *Nature Neuroscience*, *7*, 887–893.

Tillman, C. M., Thorell, L. B., Brocki, K. C., & Bohlin, G. (2008). Motor response inhibition and execution in the stop-signal task: Development and relation to ADHD behaviors. *Child Neuropsychology*, *14*(1), 42–59.

Trope, Y., & Liberman, N. (2003). Temporal construal. *Psychological Review*, *110*(3), 403–421.

Tuck, R. R., & Jackson, M. (1991). Social, neurological and cognitive disorders in alcoholics. *Medical Journal of Australia*, *155*(5), 225–229.

Verdejo-Garcia, A. J., Bechara, A., Recknor, E. C., & Perez-Garcia, M. (2006). Executive dysfunction in substance abuse dependent individuals during drug use and abstinence: An examination of the behavioral, cognitive and emotional correlates of addiction. *Journal of the International Neuropsychological Society*, *12*(3), 405–415.

Verdejo-Garcia, A. J., Lopez-Torrecillas, F., Gimenez, C. O., & Perez-Garcia, M. (2004). Clinical implications and methodological challenges in the study of the neuropsychological correlates of cannabis, stimulant, and opioid abuse. *Neuropsychology Review*, *14*(1), 1–41.

Verdejo-Garcia, A. J., Perales, J. C., & Perez-Garcia, M. (2007). Cognitive impulsivity in cocaine and heroin polysubstance abusers. *Addictive Behaviors*, *32*(5), 950–966.

Volkow, N. D., & Fowler, J. S. (2000). Addiction, a disease of compulsion and drive: Involvement of the orbitofrontal cortex. *Cerebral Cortex*, *10*(3), 318–325.

Volkow, N. D., Fowler, J. S., & Wang, G. J. (2004). The addicted human brain viewed in the light of imaging studies: Brain circuits and treatment strategies. *Neuropharmacology*, *47*(S1), 3–13.

Warriner, E. M., & Velikonja, D. (2006). Psychiatric disturbances after traumatic brain injury: Neurobehavioral and personality changes. *Current Psychiatry Reports*, *8*(1), 73–80.

Weiller, C., & Rijntjes, M. (1999). Learning, plasticity, and recovery in the central nervous system. *Experimental Brain Research*, *128*(1–2), 134–138.

Wittmann, M., Leland, D., & Paulus, M. (2007). Time and decision making: Differential contribution of the posterior insular cortex and the striatum during a delay discounting task. *Experimental Brain Research*, *179*(4), 643–653.

Yi, R., Gatchalian, K. M., & Bickel, W. K. (2006). Discounting of past outcomes. *Experimental and Clinical Psychopharmacology*, *14*(3), 311–317.

Yi, R., Johnson, M. W., & Bickel, W. K. (2005). Relationship between cooperation in an iterated prisoner's dilemma game and the discounting of hypothetical outcomes. *Learning and Behavior*, *33*(3), 324–336.

Yi, R., Mitchell, S. H., & Bickel, W. K. (in press). Addiction and discounting. In: Madden, G., and Bickel, W. K. (Eds), *Impulsivity: Theory, science, and neuroscience of discounting* Washington, DC: American Psychological Association.

Zinn, S., Stein, R., & Swartzwelder, H. S. (2004). Executive functioning early in abstinence from alcohol. *Alcoholism: Clinical and Experimental Research*, *28*(9), 1338–1346.

EXPECTATIONS MEDIATE OBJECTIVE PHYSIOLOGICAL PLACEBO EFFECTS

Anup Malani and Daniel Houser

ABSTRACT

Purpose – *A placebo effect is a (positive) change in health outcomes that is due to a (positive) change in beliefs about the value of a treatment. Placebo effects might be "behavioral," in the sense that revised beliefs lead to behavioral changes or new actions that in turn yield changes in health outcomes. Placebo effects might also include a "physiological" component, which refers broadly to non-behavioral, brain-modulated mechanisms by which new beliefs cause changes in health outcomes. Nearly all formal economic models of human behavior are consistent with behavioral placebo effects, but strongly inconsistent with their physiological counterparts. The reason is that the latter effects can imply that expectations enter, rather than multiply, state-contingent preferences. It is therefore unfortunate that little evidence exists on physiological placebo effects. We report data from novel clinical experiments with caffeine that seek to provide such evidence.*

Methods – *Subjects visit the clinic on multiple occasions. On each visit they ingest either a placebo or caffeine pill. Subjects only know the probability with which the pill includes caffeine. We obtain physiological measurements prior to ingestion and at 30, 60, and 90 min after ingestion.*

Neuroeconomics
Advances in Health Economics and Health Services Research, Volume 20, 311–327

ISSN: 0731-2199/doi:10.1016/S0731-2199(08)20013-0

Importantly, we constrain subjects to remain seated and read pre-selected magazines during the interval between treatment and outcome measurement.

Findings – *Our design provides particularly clean inference because it (i) eliminates the possibility of behavioral confounds; (ii) provides for measurements at the individual level; (iii) manipulates beliefs without deception; and (iv) uses salient rewards. We find evidence for the existence of physiological placebo effects mediated by expectations.*

Implications – *Our results are consistent with the possibility that the prefrontal cortex provides external, top-down control that modulates physiological outcomes, and make a case for the importance of research geared toward developing appropriate and tractable frameworks that accommodate non-linear relationships between expectations and preferences.*

1. INTRODUCTION

A placebo effect is a (positive) change in health outcomes that is due to a (positive) change in beliefs about the value of a treatment.[1] Placebo effects might be "behavioral," in the sense that revised beliefs lead to behavioral changes or new actions that in turn yield changes in health outcomes. Placebo effects might also include a "physiological" component, which refers broadly to non-behavioral, brain-modulated mechanisms by which new beliefs cause changes in health outcomes. Nearly all formal economic models of human behavior are consistent with behavioral placebo effects, but strongly inconsistent with their physiological counterpart. The reason is that the latter effects can imply that expectations enter, rather than multiply, state-contingent preferences. It is therefore unfortunate that little evidence exists on physiological placebo effects. We report data from novel clinical experiments with caffeine that seek to provide such evidence.

Placebo effects are clearly important to the field of medicine and health policy more generally. For example, in a situation where the placebo effects of an inert pill and the pharmacological effect of active treatment are similar, it may be more cost-effective for the healthcare system to encourage physicians to induce positive expectations about the cheap inert substance instead of prescribing the more expensive active medication (Talbot, 2000). Also, to the extent that patients are indeed affected by independently acquired scientific information about the intervention to which they have been subjected (e.g., in adherence to treatment), healthcare policy-makers should surely be interested in placebo effects.

Placebo effects have recently received attention in the economics literature. For example, Malani (2006) suggested that physiological placebo effects may cause a violation of the independence axiom in the context of blinded clinical trials. Here different treatments correspond to different states of the world. Because patients do not know their actual treatment assignment, placebo effects in any given state will depend on the subject's expected treatment assignment. Therefore, beliefs about treatment states to which a patient was not actually assigned could influence the patient's health outcomes and thus influence utility.

Building on the insight that placebo effects in blinded trials depend on potential rather than actual treatment assignments, Malani (2006) suggested that placebo effects could be estimated by manipulating the probability of assignment to different treatments while holding the subject's actual treatment constant. Specifically, Malani argued that if a treatment is subject to placebo effects, outcomes on that treatment should be improved when the probability of being assigned to the treatment (as opposed to an inferior control) is increased. To test this, Malani examined trials of medications for non-gastric ulcer and for hypercholesterolemia. When he compared the treatment group in trials offering a higher probability of assignment to treatment groups in trials with a lower probability of treatment, he found that the former had better outcomes than the latter, controlling for the actual treatment that subjects received. In addition, he found that expectations about bad outcomes also affect patient response, i.e., a nocebo effect, which we shall discuss later.

Another study that highlights the connection between beliefs and outcomes was reported by Shiv, Carmon, and Ariely (2005). They investigated placebo effects in marketing, with particular focus on whether prices can alter the realized efficacy of products to which they are applied. In a series of three experiments, it was shown that consumers who paid a discounted price for a product (an energy drink thought to increase mental acuity) derive less actual benefit (they are able to solve fewer puzzles) than consumers who purchased the same product at a regular price. The explanation was that subjects who paid a lower price inferred that the drink was of lower quality and this inference led to the subjects' completing fewer puzzles.

A limitation of both Malani (2006) and Shiv et al. (2005) is that they are unable to distinguish between physiological and behavioral placebos.

Because the clinical trials Malani examined did not either hold constant subjects' behavioral response or measure every aspect of subjects' behavioral responses to changes in the probability of assignment to treatment, he was unable to rule out that differences in subjects' expectations are responsible for differences in subjects' behavior, which in turn explain differences in subjects' outcomes. Perhaps, as Malani (2008) suggests, subjects in trials with a high probability of assignment to treatment (versus control) might be more willing to comply with treatment protocols because there is a greater likelihood compliance will have an effect on outcomes. Shiv et al. has a similar problem in tracing the chain of causation from beliefs to outcomes. There are two possible explanations for why subjects who inferred lower quality from lower price completed fewer puzzles. One explanation is that their cognitive function was lower; the other is that they did not attempt as many puzzles. Shiv et al. could not distinguish between these explanations, perhaps because it is impossible to do so.

Because behaviorally mediated placebo effects fit neatly into current economic models, while physiological placebo effects do not, it is important – when possible – to distinguish between behavioral and physiological response to expectations. That is the motivation for the laboratory study we report below. The primary goal of that experiment is to rule out the possibility of behaviorally mediated placebo effects by constraining subject behavior. The secondary purposes of the study are to (i) manipulate subjects' expectations without using deception; and (ii) measure treatment and outcomes at an individual level (as Shiv et al., 2005 do, but Malani, 2006 does not). We find compelling evidence supporting physiological placebo effects mediated by expectations.

2. BACKGROUND

2.1. Expectations and Placebo Effect

Over the past five decades, placebos and the placebo effect have been the subject of pioneering research efforts by Beecher (1955), Lasagna, Mosteller, Von Felsinger, and Beecher (1954), Shapiro (1960, 1964), and many others. These efforts have contributed to our understanding of the placebo effect and stimulated the development of the field. Parts of this work still continue to influence biobehavioral research (Olshansky, 2007). A placebo (as opposed to placebo effect) refers to "any treatment – including drugs, surgery, psychotherapy and quack therapy – used for its ameliorative effect on a symptom or disease but that is actually ineffective or not specifically effective for the condition being treated"(Shapiro & Shapiro, 1997). Some have suggested that the psychophysiological responses that placebos elicit reflect a mind/body interaction guided by subjective factors like expectations, beliefs, meaning, hope for improvement, and relational parameters (Shapiro & Shapiro, 1997).

The placebo effect is the prototype response expectancy effect but it is not the only effect of this type (Kirsch, 1997). Response expectancies are anticipations of automatic subjective and behavioral responses to particular situational cues. Their effects can be viewed as a form of self-fulfilling prophecy (Kirsch, 1985; Kirsch & Lynn, 1999). Numerous studies in health sciences (Kirsch, 1999; Kirsch & Lynn, 1999; Stewart-Williams & Podd, 2004) suggest that expectations have a mediating role in placebo effects. Essentially, when a person receives a supposedly active substance or treatment, his beliefs about the substance or treatment activate response expectancies anticipating the subjective and/or behavioral consequences of using that substance or receiving medical treatment in general. These response expectancies, along with contextual factors unrelated to the substance or treatment, lead to subjective and behavioral outcomes, or placebo effects (Shiv et al., 2005).

When discussing placebo, one must consider not only the traditional, positive *placebo* effect, but also the *nocebo* effect. The traditional *placebo* effect involves positive feelings about a therapy that contribute to improving the outcomes of that therapy. The *nocebo* effect, however, refers to the case in which a person's expectations that a therapy has certain side effects increase the likelihood that the person will subsequently develop those side effects (Malani, 2008). According to Beecher (1959), placebo effects account for 30–40% of the effect of a psychological or medical intervention (though the methodology behind that finding has been much criticized). In contrast, healthy individuals have adverse side effects to a blinded sham intervention 15–27% of the time (Liccardi et al., 2004; Olshansky, 2007).

The placebo effect can be highly domain specific, and the nature of this specificity depends on the information available to the recipient (Beauregard, 2007). Placebo effects have been studied intensely in several domains, such as pain reduction (also known as placebo analgesia) (Zubieta et al., 2005; Wager et al., 2004; Baker & Kirsch, 1991; Petrovic, Kalso, Petersson, & Ingvar, 2002), depression (Kirsch & Sapirstein, 1999; Sneed et al., 2008), sexual arousal (Palace, 1999), hypnosis (Kirsch & Lynn, 1995; Perugini et al., 1998), treatment of ulcers (Malani, 2006), hypercholesterolemia

(Malani, 2006), cardiovascular health (Olshansky, 2007), and Parkinson's disease (Benedetti et al., 2004; de la Fuente-Fernandez et al., 2001).

Nonetheless, some scholars have challenged whether placebo effects actually exist. For instance, Kienle and Kienle (1997) argue that placebo effects could be explained by the natural history of a disease, regression to the mean, concomitant treatment, observer bias, and patient bias. These authors suggest that placebo effects are grossly overrated, illusory, and the product of sloppy methodological thinking. Subsequent investigations comparing placebo to no-treatment conditions further support the view that placebo might have a negligible impact and overestimated effect (Hrobjartsson & Gotzsche, 2001, 2004, 2006). The fact that some data indicate a real response to placebo and other data do not may be explained in part by the lack of consensus regarding what actually constitutes the placebo effect (Link, Haggard, Kelly, & Forrer, 2006).

2.2. Psychological Mechanisms of Placebo Effects

One prominent hypothesis is that placebo effects result from classical conditioning (Ader, 1988; Turkkan, 1989). According to this view, active medications are unconditioned stimuli and the vehicles that deliver them (e.g., pills, capsules, syringes) are conditioned stimuli. Thus, through repeated pairings between conditioned and unconditioned stimuli, vehicles per se could come to elicit the effects of active medications as conditioned responses. From this perspective, expectations are epiphenomena rather than causes or mediators of placebo effects. A study by Montgomery (1995) seemed to contradict this view by suggesting that a conditioning's effect on responses to placebo is fully mediated by expectancy. Therefore, conditioning might be only one of the mechanisms by which stimulus and response expectancies are acquired. In turn, these expectancies might mediate placebo effects (Kirsch, 1997; Pollo et al., 2001).

Another possible mechanism for the placebo effect is based on expectancies in relation to the construction of experience. According to the work of cognitive psychologist Jerome Bruner (1957, 1986), perception is influenced not only by what actually happens, but also by expectations about what should occur. These so-called self-confirming effects of expectancies may have evolved due to their impact on the speed of action: stimulus expectancies can speed perceptual processing, although sometimes at the expense of accuracy. As most studies have suggested, placebo effects are mediated by expectancies, a fact that will be detailed later in this chapter.

Essentially, expectancies may elicit subjective and objective changes in how people respond to an intervention. It is worth noting that the explanatory mechanisms of response expectancies and conditioning may not be mutually exclusive (Price, 2000).

2.3. Behavioral versus Physiological Pathways for Placebo Effects

Malani (2006) captures one of the most important criticisms of placebo studies – that they do not control for possible effects of contingent behavior that may nonetheless be independent of the intervention. For instance, more optimistic patients who have positive expectancies related to their treatment may modify their behavior in a manner that complements their therapy. More concretely, patients with non-gastric ulcers who believe in the effects of their treatment might also change their behavior by reducing their ingestion of spicy foods. This may in turn ameliorate their ulcer. If an investigator does not control for these behavioral changes, the favorable outcomes displayed by more optimistic patients could be wrongly interpreted as indicating placebo effects.

Recent studies argue that placebo might have a physiological as well as behavioral component. That is, individual expectations about therapy might alter the outcome of that therapy not only by modifying behavior, but also by triggering physiological changes in the brain and body (Zubieta et al., 2005; Wager et al., 2004). A recent review of neuroimaging studies on placebo indicated that beliefs and expectations can substantially modulate neuropsychological and neurochemical activity in brain regions involved in perception, movement, pain, and various aspects of emotion processing (Beauregard, 2007).

Among health issues, placebo analgesia has been most extensively studied. Wager et al. (2004) carried out two experiments using functional magnetic resonance imaging to investigate the neural mechanisms underlying the effects of expectations on placebo analgesia. The results indicated that the placebo treatment significantly decreased reported pain in over 70% of volunteers. Most importantly, placebo reduced the physiological responses in some of the brain regions known to be involved in the subjective experience of pain. These regions include the right anterior cingulate cortex, the anterior insula, and parts of the thalamus (Craig, Chen, Bandy, & Reiman, 2000).

In addition, during pain, placebo-induced increases in the dorsolateral prefrontal cortex, a brain region thought to be involved in the representation and maintenance of information needed for cognitive control (MacDonald, Cohen, Stenger, & Carter, 2000), were correlated with placebo-induced reductions in the contralateral thalamus, the insula, and the right anterior cingulate cortex. Another neuroimaging study on placebo analgesia found significant placebo-induced activation of mu-opioid receptor-mediated neurotransmission in certain brain regions, including the pregenual and subgenual anterior cingulate, the dorsolateral prefrontal cortex, the insular cortex, and the nucleus accumbens (Zubieta et al., 2005). Regional activations were paralleled by lower ratings in pain intensity, coupled with reductions in its sensory and affective qualities, and reductions in the negative emotional state of the volunteers. These data strongly suggest that cognitive factors are capable of modulating physical and emotional states through the site-specific activation of mu-opioid receptor signaling in the human brain (Zubieta et al., 2005).

While these data are compelling evidence of physiological effects, they nevertheless rely on subjective evaluations and responses, leaving open the question of whether one is measuring an effect or the reporting of an effect. Our study, described in detail later, contributes to this literature by providing data on objective physiological placebo effects. In particular, we assess how exogenously manipulated caffeine expectancies impact objectively measurable physiological outcome variables – in our case, blood pressure.

3. EXPERIMENT DESIGN AND PROCEDURES

Participants were moderate caffeine users who were instructed not to drink coffee for 24 h prior to the experiment. We employed a crossover design in which participants were sequentially exposed to four possible treatments: blinded and unblinded administration of caffeine (200 mg) pill, and blinded and unblinded administration of inert pill. More precisely, each participant arrived to the clinic on four separate days. On each of the first two days (blinded visits) the participant was randomized by means of a coin flip to either a caffeine pill (200 mg, the caffeine equivalent of two cups of coffee) or an identical-looking inert pill. The participant knew the probability (0.5) that he or she would receive the caffeine pill but did not know whether he or she actually received that pill.[2] On the third day (non-blinded visit) the participant was given either a caffeine pill in a vial labeled caffeine or an inert pill in a vial labeled inert. Participants were honestly told the content of the pill they were asked to ingest. The fourth day (non-blinded visit) mirrored the third, except that if the participant received caffeine during his or her third visit, he or she received inert pill on the fourth.

On each visit, a nurse would measure the participant's diastolic and systolic blood pressure 5 min before the participant was given treatment and 30, 60, and 90 min after the participants ingested his or her pill.[3] These measurements were made by means of an automated device. Importantly, the study participant was required to remain seated and permitted only to read airline magazines during the duration of his or her visit.[4] This ensured that the behavior of participants was held constant so that any observed placebo effects were generated by physiological rather than behavioral changes over the course of the different treatments. We chose airline magazines because they are designed not to induce anxiety in readers while they are passengers on an air flight.

Our hypotheses are as follows: (i) blood pressure would be highest when subjects were given the unblinded caffeine pill, since they would experience both the pharmacological effects of caffeine and the full expectation that they were receiving caffeine; (ii) in the blinded caffeine condition participants would have the second highest blood pressure, due to the full pharmacological effects of caffeine and chance (probability 0.5) expectation of receiving a caffeine pill; (iii) the third highest level of blood pressure would be observed in participants in the blinded placebo treatment, reflecting the only the chance (0.5 probability) expectation of receiving a caffeine pill; and, finally (iv) the lowest level of blood pressure would be observed in the unblinded placebo treatment where there was no expectation of receiving caffeine.

All experiments were conducted at the National Institute Health-funded General Clinical Research Center at the University of Virginia, and all physiological measurements were obtained by their associated staff of qualified health professionals.

4. RESULTS

4.1. Descriptive Statistics

A total of 50 people participated in our experiment. Table 1 provides descriptive statistics for our overall sample (final rows), as well as by agent received on each of their first two visits. Specifically, C denotes caffeine and P placebo so that, for example, the C/P category gives statistics for the set of people who, during their first two visits, randomly received caffeine once

Table 1. Total Sample Characteristics.

Treatment	Male	Age	Smoker	White	BPs Baseline	BPs 90 min	BPd Baseline	BPd 90 min
C/P	0.25	25.91	0.36	0.78	114.67	116.03	67.72	69.47
$N = 20$	(0.44)	(9.62)	(0.49)	(0.41)	(13.27)	(12.76)	(7.09)	(7.98)
	20	20	19	19	20	20	20	20
C/C	0.46	28.12	0.15	0.75	114.02	116.93	68.84	72.12
$N = 13$	(0.51)	(13.42)	(0.37)	(0.45)	(10.43)	(13.01)	(6.3)	(8.48)
	13	13	13	12	13	13	13	13
P/P	0.23	24.36	0.18	0.68	111.08	109.33	65.46	65.75
$N = 17$	(0.43)	(6.54)	(0.40)	(0.47)	(8.71)	(6.99)	(5.95)	(6.99)
	17	17	16	16	17	17	17	17
Total	0.31	26.13	0.23	0.73	113.28	113.99	67.24	68.9
$N = 50$	(0.46)	(9.86)	(0.42)	(0.44)	(11.06)	(11.49)	(6.53)	(8.04)
	50	50	48	47	50	50	50	50

and randomly received placebo once (in either order), while C/C reports statistics for the group who randomly received caffeine on each of their first two visits, and P/P reports statistics for the group who randomly received placebo on both visits.

As seen in Table 1, our overall sample included about 1/3 males, with a mean age of 26. About a fourth smoked and that same fraction was non-white. The final four columns in the table detail information about blood pressure. Changes in blood pressure will be discussed later. For now, it suffices to notice that baseline mean blood pressure readings (both systolic and diastolic, denoted by BPs and BPd, respectively) are normal. With respect to the treatment conditions, the key thing to note is that none of the condition-specific means departs very much from the others, or from the overall average.

The analysis we report below focuses on the 32 participants (64% of the sample) who displayed any positive blood pressure response in the condition where caffeine was known to have been ingested; that is, blood pressure was higher in the non-blinded caffeine state than in the non-blinded placebo state, a result we shall call a positive non-blinded treatment effect (NTE). The reason is that the non-responsive third of the sample evidently shows no reaction or a negative to caffeine that can mask placebo effects. Moreover, focusing on those with a positive NTE does not in any way imply that physiological responses among the four treatments will satisfy our naturally ordered hypothesis.

Table 2. Positive Unblinded Caffeine Effect.

Treatment	Male	Age	Smoker	White	BPs Baseline	BPs 90 min	BPd Baseline	BPd 90 min
C/P	0.33	27.56	0.25	0.66	115.18	116.79	69.93	71.46
$N = 12$	(0.49)	(11.84)	(0.45)	(0.49)	(12.5)	(11.86)	(5.88)	(6.88)
	12	12	12	12	12	12	12	12
C/C	0.5	24.38	0.12	0.75	115.45	118.27	69.7	72.58
$N = 8$	(0.53)	(7.99)	(0.35)	(0.46)	(10.73)	(12.35)	(6.66)	(8.98)
	8	8	8	8	8	8	8	8
P/P	0.25	25.36	0.25	0.63	111.68	110.01	65.88	66.27
$N = 12$	(0.45)	(7.61)	(0.45)	(0.5)	(9.64)	(7.81)	(6.31)	(7.61)
	12	12	12	11	12	12	12	12
Total	0.34	25.94	0.21	0.67	113.93	114.62	68.35	69.79
$N = 32$	(0.48)	(9.3)	(0.42)	(0.47)	(11.81)	(10.93)	(6.34)	(7.96)
	32	32	32	31	32	32	32	32

Table 2 provides descriptive statistics for the 32 subjects analyzed below. A key point is that the non-responsive group was distributed roughly equally among treatments. In addition, the means for the retained sample do not in any case depart greatly from the means reported in Table 1. In particular, one cannot predict who will experience a positive NTE based on the sample characteristics we collected.

4.2. Blood Pressure Response to Expectations and Caffeine

Fig. 1, panels (a) and (b), details time-related mean changes in diastolic and systolic blood pressure in each of the arms of our experiment. The vertical axis is percent change in blood pressure from baseline (obtained each visit, 5 min prior to administration of a pill). The horizontal axis indicates the time at which measurements were taken. The numbers of subjects included in each mean can be inferred from Table 2, and is 32 for each of the non-blinded arms, 20 for blinded caffeine, and 24 for blinded placebo arms.

Both panels provide compelling visual evidence in favor of the ordered hypothesis advanced above. In particular, at each time point the greatest mean change in blood pressure occurs with non-blinded caffeine, the least affect occurs with non-blinded placebo. The two blinded treatments fall somewhere between, with blinded caffeine showing a greater blood pressure effect than blinded placebo.

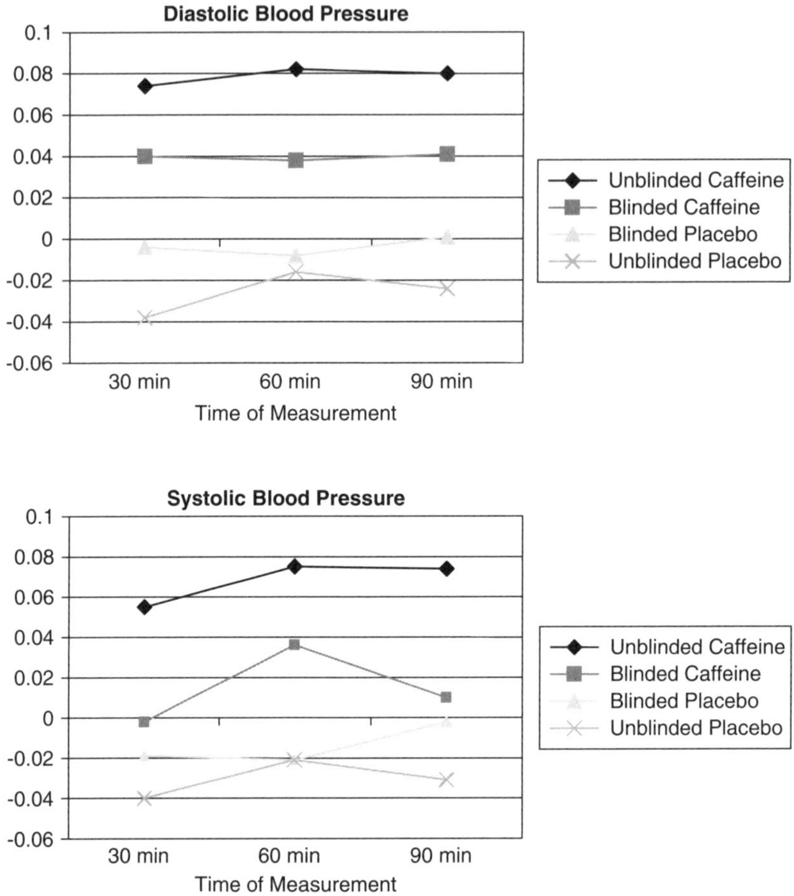

Fig. 1. Change in Diastolic and Systolic Blood Pressure in Each Arm of the Experiment.

It is worthwhile to note that, while non-monotonic, the blood pressure effects do not seem to systematically dissipate over the duration of the experiment. Indeed, in all cases mean change from baseline is roughly the same at both 30 and 90 min following ingestion of the pill. The effects at 90 min provide evidence against an anxiety-based explanation for our results: we would expect little residual anxiety following 90 min of relaxed reading of airline magazines.

To assess formally the validity of our hypothesis we conducted Jonckheere tests for ordered alternatives (Jonckheere, 1954). When $k = 2$, this test is equivalent to the well-known Wilcoxon–Mann–Whitney two-sample test for equality of medians. In our case, we test the null-hypothesis that the medians of the treatment effect distributions are the same against the alternative that the medians are ordered specifically as hypothesized above (non-blinded caffeine $\geq$ blinded caffeine $\geq$ blinded placebo $\geq$ non-blinded placebo), with at least one of the inequalities strict.[5]

We ran this test at the 90-min point for both systolic and diastolic blood pressure. We chose this point because, as noted above, it provides a control for possible anxiety effects on blood pressure outcomes. We find that the test overwhelmingly rejects the null-hypothesis in favor of our hypothesized ordering in both cases ($p < 0.001$ for both systolic and diastolic blood pressure). This result is robust to alternative measurement times. Evidence in favor of our hypothesized ordering is found for both systolic and diastolic blood pressure at the 30, 60, and 90-min measurement points ($p < 0.001$ in all cases).

5. CONCLUDING DISCUSSION

We reported data from novel clinical experiments with caffeine in order to provide evidence on the role of expectations in mediating placebo effects. In our experiment participants visited the clinic on multiple occasions. On each visit they ingested either a placebo or caffeine pill. Subjects knew only the probability with which the pill included caffeine. We obtained blood pressure measurements prior to ingestion, and provided only airline magazines to read to pass the time. Our design provides particularly clean inference because it (i) eliminates the possibility of behavioral confounds; (ii) provides for measurements at the individual level; (iii) manipulates beliefs without deception; and (iv) uses salient mechanisms to alter expectations (a coin flip). Our evidence supports the existence of physiological placebo effects, and provides compelling evidence that these effects are mediated by expectations.

Our experiment cannot identify the neural mechanisms ultimately responsible for these effects. However, our data are consistent with the possibility that the prefrontal cortex provides external, top–down control that modulates physiological outcomes (Wager et al., 2004). In addition, the proximate cause of the physiological effect (presumably hormones) is not informed by our study. In the case of blood pressure, it might be particularly challenging to document hormone levels, as the interventions (urinalysis or blood testing) to measure those levels would themselves affect blood pressure response. Nevertheless, the biological underpinnings of the responses we identify remain important areas for future research. For example, when a placebo is ingested but the probability of receiving caffeine is high, it would be very interesting to know whether the biological mechanism simulates the true pharmacological effect of caffeine or, alternatively, the effect a person believes caffeine should have.[6]

Finally, although by now something of a straw-man, our evidence raises additional questions regarding the role of expected utility analysis in understanding and predicting human behavior. It raises the possibility that expectations might not only multiply but also change the shape of the underlying utility function. Thus, our results are convergent evidence that beliefs play a complex role in economic decisions, and further the case for the importance of research geared toward developing appropriate and tractable frameworks that accommodate non-linear relationships between expectations and preferences.

NOTES

1. That treatment may or may not be an inert substance. It is possible for a pharmacologically active treatment to have placebo effects on top of what we shall call the pharmacological effects of that treatment.
2. The research pharmacy, in an off-site location, randomized the pills into bottles labeled H for heads or T for tails. The nurses administering the medication did not know this assignment. Subjects were told that either the H or the T vial contained a caffeine pill and the other contained an inert pill. A coin flip determined which vial and thus pill the subjects received. The nurse reported the H or T allocation back to the research pharmacy.
3. These timing choices were based on the half-life of caffeine, as well as its rate of absorption into the body. The rate at which a person metabolizes caffeine depends on age as well as a variety of health factors. In the case of healthy adults caffeine's half-life is around 4 h. Caffeine is typically fully absorbed into the body through the stomach and small intestine within 45 min of ingestion.
4. Bathroom breaks were regulated such that they did not occur within 5 min prior to a blood pressure measurement.
5. The Jonckheere test assumes independence among treatments, an assumption that might be violated by our data because the same subjects are observed in multiple treatments. A test that takes account of repeat measures among subjects is suggested by Page (1963). However, this test requires that all subjects participate in all treatments, which is not the case for our data (because of our randomization procedure).
6. We thank Monica Capra for this interesting suggestion.

ACKNOWLEDGMENT

The authors thank Renata Heilman for excellent research assistance.

REFERENCES

Ader, R. (1988). The placebo effect as a conditioned response. In: R. Ader, H. Weiner & A. Baum (Eds), *Experimental foundations of behavioral medicine: Conditioning approaches*. Hillside, NJ: Erlbaum.

Baker, S. L., & Kirsch, I. (1991). Cognitive mediators of pain perception and tolerance. *Journal of Personality and Social Psychology*, *61*(3), 504–510.

Beauregard, M. (2007). Mind does really matter: Evidence from neuroimaging studies of emotional self-regulation, psychotherapy, and placebo effect. *Progress Neurobiology*, *81*(4), 218–236.

Beecher, H. K. (1955). The powerful placebo. *Journal of American Medical Association*, *159*(17), 1602–1606.

Beecher, H. K. (1959). *Measurement of subjective responses: Quantitative effects of drugs*. New York, NY: Oxford University Press.

Benedetti, F., Colloca, L., Torre, E., Lanotte, M., Melcarne, A., Pesare, M., Bergamasco, B., & Lopiano, L. (2004). Placebo-responsive Parkinson patients show decreased activity in single neurons of subthalamic nucleus. *Nature Neuroscience*, *7*(6), 587–588.

Bruner, J. (1957). On perceptual readiness. *Psychological Bulletin*, *64*, 123–152.

Bruner, J. (1986). *Actual minds, possible worlds*. Cambridge: Harvard University Press.

Craig, A. D., Chen, K., Bandy, D., & Reiman, E. M. (2000). Thermosensory activation of insular cortex. *Natural Neuroscience*, *3*(2), 184–190.

de la Fuente-Fernandez, R., Ruth, T. J., Sossi, V., Schulzer, M., Calne, D. B., & Stoessl, A. J. (2001). Expectation and dopamine release: Mechanism of the placebo effect in Parkinson's disease. *Science*, *293*(5532), 1164–1166.

Hrobjartsson, A., & Gotzsche, P. C. (2001). Is the placebo powerless? An analysis of clinical trials comparing placebo with no treatment. *New England Journal of Medicine*, *344*(21), 1594–1602.

Hrobjartsson, A., & Gotzsche, P. C. (2004). Is the placebo powerless? Update of a systematic review with 52 new randomized trials comparing placebo with no treatment. *Journal of Internal Medicine*, *256*(2), 91–100.

Hrobjartsson, A., & Gotzsche, P. C. (2006). Unsubstantiated claims of large effects of placebo on pain: Serious errors in meta-analysis of placebo analgesia mechanism studies. *Journal of Clinical Epidemiology*, *59*(4), 336–338Discussion 339–341.

Jonckheere, A. R. (1954). A distribution-free k-sample test against ordered alternatives. *Biometrika*, *41*, 133–145.

Kienle, G. S., & Kienle, H. (1997). The powerful placebo effect: Fact or fiction? *Journal of Clinical Epidemiology*, *50*(12), 1311–1318.

Kirsch, I. (1985). Response expectancy as a determinant of experience and behavior. *American Psychologist*, *40*, 1189–1202.

Kirsch, I. (1997). Response expectancy theory and application: A decennial review. *Applied and Preventive Psychology*, *6*, 69–79.

Kirsch, I. (1999). *How expectancies shape experience*. Washington, DC: American Psychological Association.

Kirsch, I., & Lynn, S. J. (1995). The altered state of hypnosis: Changes in theoretical landscape. *American Psychologist*, *50*, 846–858.

Kirsch, I., & Lynn, S. J. (1999). Automaticity in clinical psychology. *American Psychologist*, *54*(7), 504–515.

Kirsch, I., & Sapirstein, G. (1999). Listening to Prozac but hearing placebo: A meta-analysis of antidepressant medication. In: I. Kirsch (Ed.), *How expectancies shape experience*. Washington, DC: American Psychological Association.

Lasagna, L., Mosteller, F., Von Felsinger, J. M., & Beecher, H. K. (1954). A study of the placebo response. *American Journal of Medicine*, *16*(6), 770–779.

Liccardi, G., Senna, G., Russo, M., Bonadonna, P., Crivellaro, M., Dama, A., D'Amato, M., D'Amato, G., Canonica, G. W., & Passalacqua, G. (2004). Evaluation of the nocebo effect during oral challenge in patients with adverse drug reactions. *Journal of Investigational Allergology Clinical Immunology*, *14*(2), 104–107.

Link, J., Haggard, R., Kelly, K., & Forrer, D. (2006). Placebo/nocebo symptom reporting in a sham herbal supplement trial. *Evaluation & the Health Professions*, *29*(4), 394–406.

MacDonald, A. W., 3rd., Cohen, J. D., Stenger, V. A., & Carter, C. S. (2000). Dissociating the role of the dorsolateral prefrontal and anterior cingulate cortex in cognitive control. *Science*, *288*(5472), 1835–1838.

Malani, A. (2006). Identifying placebo effects with data from clinical trials. *Journal of Political Economy*, *114*(2), 236–256.

Malani, A. (2008). Regulation with placebo effects. *Duke Law Journal* (forthcoming December). Available at http://works.bepress.com/anup_malani/5

Montgomery, G. H. (1995). *Mechanisms of placebo analgesia: Expectancy theory and classical conditioning*. Unpublished doctoral dissertation. University of Connecticut, Storrs, CT.

Olshansky, B. (2007). Placebo and nocebo in cardiovascular health: Implications for healthcare, research, and the doctor-patient relationship. *Journal of the American College of Cardiology*, *49*(4), 415–421.

Page, E. B. (1963). Ordered hypotheses for multiple treatments: A significance test for linear ranks. *Journal of the American Statistical Association*, *58*, 216–230.

Palace, E. M. (1999). Response expectancy and sexual dysfunction. In: I. Kirsch (Ed.), *How expectancies shape experience*. Washington, DC: American Psychological Association.

Perugini, E. M., Kirsch, I., Allen, S. T., Coldwell, E., Meredith, J., Montgomery, G. H., & Sheehan, J. (1998). Surreptitious observation of responses to hypnotically suggested hallucinations: A test of the compliance hypothesis. *International Journal of Clinical and Experimental Hypnosis*, *46*, 191–203.

Petrovic, P., Kalso, E., Petersson, K. M., & Ingvar, M. (2002). Placebo and opioid analgesia – imaging a shared neuronal network. *Science*, *295*, 1737–1740.

Pollo, A., Amanzio, M., Arslanian, A., Casadio, C., Maggi, G., & Benedetti, F. (2001). Response expectancies in placebo analgesia and their clinical relevance. *Pain*, *93*(1), 77–84.

Price, D. D. (2000). Factors that determine the magnitude and presence of placebo analgesia. In: M. Devor, M. C. Rowbotham & Z. Wiesenfeld-Hallin (Eds), *Proceedings of the 9th World Congress of Pain* (pp. 1085–1095). IASP Press: Seattle.

Shapiro, A. K. (1960). Attitudes toward the use of placebos in treatment. *Journal of Nervous and Mental Disease*, *130*, 200–211.

Shapiro, A. K. (1964). A historic and heuristic definition of the placebo. *Psychiatry*, *27*, 52–58.

Shapiro, A. K., & Shapiro, E. (1997). *The powerful placebo: From ancient priest to modern physician*. Baltimore, MD: Johns Hopkins University Press.

Shiv, B., Carmon, Z., & Ariely, D. (2005). Placebo effects of marketing actions: Consumers may get what they pay for. *Journal of marketing Research, 42*, 383–393.

Sneed, J. R., Ruthenford, B. R., Rindskopf, D., Lane, D. T., Sackeim, H. A., & Roose, S. P. (2008). Design makes a difference: A meta-analysis of antidepressant response rates in placebo-controlled versus comparator trials in late-life depression. *American Journal of Geriatric Psychiatry, 16*(1), 65–73.

Stewart-Williams, S., & Podd, J. (2004). The placebo effect: Dissolving the expectancy versus conditioning debate. *Psychological Bulletin, 130*, 324–340.

Talbot, M. (2000). The placebo prescription. *New York Times Magazine*, January 09.

Turkkan, J. S. (1989). Classical conditioning: The new hegemony. *Behavioral and Brain Sciences, 12*, 121–179.

Wager, T. D., Rilling, J. K., Smith, E. E., Sokolik, A., Casey, K. L., Davidson, R. J., Kosslyn, S. M., Rose, R. M., & Cohen, J. D. (2004). Placebo-induced changes in FMRI in the anticipation and experience of pain. *Science, 303*(5661), 1162–1167.

Zubieta, J. K., Bueller, J. A., Jackson, L. R., Scott, D. J., Xu, Y., Koeppe, R. A., Nichols, T. E., & Stohler, C. S. (2005). Placebo effects mediated by endogenous opioid activity on mu-opioid receptors. *Journal of Neuroscience, 25*(34), 7754–7762.